O G P L
OXFORD GENERAL PRACTICE LIBRARY

Women's Health

D0802923

O G P L
OXFORD GENERAL PRACTICE LIBRARY

Women's Health

Dr Carrie Sadler
General Practitioner with Special Interest
in Women's and Sexual Health,
Derbyshire, UK

Dr Jo White
General Practitioner, Dorset, UK

Dr Hazel Everitt
Clinical lecturer and General Practitioner,
University of Southampton, UK

Dr Chantal Simon
MRC Research Fellow and General
Practitioner, University of Southampton, UK

and *Series Editor*

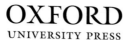

OXFORD
UNIVERSITY PRESS

OXFORD

UNIVERSITY PRESS

Great Clarendon Street, Oxford OX2 6DP

Oxford University Press is a department of the University of Oxford.
It furthers the University's objective of excellence in research, scholarship,
and education by publishing worldwide in

Oxford New York

Auckland Cape Town Dar es Salaam Hong Kong Karachi
Kuala Lumpur Madrid Melbourne Mexico City Nairobi
New Delhi Shanghai Taipei Toronto

With offices in

Argentina Austria Brazil Chile Czech Republic France Greece
Guatemala Hungary Italy Japan Poland Portugal Singapore
South Korea Switzerland Thailand Turkey Ukraine Vietnam

Oxford is a registered trade mark of Oxford University Press
in the UK and in certain other countries

Published in the United States
by Oxford University Press Inc., New York

British Library Cataloguing in Publication Data

Data available

Library of Congress Cataloging in Publication Data

Data available

Typeset by Newgen Imaging Systems (P) Ltd., Chennai, India
Printed in Italy
on acid-free paper by
Legoprint S.p.A.

ISBN 978–0–19–857138–4

10 9 8 7 6 5 4 3 2 1

Whilst every effort has been made to ensure that the contents of this book are as
complete, accurate and-up-to-date as possible at the date of writing, Oxford
University Press is not able to give any guarantee or assurance that such is the
case. Readers are urged to take appropriately qualified medical advice in all cases.
The information in this book is intended to be useful to the general reader, but
should not be used as a means of self-diagnosis or for the prescription of
medication.

Contents

Acknowledgements *vii*
Symbols and abbreviations *ix*

1	Women in society	1
2	Breast disease	41
3	Gynaecological problems	65
4	Contraception	161
5	Pregnancy	199
6	Mental health	297
7	Miscellaneous topics	327
8	Useful information and contacts	339

Index *361*

Acknowledgements

This book would not have come into being without the support and drive of the editorial and production team at Oxford University Press and we would like to say a big thank you to all of you. We would also like to thank the authors of the Oxford Handbook of General Practice for allowing us to reproduce material, and the authors and reviewers of many of the other books in the Oxford General Practice Library Series, particularly Richard Davies and Will Bolland for allowing us to use material from 'Men's health', and Francoise van Dorp for allowing us to use material from 'Child Health'. We would also like to thank Ash Monga for information provided, Clancy B for his help with the editing, proof reading and typing of amendments and Emma Gough for checking all the weblinks for us. Finally we would like to thank our major reviewers: Helen Dunkelman who reviewed the section on breast disease; Simon Crawford who reviewed the gynaecology material; and, Karen Brackley our obstetrics adviser.

All those involved in writing whilst working clinically, will be very aware that the real cost of such work is borne by families, and our families in Dorset, Hampshire and Derbyshire are no exception. We would like to thank them for their support for this project.

Symbols and abbreviations

⚠	Warning
❶	Important note
☛	Controversial point
☎	Telephone number
🖥	Website
📖	Cross reference to
±	With or without
↑	Increased/increasing
↓	Decreased/decreasing
→	Leading to
°	Degrees
$1°$	Primary
$2°$	Secondary
♂	Male
♀	Female
≈	Approximately equal
~	Approximately
%	Percent(age)
≥	Greater than or equal to
≤	Less than or equal to
>	Greater than
<	Less than
/	Per
+ve	Positive
-ve	Negative
C	Cochrane review
G	Guideline from major guideline producing body
N	NICE guidance
R	Randomized controlled trial in major journal
S	Systematic review in major journal

ND	Notifiable disease
α	Alpha
β	Beta
A&E	Accident and Emergency
ACE	Angiotensin converting enzyme
AF	Atrial fibrillation
AFP	Alpha-fetoprotein
AIDS	Acquired immune deficiency syndrome
AIS	Androgen insensitivity syndrome
ALT	Alanine-amino transferase
ANA	Anti-nuclear antibody
Anti-HBc	Anti hepatitis B core antigen
Anti-HBe	Anti-hepatitis B e antigen
Anti-HBs	Anti-hepatitis B surface antigen
AP	Antero-posterior
APH	Antepartum haemorrhage
AST	Aspartate amino transferase
bd	Twice daily
BM	Blood glucose using reagent strip
BMA	British Medical Association
BMD	Bone mineral density
BMI	Body mass index
BMJ	British Medical Journal
BNF	British National Formulary
BP	Blood pressure
bpm	Beats per minute
BSO	Bilateral salpingo-oophorectomy
BV	Bacterial vaginosis
Ca^{2+}	Calcium
CAH	Congenital adrenal hyperplasia
CBT	Cognitive behaviour therapy
CDH	Congenital dislocation of the hip
CF	Cystic fibrosis
CFS	Chronic fatigue syndrome
CHD	Coronary heart disease
CHT	Congenital hypothyroidism

CIN	Cervical intraepithelial neoplasia
CK	Creatine kinase
cm	Centimetre(s)
CMV	Cytomegalovirus
CMO	Chief Medical Officer
CNS	Central nervous system
CO_2	Carbon dioxide
COC	Combined oral contraceptive
COPD	Chronic obstructive pulmonary disease
CPN	Community psychiatric nurse
Cr	Creatinine
CRP	C-reactive protein
CS	Caesarean section
CSM	Committee on Safety of Medicines
CT	Computerized tomography
CTG	Cardiotocograph
CVD	Cardiovascular disease
CVS	Chorionic villus sampling
CXR	Chest X-ray
d	Day(s)
D&C	Dilation and curettage
DDH	Developmental dysplasia of the hip
DEXA	Dual energy X-ray absorptionometry
DIY	Do-it-yourself
dL	Decilitre
DM	Diabetes mellitus
DNA	Deoxyribonucleic acid
DoH	Department of Health
DSH	Deliberate self-harm
DT	Delirium tremens
DTB	Drugs and Therapeutics Bulletin
DVLA	Driver and Vehicle Licensing Authority
DVT	Deep vein thrombosis
DWP	Department of Work and Pensions
EBV	Epstein-Barr virus
ECG	Electrocardiograph

ECV	External cephalic version
ED	Every day
EDD	Estimated date of delivery
e.g.	For example
eGFR	Estimated glomerular filtration rate
ELISA	Enzyme-Linked ImmunoSorbent Assay
EPAU	Early pregnancy assessment unit
ERPC	Evacuation of retained products of conception
ESR	Erythrocyte sedimentation rate
etc.	Et cetera
FBC	Full blood count
FBG	Fasting blood glucose
FH	Family history
FMH	Feto-maternal haemorrhage
FSH	Follicle stimulating hormone
g	grams
GA	General anaesthetic
GAD	Generalized anxiety disorder
GBS	Group B Streptococcus
GCSE	General Certificate of Secondary Education
GGT	Gamma glutamyl transferase
GI	gastrointestinal
GMC	General Medical Council
GMS	General Medical Services
GnRH	Gonadotrophin releasing hormone
GP	General Practitioner
GPPAQ	General Practice Physical Activity Questionnaire
GTT	Glucose tolerance test
GU	Genito-urinary
GUM	Genito-urinary medicine
h	Hour(s)
Hb	Haemoglobin
HbA_{1c}	Glycosylated haemoglobin
HBcAg	Hepatitis B core antigen
HBeAg	Hepatitis B e antigen
HBsAg	Hepatitis B surface antigen

HBV	Hepatitis B
HCG or hCG	Human chorionic gonadotrophin
HCV	Hepatitis C
HDL	High density lipoprotein
HELLP	Haemolysis, Elevated liver enzymes, Low platelets
HIV	Human immunodeficiency virus
HPV	Human papilloma virus
HRT	Hormone replacement therapy
HTLV	Human T-lymphotrophic virus
ICD	International classification of disease
IDDM	Insulin dependent diabetes mellitus
Ig	Immunoglobulin
IHD	Ischaemic heart disease
IM	Intramuscular
IRT	Ummunoreactive trypsin
IT	Information technology
iu	International units
IUCD	Intrauterine contraceptive device
IUD	Intrauterine device
IUGR	Intrauterine growth restriction
IUS	Intrauterine contraceptive system
IV	Intravenous
IVF	In vitro fertilization
K^+	Potassium
Kcal	Kilocalorie(s)
kg	Kilogram(s)
l	Litre(s)
lbs	Pound(s)
LDL	Low density lipoprotein
LFTs	Liver function test
LH	Luteinizing hormone
LHRH	Luteinizing Hormone Releasing Hormone
LLETZ	Large loop excision of the transformation zone
LMP	Last menstrual period
LMWH	Low molecular weight heparin
LN	Lymph node

LSCS	Lower segment caesarean section
LSD	Lysergic acid diethylamide
m	Metres
MAOI	Monoamine oxidase inhibitor
M,C&S	Microscopy, culture and sensitivity
mcg	Micrograms
MCV	Mean cell volume
mg	Milligrams
MI	Myocardial infarct
min	Minutes
ml	Millilitres
mmHg	Millimetres of mercury
mmol	Millimole
mo	Month(s)
mph	Miles per hour
MRI	Magnetic resonance imaging
MSU	Mid-stream urine
Na^+	Sodium
NCT	National Childbirth Trust
NHS	National Health Service
NI	Northern Ireland
NICE	National Institute for Clinical Excellence
NIDDM	Non-insulin dependent diabetes mellitus
NRT	Nicotine replacement therapy
NSAID	Non-steroidal anti-inflammatory drug
NT	Nuchal translucency
O_2	Oxygen
OCD	Obsessive compulsive disorder
od	Once daily
OTC	Over-the-counter
OUP	Oxford University Press
p.	Page number
PAPP-A	Pregnancy associated plasma protein A
pp.	Pages
PCT	Primary Care Trust
PCOS	Polycystic ovarian syndrome

PE	Pulmonary embolus
PET	Pre-eclamptic toxaemia
PID	Pelvic inflammatory disease
PIH	Pregnancy-induced hypertension
PKU	Phenylketonuria
PMB	Post-menopausal bleed
PMDD	Pre-menstrual dysphoric disorder
PMH	Past medical history
PMS	Personal Medical Services or pre-menstrual syndrome
PMT	Pre-menstrual tension
po	Oral
PO_4	Phosphate
POP	Progesterone only pill
PPH	Post partum haemorrhage
PR	Per rectum or rectal examination
prn	As needed
PROM	Premature rupture of the membranes
pv or PV	Per vaginum
qds	Four times daily
QoF	Quality and outcomes framework
RA	Rheumatoid arthritis
RBCs	Red blood cells
RCGP	Royal College of General Practitioners
RCOG	Royal College of Obstetricians and Gynaecologists
RCP	Royal College of Physicians
Rh	Rhesus
RhD	Rhesus D
Rh. F	Rheumatoid factor
RTA	Road traffic accident
RUQ	Right upper quadrant
s or sec	Second (s)
s/cut	Subcutaneous
SBP	Systolic blood pressure
SERM	Selective oestrogen receptor modulator
SFH	Symphysis-fundal height
SHBG	Sex hormone binding globulin

SIGN	Scottish Intercollegiate Guidelines Network
SLE	Systemic lupus erythematosis
SNRI	Serotonin and noradrenaline reuptake inhibitor
SSRI	Selective serotonin reuptake inhibitor
STD	Sexually transmitted disease
STI	Sexually transmitted infection
T4	Thyroxine
TAH	Total abdominal hysterectomy
TB	Tuberculosis
TC	Total cholesterol
TCA	Tri-cyclic antidepressant
tds	Three times a day
TENS	Transdermal electrical nerve stimulation
TFTs	Thyroid function tests
TIA	Transient ischaemic attack
TLC	Tender-loving-care
TOP	Termination of pregnancy
TPHA	Treponema pallidum haemagglutinin test
TSH	Thyroid stimulating hormone
TV	Television or Trichomonas vaginalis
u	units
U&E	Urea and electrolytes
uE3	Oestriol
UK	United Kingdom
URTI	Upper respiratory tract infection
USS	Ultrasound scan
UTI	Urinary tract infection
VAIN	Vaginal intra-epithelial neoplasia
VDRL	Venereal disease research laboratory test
VE	Vaginal examination
VF	Ventricular fibrillation
VIN	Vulval intraepithelial neoplasia
VZ	Varicella zoster
VZ-Ig	Varicella zoster immunoglobulin
WHO	World Health Organization
wk	Week(s)
y	Year(s)

Chapter 1

Women in society

Women in society 2
Payment for women's primary health care 6
Alcohol misuse 10
Smoking 14
Drug misuse 18
Exercise 22
Obesity 26
Prevention of cardiovascular disease 32
Domestic violence 38

1

Women in society

Overall there are more women than men in the UK population (30.3×10^6 ♀ and 28.9×10^6 ♂) so health and well-being of women is extremely important. More boys than girls are born each year and there are ~20,000 more boys than girls at each age until 22y., when the number of women overtakes the number of men. This difference increases with age and by 90y. there are 3½× as many women as men (Figure 1.1).

In many ways, lives of men and women have become more similar over recent years as more and more women have entered the labour market. Despite this, differences remain.

Living arrangements
- 60% of men and women live in a couple – 50% married; 10% cohabiting.
- 81% of couples live in owner-occupied accommodation.
- Over the last 30y., the proportion of single or divorced people has ↑. Men are more likely than women to have never married, but women are more likely than men to be divorced or widowed.
- There are >3× as many widows as widowers in the population as women tend to live longer than men.
- In the last 30y., the number of single-parent families has ↑ × 2 to 6%. 90% of lone-parent families are headed by a woman.
- ~½ of lone mothers have never been married; lone fathers tend to be divorced.
- ~½ of lone mothers with dependent children live in social sector housing. Lone fathers are more likely to be owner-occupiers.
- >90% of stepfamilies consist of a couple with ≥1 child from the previous relationship of the woman only, reflecting a tendency for children to stay with the mother following the break-up of a partnership.
- There are 2½× as many women as men in residential care (269,000 ♀; 104,000 ♂) and 87% of these women are over state pension age.

Education: Girls generally perform better than boys at school:
- From key stage 1 (5–7y.) – 4 (14–16y.) girls score consistently higher than boys with the greatest difference being in English
- 58% of girls achieve ≥5 GCSE grades A*–C; 47% of boys
- 43% of girls gain ≥2 A-levels; 34% of boys
- At degree level, 58% of women gain a first or upper-second-class degree; 50% of men.

Work: 84% of men and 73% of women of employment age are working or available to work. The proportion of women in employment has ↑ over the past 20y. so the number of men and women in employment is now almost equal, but the proportion depends on the age of the woman's youngest child (Table 1.1). Almost ½ of female jobs are part-time – 40% of women with dependent children work part-time compared with 23% of those without and ~5% of men.

~¼ of female employees do administrative or secretarial work. Men are 2× as likely as women to be managers and senior officials, and far more likely to be in skilled trades (Figure 1.2). Since 1999 women's hourly pay has remained at ~80% of men's pay.

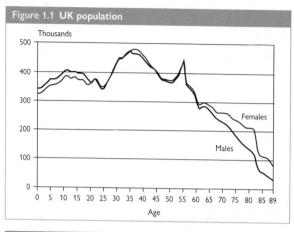

Figure 1.1 UK population

Table 1.1 Impact of children on employment of women		
Circumstance		**% in the workforce**
Women overall		73%
Women without dependent children		76%
Women with dependent children	Children aged <5y.	55%
	Youngest child aged 5–10y.	73%
	Youngest child aged 11–15y.	80%
Men with dependent children (any age)		93%

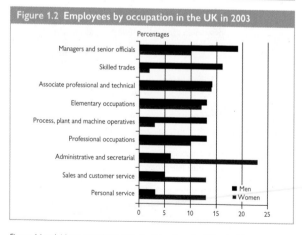

Figure 1.2 Employees by occupation in the UK in 2003

Figures 1.1 and 1.2 are reproduced with permission from the Office for National Statistics, www.statistics.gov.uk

Leisure

- Overall, men have an extra ½h. of free time each day than women.
- Women living in a couple and working full time spend ~4½h. on childcare and other activities with their children on a weekday; men spend ~3½h.
- Women spend ~2½h./d. doing housework, cooking, washing-up, cleaning and ironing – 1h. 30min. more than men.
- Both sexes spend a similar time gardening or looking after pets.
- Men spend more time than women on DIY and car maintenance.
- Women spend more time socialising than men but men spend more time than women on home entertainment, e.g. watching the TV.

Health

Life expectancy: Figure 1.3
- Girls born in 1901 could expect to live to just 49y., whereas girls born in 2004 can expect to live to 81y.
- On average, girls can expect to live 4y. longer than boys.
- Over recent years, the ↑ in life expectancy amongst older adults has been particularly dramatic. By 2004, women aged 65y. could expect to live to the age of 85y. Projections suggest that this will ↑ by another 3y. by 2021.

Healthy life
- A higher proportion of men than women in the UK report their health to be good at all ages.
- Among both sexes the proportion of people reporting good health declines with age.
- Many people in the older age groups still consider themselves to be in good health, even if they have a limiting long-term illness or disability which restricts their daily activity. 7:10 women aged 65–74y. and ¼ of women aged ≥75y. have a disability but consider themselves in good health.
- Healthy life expectancy for women in 1999 averaged 69y. compared with 67y. for men. So, while women can expect to live longer than men, they are also more likely to have more years in poor health.

Causes of death: Cancers are now the most common cause of death in women (24% deaths) – Figure 1.4. This is closely followed by circulatory disease (which includes heart disease and stroke).

Diseases: As well as conditions unique to women, such as gynaecological problems, breast disease and pregnancy, women are more likely to consult than men with autoimmune disease, mental health problems, musculoskeletal symptoms and non-specific symptoms.

GP consultations: In 2004/05, 87% of NHS GP consultations in Great Britain took place in the GPs' surgeries, 9% were over the telephone and 4% were in the home. Among adults, the proportion of GP consultations that take place in the home ↑ with age. Females are more likely than males to consult a GP – 16% of females and 11% of males did so in the 14d. before interview in the 2004/05 General Household Survey. Females have an average of 5 NHS GP consultations/y. and males have 3.

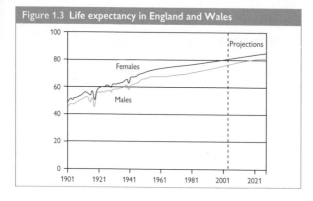

Figure 1.3 Life expectancy in England and Wales

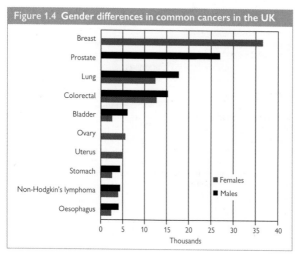

Figure 1.4 Gender differences in common cancers in the UK

5

Further information

National Statistics 🖳 www.statistics.gov.uk

Payment for women's primary health care

The General Medical Services (GMS) contract: Although there may be some differences in process in each of the four countries of the UK, the principles of the GMS contract apply to all. A total sum for GMS services is given to each primary care trust (PCT) as part of a bigger unified budget allocation. PCTs are responsible for managing the GMS budget locally.

The contract: Made between an individual practice and a PCT. All the partners of the practice, at least one of whom must be a GP, have to sign the contract. It includes:

- National terms applicable to all practices (the 'practice contract')
- Which services will be provided by that practice, i.e.
  - essential
  - additional – if not opted out
  - out-of-hours – if not opted out
  - enhanced – if opted in
- Level of quality of essential and additional services that the practice 'aspires' to
- Support arrangements, e.g. IT, premises
- Total financial resources, i.e. global sum + quality achievement payments + enhanced services payments + premises + IT + dispensing.

Essential services: All practices must undertake these services. *Include:*

- *Day-to-day medical care of the practice population:* health promotion, management of minor and self-limiting illness and referral to secondary care services and other agencies as appropriate
- *General management of patients who are terminally ill*
- *Chronic disease management*

Additional services: Services the practice will usually undertake but may 'opt out' of. If the practice opts out, the PCT takes responsibility for providing the service instead. The practice then receives a ↓ global sum payment.

Enhanced services: Commissioned by the PCT and paid for *in addition* to the global sum payment. 3 types:

- *Directed enhanced services:* services under national direction with national specifications and benchmark pricing which all PCTs must commission to cover their relevant population
- *National enhanced services:* services with national minimum standards and benchmark pricing but not directed (i.e. PCTs do not have to provide these services)
- *Services developed locally* to meet local needs (local enhanced services), e.g. enhanced care of the homeless.

Table 1.2 Payment under the GMS contract

Payment	Explanation
The global sum	Major part of the money paid to practices. Paid monthly and intended to cover practice running costs. *Includes provision for:* • Delivery of essential services and additional/out-of-hours services if not opted out • Staff costs • Career development • Locum reimbursement (e.g. for appraisal, career development and protected time).
Aspiration payments	Advance payments to allow practices to develop services to achieve higher quality standards. Aspiration payments are made monthly alongside global sum payments and amount to roughly 60% of the points achieved the previous year (for 2005/06 this was ≈2004/05 points achieved x £124.60/point x 60% x list size adjustment).
Achievement payments	Payments made for the practice's achieved number of points in the quality and outcomes framework (🕮 p.8) as measured at the start of the following year. Aspiration payments already received are deducted from the total, i.e. payment for actual points less aspiration pay.
Payment for 'extra' services	Paid to practices that provide directed enhanced services, national enhanced services and/or local enhanced services to meet local needs.
Minimum practice income guarantee (MPIG)	Protects those practices that lost out under the redistribution effect of the new resource allocation formula. Calculated from the difference between the global sum allocation (GSA) under the new GMS contract and the global sum equivalent (GSE) – the amount the practice would have earned for providing the same service under the old GMS contract ('The Red Book'). If GSA < GSE a correction factor (CF) will be applied as long as necessary so that GSA+CF = GSE.
Other payments	Payments for premises, IT and dispensing (dispensing practices only).

🕐 The Carr-Hill allocation formula is a GMS resource allocation formula for allocating funds for the global sum and quality payments. The formula takes the practice population and then makes a series of adjustments based on the profile of the local community, taking account of determinants of relative practice workload and costs.

The quality and outcomes framework: The quality and outcomes framework (QoF) was developed specifically for the new GMS contract. Financial incentives are used to encourage high quality care.

The domains: The GMS quality framework is divided into 4 domains: See Table 1.3
- Clinical
- Organizational
- Additional services
- Patient experience

Indicators: Every domain has a set of 'indicators' which relate to quality standards or guidelines that can be achieved within that domain. The indicators were developed by an expert group based on the best available evidence at the time and will be updated regularly. All data should be obtainable from practice clinical systems and Read codes have been developed to make this easier. Indicators are split into 3 types:
- *Structure:* e.g. is a disease register in place?
- *Process:* e.g. is a particular measure being recorded? Is action being taken where appropriate?
- *Outcome:* e.g. how well is the condition being controlled?

Quality points: All achievement against quality indicators converts to points. Each point has a monetary value.
- *Yes/no indicators:* All points are allocated if the result is +ve and none if –ve.
- *Range of attainment:* For most of clinical indicators it is not possible to attain 100% results (even if allowed exceptions are applied) so a range of satisfactory attainment is specified. Minimum standard is 25%. Points are allocated in a linear fashion based on comparison with attainment against a maximum standard – e.g. if the maximum % for an indicator is 90%, the minimum 40% and the practice achieves 70%, the practice will receive 30/50 (i.e. 3/5) of the available points.

Reporting on quality: Every year each practice must complete a standard return form recording level of achievement and the evidence for that. In addition there is an annual quality review visit by the PCT. Based on these, the PCT confirms level of achievement funding attained and discusses points the practice will 'aspire' to the following year (🕮 p.7). The process is confirmed in writing by the PCT and signed off by the practice. The Commission for Healthcare Audit and Inspection (or equivalents in Scotland/NI) checks PCT-wide quality against other PCTs countrywide.

The quality framework and the Personal Medical Services (PMS) contract: Mechanisms for quality delivery and the quality framework are broadly comparable for GMS and PMS practices. PMS practices can apply for aspiration payments and achievement payments in the same way as GMS practices. However, in order to reflect the local nature of the contracts, the standards that PMS practices are working to do not have to be the same as those contained in the national quality framework. Nevertheless, all standards must be rigorous, evidence based, monitored fairly, assessed against criteria agreed between PCTs and providers, and paid at appropriate and equitable rates.

Table 1.3 Calculation of points for quality framework payments

Components of total points score	Points	Way in which points are calculated
Clinical indicators	655	Achieving pre-set standards in management of: • Smoking • Dementia • CHD • Learning difficulty • Left ventricular dysfunction • Depression • AF • Mental health • Stroke and TIA • COPD • Hypertension • Asthma • Hypothyroidism • Epilepsy • DM • Cancer • Chronic kidney disease • Obesity • Palliative care
Organizational	181	Achieving pre-set standards in: • Records and information about patients • Information for patients • Education and training • Medicines management • Practice management
Additional services	36	Achieving pre-set standards in: • Cervical screening • Child health surveillance • Maternity services • Contraceptive services
Patient experience	108	Achieving pre-set standards in: • Patient survey* • Consultation length
Holistic care	20	Reflects range of achievement across clinical indicators – calculated by ranking clinical indicators in terms of proportion of points gained (1–10). Proportion of the points gained by the 3rd lowest indicator (i.e. indicator ranked 7) is the proportion of the holistic care points obtained.
Total possible	**1000**	

In 2005/06 and 2006/07 the average value of 1 point = £124.60.

* Improving Practice Questionnaire (IPQ – charge payable) – 🖵 www.cfep.co.uk or General Practice Assessment Questionnaire (GPAQ) – 🖵 www.gpaq.info

Further information
DoH The GMS contract 🖵 www.dh.gov.uk
BMA The GMS contract and supporting documents 🖵 www.bma.org.uk

Alcohol misuse

Traditionally, men have been almost 2x as likely as women to exceed the recommended daily benchmarks for consumption of alcohol. However, binge drinking amongst younger women is changing this trend. 40% of women aged 16–24y. now regularly exceed recommended limits.

Binge drinking: Defined as drinking >2x the recommended daily intake (i.e. >6u for a woman) in 1d.

Assessing drinking

Suspicious signs/symptoms: ↑ and uncontrolled BP; excess weight; recurrent injuries/accidents; non-specific GI complaints; back pain; poor sleep; tired all the time.

Ask: Assess amount, time of day, socially or alone, daily or in binges, blackouts, situations associated with heavy drinking. Consider using the CAGE questionnaire to assess dependence:
- Have you ever felt you should Cut down on your drinking?
- Have people Annoyed you by criticizing your drinking?
- Have you ever felt bad or Guilty about your drinking?
- Have you ever had a drink first thing in the morning to steady your nerves or to get rid of a hangover (Eye opener)?

Risk factors
- Previous history
- Family history
- Poor social support
- Work absenteeism
- Emotional and/or family problems
- Financial and legal problems
- Drug problems
- Alcohol associated with work, e.g. publican

Examination: Smell of alcohol; tremor; sweating; slurring of speech; ↑ BP; signs of liver damage.

Investigations: FBC (↑ MCV); LFTs (↑ GGT identifies ~25% of heavy drinkers in general practice; ↑ AST; ↑ bilirubin). Often incidental findings.

Health risk: Continuum – individual risk depends on other factors too (e.g. smoking, heart disease, pregnancy). Recommended safe level of alcohol consumption is <14u/wk. for women (Table 1.4 and 1.5).

Alcohol-related health problems: Table 1.5

Beneficial effects of alcohol: Moderate consumption (1–3u/d.) ↓ risk of non-haemorrhagic stroke, angina pectoris and MI.

Table 1.4 Health risks associated with levels of alcohol consumption		
Health risk	**Women (units/wk.)**	**Notes**
Low	<14	1 unit = 8g alcohol = ½ pint of beer (if strong beer can be as much as 1.75 units), small glass of wine/sherry, 1 measure of spirits (spirit measure in Scotland is 1.2 units). 1 bottle of 12% wine = 9 units.
Intermediate	15–35	
High	>35	

GMS contract

Specialized care of patients who are alcohol misusers may be provided by practices as a *national enhanced service*. Practices providing this service receive an annual payment plus a fee per patient per year.

Table 1.5 Alcohol-related problems

Death: ~40,000 deaths/y. in the UK are directly caused by alcohol.

Social well-being
- Marriage breakdown
- Absence from work
- Loss of work
- Social isolation
- Poverty
- Loss of shelter/home

Mental health: Anxiety, depression and/or suicidal ideas; dementia and/or Korsakoffs ± Wernicke's encephalopathy

Physical well-being
- ↓ BP
- CVA
- Sexual dysfunction
- Brain damage
- Neuropathy
- Myopathy
- Cardiomyopathy
- Infertility
- Gastritis
- Pancreatitis
- DM
- Obesity
- Fetal damage
- Haemopoietic toxicity
- Interactions with other drugs
- Fatty liver
- Hepatitis
- Cirrhosis
- Oesophageal varices ± haemorrhage
- Liver cancer
- Cancer of the mouth, larynx and oesophagus
- Breast cancer
- Nutritional deficiencies
- Back pain
- Poor sleep
- Tiredness
- Injuries due to alcohol-related activity (e.g. fights)

Advice for patients

Drinkline (government-sponsored helpline) ☎ 0800 917 8282
Alcohol Concern ⊟ www.alcoholconcern.org.uk
Alcoholics Anonymous ☎ 0845 769 7555
⊟ www.alcoholics-anonymous.org.uk

Alcohol management strategies: Figure 1.5

Patients drinking within acceptable limits: Reaffirm limits.

Non-dependent drinkers: Brief GP intervention results in ~24% reducing their drinking. Provide information about safe amounts of alcohol and harmful effects of exceeding these. If receptive to change, confirm weekly consumption using a drink diary, agree targets to ↓ consumption and negotiate follow-up.

Alcohol-dependent drinkers: Suffer withdrawal symptoms if they ↓ alcohol consumption (e.g. anxiety, fits, delirium tremens – opposite).

● If wanting to stop drinking – refer to the community alcohol team; suggest self-help organizations, e.g. Alcoholics Anonymous; involve family and friends in support.

● Detoxification in the community usually uses a reducing regimen of chlordiazepoxide over a 1wk. period (20–30mg qds on days 1 and 2; 15mg qds on days 3 and 4; 10mg qds on day 5; 10mg bd on day 6; 10mg od on day 7; then stop).

● Community detoxification is contraindicated for patients with:
   ● confusion or hallucinations
   ● history of previously complicated withdrawal (e.g. withdrawal seizures or delirium tremens)
   ● epilepsy or fits
   ● malnourishment
   ● severe vomiting or diarrhoea
   ● ↑ risk of suicide
   ● poor cooperation
   ● failed detoxification at home
   ● uncontrollable withdrawal symptoms
   ● acute physical or psychiatric illness
   ● multiple substance misuse
   ● poor home environment.

If ambivalent/unwilling to change: Provide information; reassess and re-inform on each subsequent meeting; support the family.

Vitamin B supplements: People with chronic alcohol dependence are frequently deficient in vitamins, especially thiamine – give oral thiamine indefinitely (if severe 200–300mg/d.; if mild 10–25mg/d.)[G]. During detoxification in the community – give thiamine 200mg od for 5–7d.

Relapse: Common. Warn patients and encourage them to re-attend. Be supportive and maintain contact (↓ frequency and severity of relapses[G]). Consider drugs to prevent relapse, e.g. acamprosate, disulfiram (specialist initiation only).

Further information

BMJ Addiction and dependence – II: alcohol (1997) 315 358–60
DTB Managing the heavy drinker in primary care (2000) 38(8) 60–4
SIGN The management of harmful drinking and alcohol dependence in primary care (2003) 🖳 www.sign.ac.uk

Figure 1.5 Alcohol management strategy

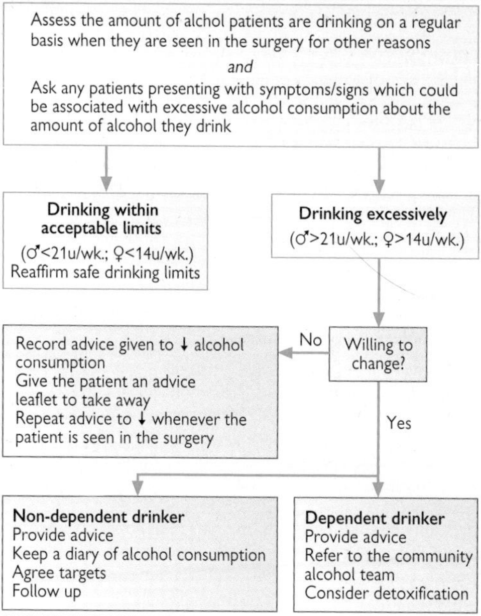

Assess the amount of alchol patients are drinking on a regular basis when they are seen in the surgery for other reasons

and

Ask any patients presenting with symptoms/signs which could be associated with excessive alcohol consumption about the amount of alcohol they drink

Drinking within acceptable limits
(♂<21u/wk.; ♀<14u/wk.)
Reaffirm safe drinking limits

Drinking excessively
(♂>21u/wk.; ♀>14u/wk.)

Willing to change? — No →

Record advice given to ↓ alcohol consumption
Give the patient an advice leaflet to take away
Repeat advice to ↓ whenever the patient is seen in the surgery

Yes

Non-dependent drinker
Provide advice
Keep a diary of alcohol consumption
Agree targets
Follow up

Dependent drinker
Provide advice
Refer to the community alcohol team
Consider detoxification

13

⚠ **Delirium tremens (DTs):** Major withdrawal symptoms usually occur 2–3 d. after an alcoholic has stopped drinking. *Features:*
- **General:** Fever, tachycardia, ↓ BP, ↑ respiratory rate
- **Psychiatric:** Vivid visual and tactile hallucinations, acute confusional state, apprehension
- **Neurological:** Tremor, fits, fluctuating level of consciousness

Action: DTs have 15% mortality and always warrant emergency hospital admission.

GP Notes: Alcohol and driving – DVLA guidance about fitness to drive for patients who misuse or are dependent on alcohol

Group 1 licence restrictions	Group 2 licence restrictions
6mo. off driving (1y. after alcohol or drug-related seizure or detoxification for alcohol dependence)	Licence revoked 1y. (3y. if alcohol dependence; 5y. if alcohol-related seizure)

ⓘ The DVLA arranges assessment prior to licence restoration.

Smoking

Facts and figures

- In the UK, 26% of women smoked in 2001.
- Prevalence is highest in the 20–24y. old age group.
- 1% school children are smokers when they enter secondary school; by 15y., 22% are smoking. 82% of smokers start as teenagers. Girls are more likely to smoke in this age group than boys.
- Government targets aim to ↓ smoking to ≤24% by 2010, and ↓ smoking among children to ≤9% by 2010.
- Surveys of smokers show 70% want to stop and 30% intend to give up in <1y. – but only ~2%/y. give up permanently.

Risks of smoking: Smoking is the greatest single cause of illness and premature death in the UK. ½ all regular smokers will eventually die as a result of smoking – 120,000 people/y.

Tobacco smoking is associated with ↑ risk of:

- *Cancers:* ~30% all cancer deaths. Common cancers include lung (>90% are smokers – incidence of lung cancer is increasing in women – Figure 1.6); lip; mouth; stomach; colon; bladder
- *Cardiovascular disease:* arteriosclerosis, coronary heart disease, stroke, peripheral vascular disease
- *Diabetes mellitus*
- *Chronic lung disease:* chronic obstructive pulmonary disease, recurrent chest infection, exacerbation of asthma
- *Dyspepsia and/or gastric ulcers*
- *Thrombosis* (especially if also on the COC pill)
- *Osteoporosis*
- *Problems in pregnancy:* pre-eclampsia, intra-uterine growth retardation, pre-term delivery, neonatal and late fetal death.

Passive smoking is associated with:

- ↑ risk of coronary heart disease and lung cancer (↑ by 25%)
- ↑ risk of cot death, bronchitis and otitis media in children.

Advice for patients: Useful contacts

Action on Smoking and Health (ASH) ☎ 020 7739 5902
🖥 www.ash.org.uk
NHS Smoking helpline: ☎ 0800 169 0 169; pregnancy smoking helpline: ☎ 0800 169 9 169 🖥 www.givingupsmoking.co.uk
Quit Helpline ☎ 0800 00 22 00 🖥 www.quit.org.uk

GMS contract			
Smoking 1	% of patients with any/combination of coronary heart disease, stroke or TIA, hypertension, diabetes, COPD or asthma whose notes record smoking status in the previous 15mo., except those who have never smoked where smoking status need only be recorded once since diagnosis	up to 33 points	40–90%
Smoking 2	% of patients with any/combination of the conditions listed in 'smoking 1' who smoke whose notes contain a record that smoking cessation advice or referral to a specialist service, where available, has been offered within the previous 15mo.	up to 35 points	40–90%
Asthma 3	% of patients with asthma between the ages of 14–19y. in whom there is a record of smoking status in the previous 15mo.	up to 6 points	40–80%
Records 22	% of patients aged >15y. whose notes record smoking status in the past 27mo., except those who have never smoked where smoking status need be recorded only once.	up to 11 points	40–90%
Information 5	The practice supports smokers in stopping smoking by a strategy which includes providing literature and offering appropriate therapy.	2 points	

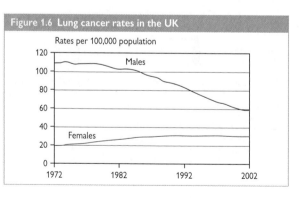

Figure 1.6 **Lung cancer rates in the UK**

Rates per 100,000 population

Males

Females

1972   1982   1992   2002

Figure 1.6 is reproduced with permission from the Office of National Statistics, www.statistics.gov.uk

Helping people to stop smoking: Advice from a GP about smoking cessation results in 2% of smokers stopping – 5% if advice is repeated[CE]. Strong motivation (often 2° to an episode of poor health directly related to smoking, e.g. myocardial infarct) is a vital factor.

Aids to smoking cessation: *BNF 4.10*

Nicotine replacement therapy (NRT)

- ↑ the chance of stopping ~1½x[N].
- All preparations are equally effective[C] and available on NHS prescription.
- Start with higher doses for patients highly dependent.
- Continue treatment for 3mo., tailing off dose gradually over 2wk. before stopping (except gum which can be stopped abruptly).
- Several preparations are now licensed for use in pregnancy if unable to stop without NRT.
- Contraindicated immediately post MI, stroke or TIA, and for patients with arrhythmia.

Bupropion (Zyban™)

- Smokers (>18y.) start taking the tablets 1–2wk. before their intended quit day (150mg od for 3d. then 150mg bd for 7–9wk.).
- Effective treatment[C] which ↑ cessation rate >2x.[N]
- *Contraindications:* epilepsy or ↑ risk of seizures, eating disorder, bipolar disorder, pregnancy/breast feeding.

Varenicline (Champix™)

- Smokers (>18y.) start taking the tablets 1wk. before intended quit day (0.5mg od for 3d., 0.5mg bd for 4d. then 1mg bd for 11wk.). Advise patients to take tablets after food and with a full glass of water. ↓ dose to 1mg od if renal impairment/elderly. If the patient has stopped smoking after 12wk., consider prescribing a further 12wk. treatment to ↓ chance of relapse.
- Effective treatment which ↑ cessation rate >2x.
- *Contraindications:* Caution in men with psychiatric illness.

Alternative therapies: There is some evidence hypnotherapy is helpful in some cases[C].

Support: In many areas 'smoke stop' services are provided by PCTs. These programmes vary from area to area but generally consist of a combination of group education, counselling and support ± individual support in combination with nicotine replacement or bupropion. There is very little evidence this type of support increases smoking cessation rates over and above rates achieved using medication alone[C].

Further information

Clinical evidence Thorogood *et al.* Cardiovascular disorders: changing behaviour (2003) Accessed via 🖳 www.library.nhs.uk
NICE 🖳 www.nice.org.uk

- Nicotine replacement therapy and bupropion for smoking cessation (2002)
- Brief interventions and referral for smoking cessation in primary care and other settings (2006)
- Guidance on prescribing of varenicline – expected in 2007

Figure 1.7 Management plan for smokers in the surgery

Remind smokers of the importance of stopping smoking with leaflets and posters around the surgery
Assess smoking status of all patients at least 1x/y. if possible

If smoking

Advise smokers to stop
Assess willingness to change

If the patient does not want to stop

If the patient wants to stop

Record advice given to stop smoking
Give the patient an advice leaflet to take away
Repeat advice to stop whenever the patient is seen in the surgery

Offer to refer to the smoke stop clinic (for equivalent alternative)
Help the patient to set a quit date and stick to it
Advise the patient to stop smoking completely on the quit date – 'not even one puff'
Recommend nicotine replacement therapy, bupropion or varenicline
Consider offering a follow-up appointment to check progress
Support the information given with an advice sheet

GP Notes:

⚠ Prescibe *only* for smokers who commit to target stop date. Initially prescribe only enough to last 2wk. after the target stop date, i.e. 2wk. nicotine replacement therapy or 3–4wk. bupropion. Only offer a 2nd prescription if the smoker demonstrates continuing commitment to stop smoking.

🛈 If unsuccessful the NHS will not fund another attempt for ≥6mo.

Smoking cessation in pregnancy: Individual/group sessions and behavioural therapy are preferable to NRT. Only use NRT if risk of smoking outweighs risk of treatment and only use for 2–3mo., preferably using an intermittent form (e.g. gum). If using patches, remove at night.

Drug misuse

In England and Wales, ~1:5 women aged 16–24y. have used cannabis in the past year. Other common drugs include amphetamines, ecstasy and cocaine. Class A drugs were used by ~5% of young women and, of those presenting for treatment, opioids are the main drugs of abuse (heroin – 54%; methadone – 13%). 3 factors are important:
- availability of drugs
- vulnerable personality
- social pressures, particularly from peers.

Detection: Warning signs suggesting drug misuse include the following.

Use of services: suspicious requests for drugs of abuse (e.g. no clear medical indication, prescription requests are too frequent).

Signs and symptoms
- Inappropriate behaviour
- Lack of self-care
- Unexplained nasal discharge
- Unusually constricted or dilated pupils
- Evidence of injecting (e.g. marked veins)
- Hepatitis or HIV infection

Social factors: family disruption, criminal history

Assessment: Assess on >1 occasion before deciding how to proceed. Exceptions are severe withdrawal symptoms and/or evidence of an established regime requiring continuation. Points to cover:

General information
- Check identification (ask to see an official document)
- Contact with other agencies (including last GP) – check accuracy
- Current residence; family – partner, children
- Employment and finances
- Current legal problems
- Criminal behaviour – past and present

History of drug use/risk taking behaviour
- Reason for consulting now and willingness to change
- Current and past usage
- Knowledge of risks
- Unsafe sexual practices

Medical and psychiatric history
- Complications of drug abuse, e.g. HIV, hepatitis, accidents
- General medical and psychiatric history and examination
- Overdoses – accidental or deliberate
- Alcohol abuse

Investigations
- Consider urine toxicology to confirm drug misuse.
- Consider blood for FBC, LFTs, and Hepatitis B, C & HIV serology (with consent and counselling), and other tests according to medical history/examination.

GMS contract

Specialized care of patients suffering from drug misuse may be provided by practices as a *national enhanced service*. Practices providing this service receive an annual payment plus a fee per patient per year.

Advice for patients: Advice and support for drug misusers

'Talk to FRANK' (England and Wales) Government-run information, advice and referral service ☎ (24h.) 0800 77 66 00 🖳 www.talktofrank.com
Drugscope Information about drug abuse and how to get treatment 🖳 www.drugscope.org.uk
Drugs-info Information about substance abuse for families of addicts 🖳 www.drugs-info.co.uk
ADFAM Support for families of addicts ☎ 020 7928 8898 🖳 www.adfam.org.uk
Ecstasy 🖳 www.ecstasy.org
Benzodiazepines 🖳 www.benzo.org.uk
Solvent abuse ☎ 0808 800 2345 🖳 www.re-solv.org
National Treatment Agency for Substance Abuse 🖳 www.nta.nhs.uk
Substance Misuse Management in General Practice (SMMGP) 🖳 www.smmgp.org.uk

GP Notes:

DVLA guidance about fitness to drive for patients with substance misuse problems

	Group 1 licence restrictions	Group 2 licence restrictions
Drug or alcohol misuse or dependency	6mo. off driving (1y. after alcohol- or drug-related seizure or detoxification for alcohol, opiate, cocaine or benzodiazepine dependence).	Licence revoked 1y. (3y. if alcohol dependence or misuse of opiates, cocaine or benzodiazepines; 5y. if alcohol- or drug-related seizure).
	DVLA arranges assessment prior to licence restoration.	DVLA arranges assessment prior to licence restoration.

Travelling with controlled drugs: Patients travelling abroad with controlled drugs may require an export licence. Further details can be obtained from the Home Office (☎ 020 7273 3806). Patient applications must be accompanied by a doctor's letter giving details of: patient's name and current address; quantities of drugs to be carried; strength and form of drugs; dates of travel. A 'To whom it concerns' letter from prescriber is advisable in all other cases.
For clearance to import the drug into the country of destination, contact the Embassy or High Commission of that country prior to departure.

Management of drug misuse: *Aims to*:
- ↓ risk of infectious diseases
- ↓ drug-related deaths
- ↓ criminal activity used to finance drug habits.

The GP and primary health care team have a vital role in:
- identifying drug misusers
- assessing their health and willingness to modify drug-abusing behaviour
- routine screening and prevention (e.g. cervical screening, contraception).

General measures: At each meeting consider the following.

Education
- Safer routes of drug administration
- Risks of overdose
- Condom use
- Driving and drug misuse (🕮 p.19)

Hepatitis B immunization: For injecting drug misusers not already infected/immune and close contacts of those already infected.

Treatment of dependence
- Set realistic goals.
- Responsibility contracts signed by GP, patient ± community pharmacist can be helpful.
- Review regularly.
- Give contact numbers for community support organizations (🕮 p.19).
- Seek advice and/or refer to a community substance misuse team as needed.

Specific drugs: Table 1.6

Solvent abuse
- Common amongst teenagers as solvents are easily obtained and cheap.
- Initial effects of inhalation are euphoria, incoordination, blurred vision and slurring of speech.
- Rarely the solvent may cause bronchoconstriction or arrhythmia and deaths, when they occur, are usually due to hypoxia, VF or accidents whilst intoxicated.
- Symptoms to look for in the surgery are changes in behaviour (e.g. drop in school performance or attendance, irritability, mood swings) and local changes due to inhalation (e.g. cough, headaches, conjunctivitis).
- If detected, refer to the youth support agencies.

GP Notes:

The RCGP Substance Misuse Unit provides certificate courses in management of drug abuse. 🖥 www.rcgp.org.uk

Table 1.6 Withdrawal of common drugs

Drug class	Drug withdrawal effects	Action
Opiates	*Symptoms:* Sweating Running eyes/nose Hot and cold turns ± goose-flesh GI problems – anorexia, nausea, vomiting, diarrhoea, abdominal pain Restlessness and tremor Insomnia Aches and pains Tachycardia ± hypertension Untreated heroin withdrawal reaches a peak 36–72h. after the last dose (methadone – 4–6d.) Symptoms subside by 5d. (methadone – 10–12d.)	Refer to substance abuse team
Benzodiazepines	*Symptoms:* Rebound anxiety Tremor Tachycardia Tachypnoea Nausea and/or diarrhoea Abdominal and muscular cramps Rarely perceptual disturbances and seizures	Taper dosage over weeks Seek specialist advice if the patient has any chronic debilitating condition or heart disease
Stimulants (e.g. amphetamines, cocaine, ecstasy)	Some patients experience insomnia and depression May require antidepressant drugs after withdrawal	Can be stopped abruptly
Hallucinogenic drugs (e.g. LSD)		Can be stopped abruptly
Barbiturates	Sudden cessation may cause fits ± death	Admit to hospital for supervised withdrawal

Further information

DoH Drug misuse and dependence – guidelines on clinical management (1999) 🖥 www.dh.gov.uk
NICE 🖥 www.nice.org.uk
• Substance misuse interventions (2007)
• Drug misuse: opioid detoxification (2007)
• Drug misuse: psychosocial interventions (2007)

Exercise

In the UK, 70% of women are not active enough to benefit their health.

> **Recommended amounts of activity (DoH):**
> - *Adults:* ≥30min. moderate-intensity exercise across the day on ≥5d./wk.
> - *Children:* ≥1h. moderate-intensity exercise across the day every day.

Dimensions of exercise
- *Volume or quantity* – quantity of activity, usually expressed as kcal per day or week. Can also be expressed as MET hours per day or week, where 1 MET = resting metabolic rate.
- *Frequency* – number of sessions per day or week.
- *Intensity* – light, moderate or vigorous. Light intensity = <4 METS (e.g. strolling); moderate = 4–6 METS (e.g. brisk walking); vigorous = 7+ METS (e.g. running).
- *Duration* – time spent on a single bout of activity.
- *Type or mode*, e.g. brisk walking, dancing or weight training.

 Use a validated tool to assess levels of physical activity, e.g. General Practitioner Physical Activity Questionnaire (GPPAQ – Box 1.1).

Exercise is beneficial: Regular physical activity:

↓ risk of:
- Cerebrovascular disease – physically inactive people have ~2x ↑ risk of coronary heart disease and ~3x ↑ risk of stroke[S]
- Diabetes mellitus – through ↑ insulin sensitivity[S]
- Obesity[S] – p.26
- Osteoporosis – exercise ↓ risk of hip fractures by ½[S]
- Cancer – ↓ risk of colon cancer ~40%. There is also evidence of a link between exercise and ↓ risk of breast and prostate cancers[S].

Is a useful treatment for
- ↑ BP – can result in 10mmHg drop of systolic and diastolic BP; can also delay onset of hypertension[S]
- Hypercholesterolaemia – ↑ high-density lipoprotein (HDL), ↓ low density lipoprotein (LDL)[C]
- Post-myocardial infarct[C]
- DM – improves insulin sensitivity and favourably affects other risk factors for DM including obesity, HDL/LDL ratio and ↑ BP
- HIV – ↑ cardiopulmonary fitness and psychological well-being[C]
- Arthritis and back pain – maintains function[C]
- ↓ intensity of depression; ↓ anxiety[S].

Benefits the elderly
- Maintains functional capacity
- ↓ levels of disability
- ↓ risk of falls & hip fracture
- Improves quality of sleep[C].

Box 1.1 General Practitioner Physical Activity Questionnaire (GPPAQ)

1) *Please tell us the type and amount of physical activity involved in your work*

Please mark one box only

(a) I am not in employment (e.g. retired, retired for health reasons, unemployed, full-time carer etc.) ☐

(b) I spend most of my time at work sitting (such as in an office) ☐

(c) I spend most of my time at work standing or walking. However, my work does not require much intense physical effort (e.g. shop assisstant, hairdresser, security guard, childminder, etc.) ☐

(d) My work involves definite physical effort including handling of heavy objects and use of tools (e.g. plumber, electrician, carpenter, cleaner, hospital nurse, garderner, postal delivery workers etc.) ☐

(e) My work involves vigorous physical activity including handling of very heavy objects (e.g. scaffolder, construction worker, refuse collector, etc.) ☐

2) *During the <u>last week</u>, how many hours did you spend on each of the following activities?*

		None	Some but <1h.	≥1h. but <3h.	≥3h.
(a)	Physical exercise e.g. swimmimg, jogging, aerobics, football, tennis, gym workout etc.				
(b)	Cycling, including cycling to work and during leisure time				
(c)	Wlaking, including walking to work, shopping, for pleasure etc.				
(d)	Housework/Childcare				
(e)	Gardening/DIY				

3) *How would you describe your usual walking pace?*

🔵 *Please mark one box only.*

Slow pace (<3mph)	Steady average pace	Brisk pace	Fast pace (>4mph)

Scoring: Table 1.7, 📖 p.25

Box 1.1 is reproduced with permission from the Department of Health 🖳 www.dh.gov.uk

Effective interventions

- *Healthcare:* ↑ physical activity for 1° and 2° prevention is effective in the short term – no evidence effects are maintained long-term. Counselling for physical activity is as effective as more structured exercise sessions.
- *Workplace:* Interventions to ↑ rates of walking to work are effective.
- *Schools:* Appropriately designed and delivered physical education curricula can enhance physical activity levels. A whole-school approach to physical activity promotion is effective.
- *Transport:* Well-designed interventions ↑ walking and cycling to work.
- *Communities:* Community-wide approaches to physical activity promotion → ↑ activity.

Negotiating change: It is possible to encourage people to ↑ activity levels. As with all lifestyle interventions the patient must want to change.

- If exercise levels are satisfactory (i.e. 'active' in Table 1.7), congratulate and inform about the benefits of exercise.
- If levels are unsatisfactory, explain the benefits of a higher level of physical activity and support with health education leaflets.
- Once the patient has agreed to increase activity levels, advise and agree ways to do that. Provide information about local opportunities for exercise. Set goals.
- Follow up at intervals over a 3–6mo. period.

You are more likely to be successful if:

- Exercise recommended is moderate, does not require attendance at a special facility and can be incorporated into daily life routines, e.g. walking/cycling to work.
- You suggest a graduated programme of exercise for sedentary patients (there is an ↑ risk of sudden cardiac death associated with sudden vigorous exercise).

🛈 When providing advice, always take into account the individual's needs, preferences and circumstances.

Exercise schemes

- *Specialist rehabilitation schemes* (e.g. cardiac, respiratory) are in operation in many areas – they are usually operated in association with specialist services and incorporate exercise and education for patients with specific conditions, e.g. post-MI.
- *Exercise prescription schemes:* Collaboration between community medical services and local sports facilities. They offer low-cost, supervised exercise for patients who might otherwise find it unacceptable to visit a gym, and are accessed via GP 'prescription'.
- *Local sports centres:* Many sports facilities also offer special sessions both on dry land and in the swimming pool for pregnant women, the over 50s and people with disability.

Further information

NICE Physical activity guidance (2006) 🖳 www.nice.org.uk
DoH The General Practice Physical Activity Questionnaire (2006) 🖳 www.dh.gov.uk

Table 1.7 Physical activity index (PAI) derived from the GPPAQ

Physical exercise and/or cycling (h/wk.)	Occupation			
	Sedentary	Standing	Physical	Heavy manual
0	Inactive	Moderately inactive	Moderately active	Active
Some but <1	Moderately inactive	Moderately active	Active	Active
1–2.9	Moderately active	Active	Active	Active
≥3	Active	Active	Active	Active

ⓘ Responses to questions 2 c, d & e and question 3 on the GPPAQ are not used to calculate the PAI

Figure 1.8 Management plan for increasing activity levels

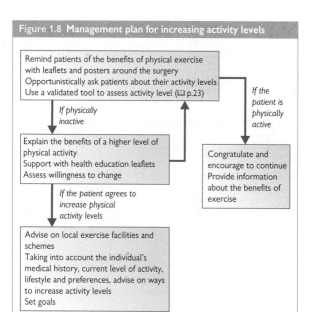

Remind patients of the benefits of physical exercise with leaflets and posters around the surgery
Opportunistically ask patients about their activity levels
Use a validated tool to assess activity level (□ p.23)

If physically inactive

If the patient is physically active

Explain the benefits of a higher level of physical activity
Support with health education leaflets
Assess willingness to change

If the patient agrees to increase physical activity levels

Congratulate and encourage to continue
Provide information about the benefits of exercise

Advise on local exercise facilities and schemes
Taking into account the individual's medical history, current level of activity, lifestyle and preferences, advise on ways to increase activity levels
Set goals

Table 1.7 is reproduced with permission from the Department of Health 🖳 www.dh.gov.uk

Obesity

The best measure of obesity is body mass index (BMI). Recent evidence shows obesity is increasing and it is set to take over from smoking as the number one preventable cause of disease in the UK. In 2001, >1:5 adults in the UK were classified as obese ($\male$ = $\female$). Rarely obesity has an underlying endocrine cause.

Classification: BMI (weight in kg ÷ (height in m)^2):

- 18.5–24.9kg/m^2 – normal
- 25–29.9kg/m^2 – overweight
- 30–39.9kg/m^2 – obese
- >40kg/m^2 – morbid obesity

Health risks of obesity

- Death (BMI >30kg/m^2 carries 3x ↑ risk of mortality)
- Ischaemic heart disease
- Hypercholesterolaemia
- ↑ BP
- Cerebrovascular disease
- Type 2 diabetes mellitus
- Gallbladder disease
- Complications after surgery
- Sleep apnoea
- Psychological problems
- Cancer of cervix, uterus, ovary and breast
- Musculoskeletal problems and arthritis
- Ovulatory failure
- Menstrual irregularities
- Complications in pregnancy (gestational diabetes, ↑ BP, pre-eclampsia), labour and delivery
- Stress incontinence

Waist circumference: An alternative indirect measurement of body fat that reflects the intra-abdominal fat mass. Strongly correlated with coronary heart disease risk, diabetes, hyperlipidaemia and ↑ BP (Table 1.8). Measured halfway between the superior iliac crest and the rib cage in the mid-axillary line.

Risk factors

- Genetic predisposition (accounts for about $^1/_3$ obesity)
- Endocrine disease, e.g. hypothyroidism, PCOS, Cushing's syndrome
- Previous obesity and successful dieting
- Physical inactivity
- Low education
- Smoking cessation

Investigation: Only investigate if other symptoms/signs of endocrine disease.

Prevention: Begins in childhood by instilling healthy patterns of exercise and diet.

🛈 There is little evidence to show that dietary advice by GPs or practice nurses is heeded. Most influence on diet comes from national food policy, price of food, advertising, general education and cultural influences.

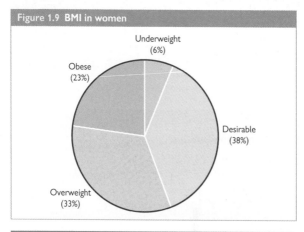

Figure 1.9 BMI in women

Underweight (6%)

Obese (23%)

Desirable (38%)

Overweight (33%)

Table 1.8 Association of waist circumference with risk of coronary heart disease and diabetes mellitus

	Waist circumference	
	White Caucasians	*Asians*
♂	≥102cm (40 inches)	≥90cm (36 inches)
♀	≥88cm (35 inches)	≥80cm (32 inches)

Further information

National Audit Office Tackling obesity in England (2001)
🖥 www.nao.org.uk

NICE 🖥 www.nice.org.uk
- Guidance on the use of sibutramine for the treatment of obesity in adults (2001)
- Orlistat for treatment of obesity in adults (2001)
- Rimonabant for the treatment of overweight and obese patients – in preparation
- Obesity: the prevention, identification, assessment and management of overweight and obesity in adults and children (2006)

National Obesity Forum 🖥 www.nationalobesityforum.org.uk
- Guidelines on the management of adult obesity and overweight in primary care (2002)
- An approach to weight management in children and adolescents (2–18 years) in primary care (2003)

SIGN Management of obesity in children and young people (2003)
🖥 www.sign.ac.uk

Counterweight Project 🖥 www.counterweight.org

Figure 1.10 BMI ready reckoner

Height in metres

Weight in kilograms	1.36	1.40	1.44	1.48	1.52	1.56	1.60	1.64	1.68	1.72	1.76	1.80	1.84	1.88	1.92	1.96	2.00
125	68	64	60	57	54	51	49	46	44	42	40	39	37	35	34	33	31
123	67	63	59	56	53	51	48	46	44	42	40	38	36	35	33	32	31
121	65	62	58	55	52	50	47	45	43	41	39	37	36	34	33	31	30
119	64	61	57	54	52	49	46	44	42	40	38	37	35	34	32	31	30
117	63	60	56	53	51	48	46	44	41	40	38	36	35	33	32	30	29
115	62	59	55	53	50	47	45	43	41	39	37	35	34	33	31	30	29
113	61	58	54	52	49	46	44	42	40	38	36	35	33	32	31	29	28
111	60	57	54	51	48	46	43	41	39	38	36	34	33	31	30	29	28
109	59	56	53	50	47	45	43	41	39	37	35	34	32	31	30	28	27
107	58	55	52	49	46	44	42	40	38	36	35	33	32	30	29	28	27
105	57	54	51	48	45	43	41	39	37	35	34	32	31	30	28	27	26
103	56	53	50	47	45	42	40	38	36	35	33	32	30	29	28	27	26
101	55	52	49	46	44	42	39	38	36	34	33	31	29	28	27	26	25
99	54	51	48	45	43	41	39	37	35	33	32	31	29	28	27	26	25
97	52	49	47	44	42	40	38	36	34	33	31	30	28	27	26	25	24
95	51	48	46	43	41	39	37	35	34	32	31	29	28	27	26	25	24
93	50	47	45	42	40	38	36	35	33	31	30	29	27	26	25	24	23
91	49	46	44	42	39	37	36	34	32	31	29	28	27	26	25	24	23
89	48	45	43	41	39	37	35	33	32	30	29	27	26	25	24	23	22
87	47	44	42	40	38	36	34	32	31	29	28	27	26	25	24	23	22
85	46	43	41	39	37	35	33	32	30	29	27	26	25	24	23	22	21
83	45	42	40	38	36	34	32	31	29	28	27	26	25	23	23	22	21
81	44	41	39	37	35	33	32	30	29	27	26	25	24	23	22	21	20
79	43	40	38	36	34	32	31	29	28	27	26	24	23	22	21	21	20
77	42	39	37	35	33	32	30	29	27	26	25	24	23	22	21	20	19
75	41	38	36	34	32	31	29	28	27	25	24	23	22	21	20	20	19
73	39	37	35	33	32	30	29	27	26	25	24	23	22	21	20	19	18
71	38	36	34	32	31	29	28	26	25	24	23	22	21	20	19	18	18
69	37	35	33	32	30	28	27	26	24	23	22	21	20	20	19	18	17
67	36	34	32	31	29	28	26	25	24	23	22	21	20	19	18	17	17
65	35	33	31	30	28	27	25	24	23	22	21	20	19	18	18	17	16
63	34	32	30	29	27	26	25	23	22	21	20	19	18	17	17	16	16
61	33	31	29	28	26	25	24	23	22	21	20	19	18	17	17	16	15
59	32	30	28	27	26	24	23	22	21	20	19	18	17	17	16	15	15
57	31	26	27	26	25	23	22	21	20	19	18	17	16	16	15	15	14
55	30	30	27	25	24	23	21	20	19	18	17	16	16	15	14	14	14
53	29	29	26	24	23	22	21	20	19	18	17	16	15	15	14	14	13
51	28	26	25	23	22	21	20	19	18	17	16	16	15	14	14	13	13
49	26	25	24	22	21	20	19	18	17	16	16	15	14	14	13	13	12
47	25	24	23	21	20	19	18	17	17	16	15	14	13	13	12	12	12
45	24	23	22	21	19	18	18	17	16	15	15	14	13	13	12	12	11
43	23	22	21	20	19	18	17	16	15	15	14	13	13	12	11	11	11

- BMI <18.5 – underweight
- BMI 18.5–24.9 – acceptable weight
- BMI 25–29.9 – overweight
- BMI 30–39.9 – obese
- BMI ≥40 – morbid obesity

Figure 1.10 is reproduced from Simon, C. et al. (2005) Oxford Handbook of General Practice 2nd ed., p. 229, with permission from Oxford University Press.

GMS contract

Obesity 1	The practice can produce a register of patients ≥16y. with a BMI ≥30kg/m² in the previous 15mo.	8 points	
Diabetes 2	% of patients with DM whose notes record BMI in the previous 15mo.	up to 3 points	40–90%

29

Figure 1.11 The plate model. Developed nationally to communicate current recommendations for healthy eating. It shows rough proportions of the various food groups that should make up each meal

Fruits and vegetables

Bread, other cereals, and potatoes

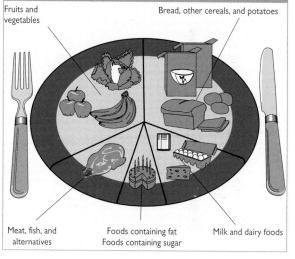

Meat, fish, and alternatives

Foods containing fat
Foods containing sugar

Milk and dairy foods

Figure 1.11 is reproduced from Simon, C. et al. (2005) Oxford Handbook of General Practice 2nd ed., p. 229, with permission from Oxford University Press.

Treatment: When the body's intake is > output over a period of time, obesity results. Management of obesity aims to reverse this trend on a long-term basis.

Healthy diet: Encourage all patients to ↓ fat intake; ↑ proportion of unrefined carbohydrate; eat 5 portions of fruit and vegetables/d.; ↓ hidden sugars (alcohol, prepared foods); ↑ fibre – Figure 1.11, 📖 p.29.

Low calorie diets
- All obese people lose weight by reducing energy intake.
- A realistic goal is weight loss of 1–2lbs (0.5–1kg)/wk. and is achievable using diets of 1000–1500kcal/d. intake.
- Rates of weight loss >1kg/wk. involve loss of lean tissue rather than fat.
- Aim for a BMI of 25. There is no health benefit of weight ↓ below this.
- Weight loss in the first few weeks may be higher due to water and glycogen depletion.
- If simple diet sheets are not effective, refer to a dietician.

Very low calorie diets (<800kcal/day): Only limited place in management as this pattern of eating cannot be maintained and rebound weight gain is seen on stopping. Only use to treat morbid obesity under strict supervision.

Exercise: Regular aerobic exercise helps ↓ weight and improve health. Tailor advice to the individual and local facilities.

Drug therapy (BNF 4.5)
- Drugs specifically licensed for the treatment of obesity are orlistat (120mg tds with food) which acts by ↓ fat absorption from the GI tract, and centrally acting appetite suppressants sibutramine (10–15mg od – monitor BP and pulse rate closely) and rimonabant (20mg mane)
- Consider if BMI ≥30kg/m^2 or ≥27kg/m^2 in the presence of co-morbidity, e.g. diabetes, hypercholesterolaemia, hypertension.
- There is little evidence to guide selection but it is logical to choose orlistat for those who have a high intake of fats and sibutramine for those who cannot control their eating.
- Combination therapy involving >1 anti-obesity drug is contraindicated.

Group therapy: Group activities, e.g. Weight Watchers, seem to have a higher success rate in producing and maintaining weight loss.

Behavioural therapy: Shown to be effective individually and in groups when combined with low calorie diets. In simplest form involves advice to avoid situations that tempt overeating.

Surgery: Only consider referral as a last resort if behavioural and dietary modification have failed and BMI >40. Gastroplasty is the most common procedure. Mortality is high.

Follow-up: on a regular basis is essential to maintain motivation.

Maintenance of weight loss: Once a patient has lost weight, diet still needs to be monitored. Ongoing follow-up has been shown to help sustain weight loss. Weight fluctuation (yo-yo dieting) may be harmful.

Use of orlistat

Warn patients about common side-effects: The major problems patients experience are GI side-effects – oily leakage from rectum, flatulence, faecal urgency, liquid or oily stools, faecal incontinence, abdominal distension and pain. GI side-effects are minimized by reduced fat intake.

NICE guidance: NICE has recommended (2001) that treatment with orlistat should be continued >6mo. only if ≥10% of starting weight has been lost since the start of treatment.

Use of sibutramine

Contraindications/cautions

- *History of psychiatric illness:* psychosis, major eating disorders, Tourette's syndrome (use with caution if family history of motor or vocal tics), drug or alcohol abuse, use with caution in depression
- *Cardiovascular disease:* avoid if history of coronary artery disease, congestive heart failure, tachycardia or other arrhythmia, peripheral arterial occlusive disease, cerebrovascular disease, uncontrolled ↑ BP
- *Endocrine disease:* hyperthyroidism or phaeochromocytoma
- *Prostatic hypertrophy*
- *Glaucoma:* avoid in angle closure glaucoma; use with caution if open angle glaucoma or history of ocular hypertension
- *Sleep apnoea:* use with caution – may cause ↑ BP – stop if does
- *Hepatic or renal failure:* use with caution if mild – avoid if severe
- *Pregnancy or breast feeding:* avoid
- *Epilepsy:* use with caution
- *Warfarin use or bleeding tendency:* use with caution

NICE guidance: NICE has recommended that sibutramine should be prescribed only for individuals who have attempted seriously to lose weight by diet, exercise and other behavioural modification. In addition, arrangements should exist for appropriate health-care professionals to offer specific advice, support and counselling on diet, physical activity and behavioural strategies to those receiving sibutramine.

Monitoring: Monitor BP and pulse rate:

- every 2wk. for the first 3mo. *then*
- monthly for 3mo. *then*
- at least every 3mo.

Discontinue if blood pressure >145/90mmHg *or* if systolic or diastolic pressure raised by >10mmHg *or* if pulse rate raised by 10 bpm at 2 consecutive visits.

Discontinue treatment if:

- weight loss after 3mo. is <5% of initial body weight
- weight loss stabilizes at <5% less than initial body weight
- individuals regain ≥3kg after previous weight loss

In individuals with co-morbid conditions, treatment should be continued only if weight loss is associated with other clinical benefits.

Prevention of cardiovascular disease

Coronary heart disease (CHD) is the most common cause of death in the UK (1:4 deaths) among men and women. Mortality is falling but morbidity rising. With an ageing population, prevention is very important both to preserve lifestyle in old age and also to ↓ health and social care costs of looking after patients with cardiovascular disease (CVD).

Risk factors for heart disease: Table 1.9, 📖 p.34

Primary prevention: Aims to stop coronary, cerebrovascular and peripheral vascular disease developing in a population. *Strategies:*
- *Population strategy:* Influences the factors which ↑ risk of CVD in an entire population, e.g. anti-smoking campaigns. GPs can do this by displaying health education posters/literature where all patients have access (waiting room, practice leaflet).
- *High-risk strategy:* Identifies individuals at high risk and attempts to ↓ their risk. Selection of patients is based on overall risk which depends on the combination of risk factors a patient has and can be estimated using tables (Figure 1.12 and 🖥 www.bhsoc.org). Only small benefit is gained by screening an entire population and population screening is not cost-effective[R]. An opportunistic strategy targeting high-risk individuals is preferable.

Secondary prevention: *Objective:* To stop progression of symptomatic CVD. 46% people who die from MI are already known to have CHD. There is strong evidence that targeting patients with CVD for risk-factor modification is effective in ↓ risk of recurrent CVD[S].

The GP's role: GPs have a role in:
- identification of patients who would benefit from 1° prevention through opportunistic risk factor screening or routine checks (e.g. new patient checks). Quality and outcome framework points (and thus payments) are available for doing this
- ensuring patients who have proven atherosclerotic disease have ongoing follow-up (through disease registers, routine recall and follow-up by the practice, PCT and/or 2° care services and monitoring of drug prescriptions)
- points gained for meeting secondary prevention targets contained within the quality and outcome framework reward practices for secondary prevention – 📖 pp.35–6
- promoting lifestyle modification in at-risk patients
- ensuring current best care guidelines are followed and treatment regimes are updated as policies change
- checking the process through audit.

Further information

DoH National Service Framework: coronary heart disease (2000 and update 2005) 🖥 www.dh.gov.uk
JBS2: Joint British Societies guidelines on prevention of cardiovascular disease in clinical practice (2005) 🖥 www.bcs.com
NICE MI: Secondary prevention (2007) 🖥 www.nice.org.uk

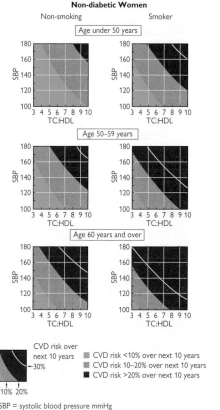

Figure 1.12 Cardiovascular risk chart for non-diabetic women

Non-diabetic Women

Non-smoking   Smoker

Age under 50 years

Age 50–59 years

Age 60 years and over

CVD risk over next 10 years ~30%

■ CVD risk <10% over next 10 years
■ CVD risk 10–20% over next 10 years
■ CVD risk >20% over next 10 years

10% 20%

SBP = systolic blood pressure mmHg
TC:HDL = serum total cholesterol to HDL cholesterol ratio

⚠ These charts are not appropriate for use with patients with pre-existing CVD, familial hypercholesterolaemia, chronic renal dysfunction or DM.

ⓘ Patients in the following groups have ↑ risk:
• Family history of premature CHD or stroke (multiply risk by 1.5x)
• Originate from the Indian subcontinent (multiply risk by 1.5x)
• ↑ triglycerides, premature menopause, or impaired glucose tolerance.

Advice for patients: Information for patients on coronary prevention

British Heart Foundation ☎ 0845 0708 070 🖳 www.bhf.org.uk

Figure 1.12 is reproduced with permission from the University of Manchester

33

GMS contract

Primary prevention

Records 11	BP of patients aged ≥45y. is recorded in the preceding 5y. for ≥65% of patients	10 points	
Records 17	BP of patients aged ≥45y. is recorded in the preceding 5y. for ≥80% of patients	5 points	
Records 22	% of patients aged >15y. whose notes record smoking status in the past 27mo., except those who have never smoked where smoking status need only be recorded once	up to 11 points	40–90%
Information 5	The practice supports smokers in stopping smoking by a strategy which includes providing literature and offering appropriate therapy	2 points	
Obesity 1	The practice can produce a register of patients aged ≥16y. with a BMI ≥30 in the previous 15mo.	6 points	

Table 1.9 Risk factors for heart disease

Non-modifiable	Modifiable (proven benefit)	Modifiable (unproven benefit)
Age – ↑ with age Sex – ♂>♀ in those <65y. Ethnic origin – in the UK people who originate from the Indian subcontinent have ↑ risk, Afro-Caribbeans have ↓ risk Socio-economic position Personal history of CHD Family history of CHD – <55y. ♂; <65y. ♀ Low birth weight (IUGR) – 🕮 p.260	Smoking – 🕮 p.14 Hyperlipidaemia (target cholestreol ≤5mmol/l) Hypertension (BP ≤150/90 or ≤145/85 if diabetic) DM (HbA$_{1c}$ ≤7.5) Diet – 🕮 p.30 Obesity (BMI <30) – 🕮 p.26 Physical inactivity – 🕮 p.22 Left ventricular dysfunction/heart failure (2° prevention) Coronary prone behaviour – competitiveness, aggression and feeling under time pressure (2° prevention) – behaviour modification is associated with ↓ risk	Haemostatic factors – ↑ plasma fibrinogen Apolipoproteins – ↑ lipoprotein(a) Homocysteine – ↑ blood homocysteine Vitamin levels – ↓ blood folate, vitamin B$_{12}$ and B$_6$ Depression

ⓘ Targets quoted are those needed for quality and outcomes framework points:

Primary or secondary prevention

Hypertension indicators

BP 1	The practice can produce a register of patients with established hypertension	6 points	
BP 4	% of patients with ↑ BP in whom there is a record of BP in the previous 9mo.	up to 20 points	40–90%
BP 5	% of patients with ↑ BP in whom the last BP (measured in the previous 9mo.) is ≤150/90	up to 57 points	40–70%
BP 5	The practice can produce a register of patients with established hypertension	6 points	

Diabetes indicators

DM 19	The practice can produce a register of all patients aged ≥17y. with DM, which specifies whether the patient has type 1 or type 2 diabetes	6 points	
DM 2	% of patients with DM whose notes record BMI in the previous 15mo.	up to 3 points	40–90%
DM 5	% of diabetic patients who have a record of HbA_{1c} or equivalent in the previous 15mo.	up to 3 points	40–90%
DM 20	% of patients with DM in whom the last HbA_{1c} is ≤7.5 (or equivalent test/reference range depending on local laboratory) in the previous 15mo.	up to 17 points	40–50%
DM 7	% of patients with DM in whom the HbA_{1c} is ≤10 (or equivalent test/reference range depending on local laboratory) in the previous 15mo.	up to 11 points	40–90%
DM 9	% of patients with DM with a record of the presence or absence of peripheral pulses in the previous 15mo.	up to 3 points	40–90%
DM 11	% of patients with DM who have a record of BP in the previous 15mo.	up to 3 points	40–90%
DM 12	% of patients with DM in whom the last BP is ≤145/85	up to 18 points	40–60%
DM 16	% of patients with DM who have a record of total cholesterol in the previous 15mo.	up to 3 points	40–90%
DM 17	% of patients with DM whose last measured total cholesterol within the previous 15mo. is ≤5mmol/l	up to 6 points	40–70%

Secondary prevention

Smoking indicators

Smoking 1	% of patients with any/combination of coronary heart disease, stroke or TIA, hypertension, diabetes, COPD or asthma whose notes record smoking status in the previous 15mo., except those who have never smoked where smoking status need only be recorded once since diagnosis	up to 33 points	40–90%
Smoking 2	% of patients with any/combination of the conditions listed in 'smoking 1' who smoke whose notes contain a record that smoking cessation advice or referral to a specialist service, where available, has been offered within the previous 15mo.	up to 35 points	40–90%

Coronary heart disease (CHD) indicators

CHD 1	The practice can produce a register of patients with CHD	4 points	
CHD 5	% of patients with CHD who have a record of BP in the previous 15mo.	up to 7 points	40–90%
CHD 6	% of patients with CHD in whom the last BP (measured in the previous 15mo.) is ≤150/90	up to 19 points	40–70%
CHD 7	% of patients with CHD whose notes have a record of total cholesterol in the previous 15mo.	up to 7 points	40–90%
CHD 8	% of patients with CHD whose last measured total cholesterol (measured in the previous 15mo.) is ≤5mmol/l	up to 17 points	40–70%
CHD 9	% of patients with CHD with a record in the previous 15mo. that aspirin, an alternative antiplatelet therapy or anticoagulant is being taken (unless a contraindication or side-effects are recorded)	up to 7 points	40–90%
CHD 10	% of patients with CHD who are currently treated with a β-blocker (unless a contraindication or side-effects are recorded)	up to 7 points	40–60%
CHD 11	% of patients with a history of MI (diagnosed after 1.4.2003) who are currently treated with an ACE inhibitor or angiotensin II antagonist	up to 7 points	40–80%

Stroke and transient ischaemic attack (TIA) indicator			
Stroke 1	The practice can produce a register of patients with stroke or TIA	2 points	
Stroke 5	% of patients with stroke/TIA who have a record of BP in the notes in the preceding 15mo.	up to 2 points	40–90%
Stroke 6	% of patients with stroke/TIA in whom the last BP (measured in the previous 15mo.) is ≤150/90	up to 5 points	40–70%
Stroke 7	% of patients with stroke/TIA who have a record of total cholesterol in the last 15mo.	up to 2 points	40–90%
Stroke 8	% of patients with stroke/TIA whose last measured total cholesterol (measured in the previous 15mo.) is ≤5mmol/l	up to 5 points	40–60%
Stroke 12	% of patients with stroke shown to be non-haemorrhagic, or history of TIA, who have a record that an antiplatelet agent (aspirin, clopidogrel, dipyridamole or a combination) or an anticoagulant is being taken (unless a contraindication or side-effects are recorded)	up to 4 points	40–90%
Depression indicator			
Depression 1	% of patients on the coronary heart disease and/or diabetes register for whom case finding for depression has been undertaken on one occasion in the preceding 15mo. using 2 standard screening questions*	up to 8 points	40–90%
Depression 2	For those patients with a new diagnosis of depression in the previous 12mo., the % of patients with an assessment of severity, using an assessment tool validated for use in primary care, recorded in the patient record at the start of treatment	up to 25 points	40–90%

* Standard screening questions:
- During the last month, have you often been bothered by feeling down, depressed or hopeless?
- During the last month, have you often been bothered by having little interest or pleasure in doing things?

Patients replying 'yes' to either question require further mood assessment.

Domestic violence

Used to describe physical, emotional and mental abuse of women by male partners. Affects ~1:4 women – the most common form of interpersonal crime. 60% – current partner; 21% – former partners. ½ suffer >1 attack. $^1/_3$ have been attacked repeatedly.

General practice is often the first place in which women seek formal help but only ¼ actually reveal that they have been beaten. Without appropriate intervention, violence continues and often ↑ in frequency and severity. By the time the woman's injuries are visible, violence may be a long-established pattern. On average, a woman will be assaulted 35 times before reporting it to the police.

Effects: High incidence of psychiatric disorders, particularly depression, and self-damaging behaviours including drug and alcohol abuse, suicide and parasuicide.

Factors preventing the woman leaving the abusive situation

- Loss of self-esteem makes women think they are to blame
- Fear of partner
- Disruption of the family and children's relationship with their father
- Loss of intimate relationship with partner
- Fall in income
- Risk of homelessness
- Fear of the unknown

Guidelines for care

- Consider the possibility of domestic violence – ask directly.
- Emphasize confidentiality.
- Document – accurate, clear documentation, over time at successive consultations, may provide cumulative evidence of abuse, and is essential for use as evidence in court, should the need arise.
- Assess the present situation – gather as much information as possible.
- Provide information and offer help in making contact with other agencies.
- Devise a safety plan – give the phone number of local women's refuge; advise to keep some money and important financial and legal documents hidden in a safe place in case of emergency; help plan an escape route in case of emergency.

ⓘ Do not pressurize women into any course of action. If the patient decides to return to the violent situation, she will not forget the information and support given. In time this might give her the confidence and back-up she needs to break out of her situation.

⚠ If children are likely to be at risk, you have a duty to inform social services or the police, preferably with the patient's consent.

Elder abuse: Defined as 'A single or repeated act or lack of appropriate action, occurring within any relationship where there is an expectation of trust, which causes harm or distress to an older person'.

Older people may report the abuse but often do not. May take several forms which may co-exist:

* *Physical:* e.g. cuts, bruises, unexplained fractures, dehydration/malnourishment with no medical explanation, burns
* *Psychological:* e.g. unusual behaviour, unexplained fear, appears helpless or withdrawn
* *Financial:* e.g. removal of funds by carers, new will in favour of carer
* *Sexual:* e.g. unexplained bruising, vaginal or anal bleeding, genital infections
* *Neglect:* e.g. malnourished, dehydrated, poor personal hygiene, late requests for medical attention.

Prevalence (in own home): Physical abuse – 2%; verbal abuse – 5%; financial abuse – 2%.

Signs: Inconsistent story from patient and carer, inconsistencies on examination; fear in presence of carer; frequent attendance at A&E; frequent requests for GP visits; carer avoiding GP.

Management: Talk through the situation with the patient, carer and other services involved in care. Assess the level of risk. Consider admission to a place of safety – contact social services and/or police as necessary; seek advice from Action on Elder Abuse.

Further information

DoH Domestic violence: a resource manual for health care profession-als. Available from 🖳 www.dh.gov.uk
Home Office 🖳 www.homeoffice.gov.uk/crime-victims/reducing-crime/domestic-violence
RCGP Heath I. Domestic violence 🖳 www.rcgp.org.uk
BMJ Ramsay J et al. Should health professionals screen women for domestic violence? Systematic review (2002) 325: 314

Useful contacts

Womens' Aid ☎ 0808 2000 247 🖳 www.womensaid.org.uk
Action on Elder Abuse ☎ 0808 808 8141 🖳 www.elderabuse.org.uk
Police domestic violence units ☎ 0845 045 45 45
Local authority social services departments
Local authority housing departments

GP Notes:

Domestic violence may start or escalate in pregnancy – estimated prevalence is 17%. It ↑ risk of pre-term birth, antepartum haemor-rhage and perinatal mortality. Ask routinely about domestic violence as part of usual antenatal care.

Chapter 2

Breast disease

Assessment of breast disease 42
Benign breast disease 48
Breast cancer screening 52
Breast cancer 56

Assessment of breast disease

Encourage all women to be breast aware (see opposite) to minimize delay in presentation of symptoms. Treat all women presenting with breast symptoms with sensitivity as most will be worried about the possibility of breast cancer. Even if their worries are unfounded, a bad experience may delay future presentation.

History: Malignancy is rare <30y.

Presenting complaint
- **Lump** – how and when noticed, relationship to menstrual cycle, pain/tenderness, change in size/shape since noticed
- **Skin changes** – ulceration, eczema, dimpling
- **Nipple discharge** – both sides or just one, colour, any associated lumps
- **Nipple inversion** – new or long-standing
- **Other symptoms** – weight loss, anorexia/nausea, breathlessness, sweats, bone pain, neurological symptoms

Past medical history
- **Previous breast disease** – breast cyst or other benign breast disease, breast cancer, breast trauma, breast imaging, breast surgery or radiotherapy
- **Gynaecological history** – age of menarche/menopause, number of children and age at first pregnancy, history of breast feeding

Treatment/drug history: HRT, oral contraceptive

Family history: breast cancer.

Examination
Look: With the patient seated, with arms at her sides, above her head and pressing on her lips, look at:
- **Size and shape of breasts** – breasts enlarge during pregnancy and with weight gain. Acute change in 1 breast is likely to reflect pathology e.g. tumour or cyst.
- **Skin contour** – are any lumps visible? Is there any skin dimpling?
- **Skin changes** – eczema, ulceration, colouration, arm swelling. Suspect underlying breast cancer if there is eczema of the nipple (p.58).
- **Nipple changes** – inversion, discharge, excoriation or eczema. The nipple usually points downwards and laterally. If it points inwards/upwards, suspect underlying disease.

Palpate
- Seat the woman at 45° supported on a couch.
- Ask the woman to point to the painful area or find the lump.
- Ask her to place the hand on the side being examined behind her head. Examine both breasts starting with the normal side.
- Palpate each quadrant of the breast with a flat hand. Check the tail of the breast in the axilla.
- If a lump is found assess shape, size, surface, edge, consistency, mobility and attachments.
- Check local lymph nodes in the axilla and supraclavicular region.

Advice for patients:

Breast awareness: Breast awareness means knowing what your breasts look and feel like normally. Evidence suggests that there is no need to follow a specific or detailed routine such as breast self-examination, but you should be aware of any changes in your breasts.

The breast awareness 5-point code

1. Know what is normal for you
2. Know what changes to look and feel for
3. Look and feel
4. Report any changes to your GP without delay
5. Attend for routine breast screening if you are aged 50 or over

Changes to be aware of

- *Size* – if one breast becomes larger, or lower
- *Nipples* – if a nipple becomes inverted (pulled in) or changes position or shape
- *Rashes* – on or around the nipple
- *Discharge* – from one or both nipples
- *Skin changes* – puckering or dimpling
- *Swelling* – under the armpit or around the collar-bone (where the lymph nodes are)
- *Pain* – continuous, in one part of the breast or armpit
- *Lump or thickening* – different to the rest of the breast tissue

What should I do if I notice a change? If you do notice a change in your breasts, try not to worry but see your GP as soon as you can. Your GP may ask you to come back at a different time in your menstrual cycle, or send you to a breast clinic for a more detailed examination.

ℹ️ Remember that most breast changes are not cancer, even if they need follow-up treatment or further investigation.

Further information

Breast Cancer Care 🖳 www.breastcancercare.org.uk
NHS Cancer Screening 'Be breast aware' leaflet and other information 🖳 www.cancerscreening.org.uk/breastscreen/breastawareness.html

Reproduced with permission from 🖳 www.breastcancercare.org.uk

Consider general examination for disseminated disease
- Respiratory – shortness of breath, effusion
- Abdomen – hepatomegaly, ascites
- Musculoskeletal – pain, tenderness, ↓ movement
- Neurology – headache, weakness, sensory disturbance, ataxia

Breast lump
Differential diagnosis
- Breast cancer 📖 p.56
- Fibroadenoma 📖 p.48
- Breast cyst 📖 p.50
- Mammary duct ectasia/periductal mastitis 📖 p.51
- Fat necrosis 📖 p.50
- Phyllodes tumour 📖 p.50
- Intraductal papilloma 📖 p.51
- Lipoma
- Sebaceous cyst

Management
- **No lump:** Reassure. Educate the woman about breast awareness (📖 p.43). Consider reviewing in 6wk.
- **Discrete lump:** Refer.
- **Asymmetrical nodularity**
  - <30y. old with family history of breast cancer or ≥30y. – non-urgent referral.
  - <30y. and no family history – review in 6wk. If the nodularity has gone reassure, otherwise refer.

⚠ Any patient being referred with a breast lump will be concerned about the possibility of breast cancer even though most will not have cancer. Talk to the patient about these worries and the information they need.

Discharge from the nipple: 90% of pre-menopausal women can express milky, multiple duct discharge. Ask about colour, quantity and whether the discharge is unilateral/bilateral. Examine to check there are no lumps. Note colour/quantity of discharge and whether the discharge is coming from multiple or a single duct.

Differential diagnosis
- Physiological (e.g. pregnancy)
- Mammary duct ectasia 📖 p.51
- Breast cancer 📖 p.56
- Periductal mastitis 📖 p.51
- Intraduct papilloma 📖 p.51

Management
- Refer urgently if unilateral, spontaneous bloody discharge.
- Refer if >50y. or features suggesting pathological cause (Table 2.1).

Breast pain or mastalgia: Most common in women aged 30–50y. Use a pain chart for >2mo. to distinguish cyclical from non-cyclical pain.

Cyclical breast pain: Common – ~2/3 of women >35y. have cyclical mastalgia which causes distress or interferes with lifestyle. Symptoms are often long-standing:
- usually bilateral though may not be the same intensity in both breasts
- pain is generally felt over the lateral side of the breast, increases from mid-cycle onwards and is relieved by menstruation.

Examination may reveal tenderness ± areas of nodularity/lumpiness.

Urgent referral of patients with breast disease[N]

Encourage all female patients to be breast aware (📖 p.43).

Refer any patient who presents with symptoms suggestive of breast cancer urgently (to be seen in <2wk.) to a team specializing in the management of breast cancer.

Urgent referral (to be seen in <2wk.) is always required for

Lump
- Any age with a discrete, hard lump with fixation ± skin tethering
- Any age with a past history of breast cancer presenting with a further lump or other suspicious symptoms
- Aged ≥30y. with a discrete lump that persists after the next period, or presents after menopause
- Aged <30y.
  - with a lump that enlarges
  - with a lump that is fixed and hard
  - in whom there are other reasons for concern such as family history.

Nipple changes
- Unilateral eczematous skin or nipple change that does not respond to topical treatment
- Nipple distortion of recent onset
- Spontaneous unilateral bloody nipple discharge

Consider a non-urgent referral if:
- Woman is aged <30y. and has a lump which has no suspicious features and is not enlarging
- Breast pain and no palpable abnormality, when initial treatment fails and/or symptoms persist (use of mammography is not recommended)

⚠ In patients presenting with symptoms and/or signs suggestive of breast cancer, investigation prior to referral is not recommended.

Referral of patients with family history of breast cancer
📖 p.57

Further information
NICE Referral guidelines for suspected cancer (2005).
🖥 www.nice.org.uk

Table 2.1 Features of nipple discharge which suggest physiological or pathological cause

Physiological cause likely	Pathological cause likely – refer
• Bilateral	• Unilateral
• Multiple ducts	• Single duct
• On expression only	• Spontaneous
• Green, milky	• Red, brown, black
• Stains only	• Profuse and watery

Differential diagnosis
- Physiological
- Mammary duct ectasia/periductal mastitis 📖 p.51
- Breast cancer 📖 p.56
- Sclerosing adenosis 📖 p.50
- Mastitis 📖 p.276
- Breast abscess 📖 p.51
- Referred pain (e.g. cervical root pressure)

Management of mild/moderate cyclical pain: 85% patients. Reassure that breast pain is a very *unusual* symptom of breast cancer. Explain the hormonal basis of symptoms. Consider:
- *Diet* – reducing saturated fats and caffeine may help.
- *Support* – advise the woman to try wearing a soft, support bra at night
- *OTC medication* – try simple analgesia (e.g. paracetamol 1g qds prn) and/or NSAID (e.g. ibuprofen 200–400mg tds prn). Some women also find oil of evening primrose (gamolenic acid) is effective but it may take 4mo. to work.
- *Changing/stopping hormonal contraceptives or HRT.*

Management of severe cyclical pain: Defined as pain for >7d./mo. for >6mo. which interferes with lifestyle. 15% patients. Try measures for management of mild/moderate cyclical pain first. If they fail, consider:
- *Danazol* – 100mg tds for 3–6mo. Start on day 1 of the menstrual cycle. Acne, weight gain, menorrhagia and muscle cramps are common side-effects. Withdraw if virilization.
- *Bromocriptine* – 1–1.25mg nocte increased slowly to 2.5mg bd. Acts in <2mo. but associated with pulmonary, retroperitoneal and pericardial fibrotic reactions (CSM advises checking CXR and blood for ESR and Cr prior to treatment and monitoring for dyspnoea, persistent cough, chest pain, cardiac failure and abdominal pain/tenderness). May also cause hypotensive reactions and/or sleepiness – warn not to drive or operate machinery if affected.
- *Tamoxifen* (unlicensed) – 20mg on days of the cycle when symptoms are predicted. Common side-effects include hot flushes and vaginal discharge. Associated with ↑ risk of DVT. Advise patients to report sudden breathlessness or unilateral calf pain. Also associated with endometrial changes including hyperplasia, polyps and cancer. Advise patients to report menstrual irregularities, abnormal discharge and/or pelvic pain/pressure.
- *LHRH analogues*, e.g. goserelin – occasionally used in specialist settings.

Drug treatment helps ~80% of women. Review treatment after 3–6mo. and continue if necessary. After stopping, symptoms recur in ~½, but are often less severe. Refer if treatment fails.

Non-cyclical breast pain: Pain which is either continuous, or intermittent but with no relationship to the menstrual cycle. Treat the cause. Ask if the pain is localized or diffuse:
- *Well localized/point specific* – consider breast cyst, breast abscess, mastitis, breast cancer (rarely presents with pain), chest wall causes, e.g. costochondritis
- *More generalized* – usually referred pain. Consider nerve root pain, post-herpetic neuralgia, lung disease.

GP Notes: Breast calcifications/microcalcifications

Common, usually harmless spots of calcium salts that develop naturally as the breast ages and changes. Associations:

- benign breast disease, e.g. fibroadenomas, cysts
- inflammation/foreign bodies, e.g. implants, stitches
- breast cancer.

Usually detected as 'white spots' on mammograms. Depending on the pattern of the calcifications, a stereotactic biopsy may be needed to exclude cancer. Once cancer is excluded no further action is required.

Figure 2.1 Cross-section of the female breast

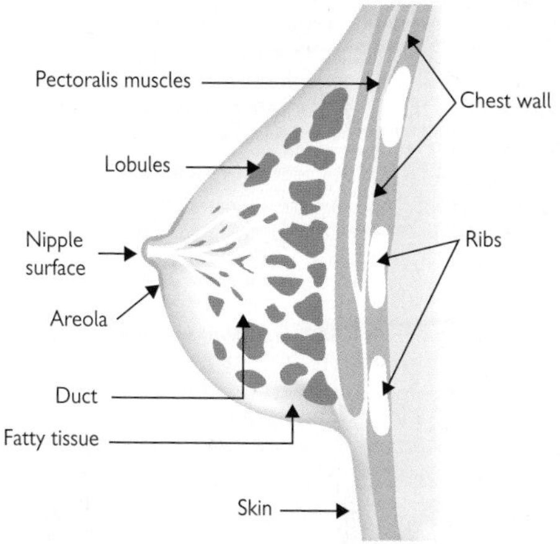
Pectoralis muscles
Chest wall
Lobules
Nipple surface
Ribs
Areola
Duct
Fatty tissue
Skin

Further information

NICE Referral guidelines for suspected cancer (2005)
🖫 www.nice.org.uk
Cancer Research UK Guidelines for referral of patients with breast problems (2003). Available from NHS Responseline ☎ 08701 555 455; e-mail: doh@prolog.uk.com 🖫 www.cancerscreening.nhs.uk
Clinical evidence Bundred N. Breast pain (2005)
🖫 www.clinicalevidence.com

Figure 2.1 is reproduced with permission from 🖫 www.training.seer.cancer.gov; which is funded by the U.S. National Cancer Institute's Surveillance, Epidemiology and End Results (SEER) Program with Emory University, Atlanta SEER Cancer Registry, Georgia, U.S.A.

Benign breast disease

Most breast complaints are benign in nature and have a physiological basis. For this reason they are often termed anomalies of normal development and involution (ANDI). Despite this, most women with breast complaints 'assume the worst' when a new problem is discovered. In most cases reassurance that there is nothing sinister underlying their symptoms is all that is required.

Assessment: 📖 p.42 and Figure 2.2

Calcifications: 📖 p.47

Mastalgia: 📖 p.44

Nodularity: Some women have more nodular breasts than others. Most common among teenagers and women aged 40–60y. and often associated with a history or premenstrual mastalgia. Patients may notice a lump or diffuse lumpiness which may be tender/painful. Lumps may change through the cycle becoming larger prior to menstruation and smaller afterwards.

Examination: Isolated lump or several diffuse areas of thickening scattered throughout both breasts. Characteristically lumps are diffuse, difficult to define, not fixed and not associated with skin changes/skin tethering.

Management
- *Discrete lump:* Refer all lumps for specialist assessment (📖 pp.44–5).
- *Asymmetrical nodularity:* If <30y. and no family history, review in 6wk. If the nodularity has gone reassure, otherwise refer. If ≥30y. or family history of breast cancer, refer.
- *Diffuse symmetrical lumpiness:* Review regularly until you are sure there is no enlarging mass.

Fibroadenoma: An aberration of normal lobular development. Peak age 16–24y. 3 types:
- common
- giant (>5cm diameter)
- juvenile (in adolescent girls).

Presentation: Present with a discrete, firm, non-tender and highly mobile lump ('breast mouse'). Account for 13% of breast lumps.

Management: Refer for confirmation of diagnosis – urgently if ≥30y., any personal/family history of breast cancer or any sinister features (📖 p.45). Diagnosis is confirmed with a combination of USS, mammography and fine-needle aspirate/core biopsy. In women >40y. or if the lump is large (>4cm), the fibroadenoma is usually excised. In other groups, conservative management is usual and women are advised to return if progressive symptoms. 95% fibroadenomas do not enlarge after diagnosis and 25% reduce in size or disappear with time.

🕛 Fibroadenomas may calcify in older women and give a characteristic appearance in mammograms.

Figure 2.2 Algorithm for management of breast symptoms

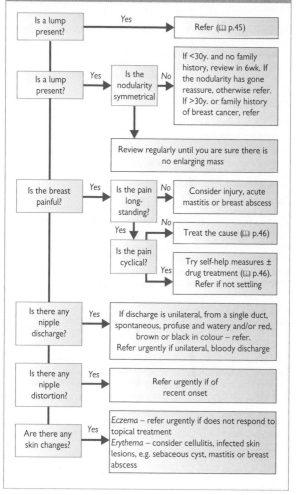

Sclerosing adenosis: Benign condition resulting from over-proliferation of the terminal duct lobules. It can cause recurring pain and/or result in a small, firm lump in the breast. Often detected incidentally on mammography as a calcified, 'stellate' abnormality. Always refer for confirmation of diagnosis. Following a clear diagnosis, treatment is symptomatic.

Phyllodes tumour: Rare breast tumour. Peak age 40–50y. 3 types:
- Benign – most common
- Borderline malignant – uncommon
- Malignant – rare.

Presentation and management: Presents with a breast lump. Refer for confirmation of diagnosis through a combination of USS, mammography and fine-needle aspirate/core biopsy. Treatment is always surgical with wide excision of the lump. Recurrence may occur.

Fat necrosis: Usually history of injury ± bruising. As bruising settles, scarring results in a firm lump in the breast ± puckering of skin. Most common in women with large breasts. Always refer to a breast surgeon for triple assessment (USS, mammography and fine-needle aspiration/core biopsy). Once diagnosis is confirmed, no treatment is needed. The lump often disappears spontaneously.

Breast cyst: Benign fluid-filled sac caused by coalescence of breast acini. Cysts may be of any size, single or multiple. Most common >35y. Usually pre-menopausal women but may occur in post-menopausal women taking HRT.

Examination: Firm, rounded lump which is not fixed and not associated with skin changes/skin tethering.

Management
First breast cyst: Refer for exclusion of malignancy – urgently if ≥30y., family history of breast cancer or other suspicious features. Diagnosis is confirmed with a combination of mammography, USS and aspiration.

Past history of breast cysts: 30% of patients who have had a breast cyst develop another at a later date. If the lump is accessible it is reasonable to attempt aspiration. There is no need to send aspirated fluid for cytology if the fluid is *not* bloodstained and lump completely resolves. Refer if:
- fluid aspirated is bloodstained
- lump does not disappear completely
- cyst refills
- aspiration fails
- cytology reveals malignant or suspicious cells.

⚠ Do not attempt aspiration if you have not been trained to do so as there is a small but significant risk of pneumothorax.

Galactocoele: Milk-containing cyst which arises during pregnancy. Refer any new lump arising in pregnancy to a breast surgeon. Once diagnosis is confirmed repeated aspiration may be needed. Resolves spontaneously.

Mastitis in lactating women: 📖 p.276

Duct ectasia: Occurs around the menopause. Ducts become blocked and secretions behind 'stagnant'.

Presentation
- Peri-menopausal woman
- Discharge from ≥1 duct which may be bloodstained ± breast lump ± nipple retraction ('transverse slit' appearance) ± breast pain.

Management: Refer for confirmation of diagnosis – urgently if lump and/or bloodstained nipple discharge and/or nipple retraction. Usually no treatment is needed though surgery may be required to confirm diagnosis, if discharge is troublesome, or to evert the nipple.

Periductal mastitis: Infected subareolar ducts. Affects younger women than duct ectasia with peak age 32y.

Presentation: Breast tenderness ± inflammation in areolar area. May also have nipple discharge and/or retraction and/or an associated inflammatory mass/abscess.

Management
- Treat with antibiotics e.g. co-amoxiclav 250/125 tds. Advise smokers that smoking can slow the healing process.
- If an abscess is present, refer for drainage – mammary duct fistula is a complication.
- Refer if any residual inflammation or masses following treatment to exclude cancer.
- If recurrent infection, refer for consideration of surgery to remove the blocked duct.

Intraductal papilloma: Benign wart-like lump that forms within a duct just behind the areola. Peri-menopausal women are more likely to have a single intraductal papilloma; younger women often have >1. May be bilateral.

Presentation: Nipple discharge which may be bloodstained ± a subareolar lump/nodule (30%).

Management: Refer for confirmation of diagnosis – urgently if lump and/or bloodstained discharge. Usually treated by excision.

Breast abscess: Usually occurs in a lactating breast following mastitis; occasionally in a non-lactating breast in association with indrawn nipple, mammary duct ectasia or local skin infection.

Presentation: Gradual onset of pain in 1 breast segment with hot, tender swelling of the affected area.

Management: Refer for surgical assessment. May be treated with repeated aspiration under ultrasound guidance or surgical incision and drainage.

Mamary duct fistula: Fistula between a mammary duct and the skin. Usually a complication of a breast abscess. Refer for surgical excision.

Breast cancer screening

In the UK there has been a national screening programme for breast cancer since 1988. The aim of the screening programme is to detect breast cancer at an early stage in order to ↑ survival chances (stage I tumours – 84% 5y. survival; stage IV tumours – 18% 5y. survival) – Figure 2.3.

Breast awareness: Trials of breast self-examination have not demonstrated ↓ mortality. Instead less formal 'breast awareness' is advocated – 📖 p.43.

Screening test: 2-view mammographic screening performed 3-yearly. Screening detects 85% of cancers in women aged >50y. (60% of which are impalpable) and ~70–80% screening-detected cancers have good prognosis. Screening more frequently does not ↓ mortality[R]. Organization of breast cancer screening in the UK – Figure 2.4 (📖 p.54).

Interval cancers: Cancer occurring in the interval between screens. Can occur through failure to detect a cancer at screening or as a result of a new event after screening took place. In the 1st year after screening, 20% of breast cancers are interval cancers. This ↑ to ~60% in the 3rd year.

Screening population: Available to women aged 50–70y. Older women can request screening 1x/3y. In addition, annual screening with mammography is offered to women aged 40–49y. with a strong family history of breast cancer (📖 p.57). Women with a strong family history may also benefit from genetic screening (📖 p.56).

Acceptability of screening: 81% women find mammography uncomfortable but 90% return for subsequent screens. GPs have an important role – sending personalized invitations for screening to women from their GPs increases uptake rates[R].

Anxiety due to screening: False-positive results cause anxiety as well as prompting further invasive investigations. Anxiety levels in women who are recalled and then found to be disease free are higher during the year after their recall appointment than women who receive negative results at screening.

Patient choice: The breast screening programme has designed a leaflet for women – 'Breast screening: the facts' – to facilitate informed choice. Copies can be obtained from the NHS response line ☎ 08701 555 455 or by e-mail from dh@prolog.uk.com. Alternatively the leaflet is available online at 🖥 www.cancerscreening.org.uk/breastscreen.

Further information

NHS Breast Screening 🖥 www.cancerscreening.org.uk
Cancer Research UK Breast Screening – UK (2003) Available from 🖥 http://info.cancerresearchuk.org/cancerstats
NICE Classification and care of women at high-risk of familial breast cancer in primary, secondary and tertiary care (2004) 🖥 www.nice.org.uk

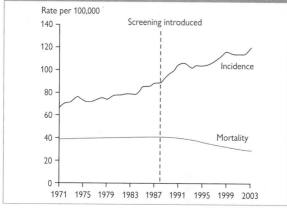

Figure 2.3 Breast cancer incidence and mortality since introduction of breast cancer screening in the UK

Table 2.2 Pros and cons of breast cancer screening

Benefits	Adverse effects
• Earlier diagnosis • Improved prognosis and lower mortality • Less radical and invasive treatment needed • Reassurance for those with a negative result	• Discomfort and inconvenience of screening • Radiation risks of screening (very small) • Reassurance to those women who have false-negative result • Reassurance to those who develop an interval cancer and possibly later presentation due to a false sense of security • Anxiety and adverse effects of further investigation for those with false-positives • Overdiagnosis of minor abnormalities that would never develop into breast cancer • Earlier knowledge of disease and overtreatment for those in whom, despite early diagnosis, the prognosis is unchanged

53

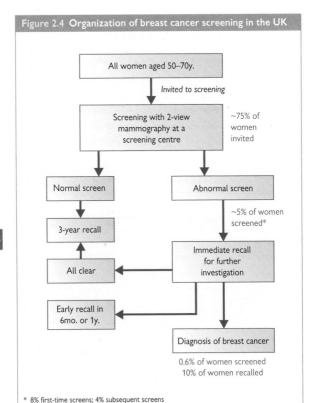

Figure 2.4 Organization of breast cancer screening in the UK

All women aged 50–70y.

Invited to screening

Screening with 2-view mammography at a screening centre

~75% of women invited

Normal screen

Abnormal screen

~5% of women screened*

3-year recall

All clear

Immediate recall for further investigation

Early recall in 6mo. or 1y.

Diagnosis of breast cancer

0.6% of women screened
10% of women recalled

* 8% first-time screens; 4% subsequent screens

Frequently asked questions about breast cancer screening

I haven't been called for breast screening even though I'm over 50 – do I need to contact anyone? The NHS Breast Screening Programme is a rolling one which calls women from doctors' practices in turn. This means not every woman receives her invitation as soon as she is 50. It will be sometime between the ages of 49 and 52. If you are registered with a GP and the practice has your correct details, then you will automatically receive an invitation. You don't need to contact anyone but you might like to check your surgery has your correct contact details and ask them when the women on their list are next due for screening.

I'm worried that I might have breast cancer. Can I walk into the mobile breast screening unit and request a mammogram? The NHS Breast Screening Programme is a population screening programme which invites all women aged 50 to 70 as a matter of routine. It is not aimed at women who already have symptoms. So if you have found something that worries you or are concerned about your breast health, you should see your GP in the usual way. He or she will decide whether or not you need to be referred for further investigations or treatment.

Why doesn't the NHS screen younger women? Mammograms are not as effective in younger women because the density of the breast tissue makes it more difficult to detect problems and also because the incidence of breast cancer is lower. The average age of the menopause in the UK is 50 and so this is the age when women join the NHS Breast Screening Programme. As women past the menopause, the glandular tissue in their breast "involutes" and the breast tissue is increasingly made up of only fat. This is clearer on the mammogram and makes interpretation more reliable.

Why does breast screening stop at 70? It doesn't. Although women over 70 are not routinely invited for breast screening, they are encouraged to call the local unit to request breast screening every 3 years. Cards have been produced to help them remember and these are handed out at their last routine breast screening appointment.

Women abroad get more frequent breast screening. Why doesn't this happen in the UK? A large research trial in 2002 concluded that the NHS Breast Screening Programme has got the interval between screening and invitations about right at 3 years, compared with more frequent screening.

Further information

Breast screening – the facts. Available from
🖥 www.cancerscreening.org.uk
Over 70? You are still entitled to breast screening. Available from
🖥 www.cancerscreening.org.uk

Reproduced with permission in modified format from the NHS Cancer Screening Programmes 🖥 http://cancerscreening.org.uk/breastscreen/faqs.html

Breast cancer

Breast cancer is now the most common cancer in the UK – >100 women/d. are diagnosed with the disease (1:9 women). Men can also get breast cancer but it is rare.

Risk factors

Geography: More common in the developed world – migrants assume the risk of the host country within 2 generations.

Personal characteristics

- *Age* – ↑ with age – ~80% of breast cancers occur in women >50y.
- *Socio-economic status* – higher incidence in more affluent social classes
- *Physical characteristics* – taller women have ↑ risk; women with denser breasts have 2–6x ↑ risk

Lifestyle factors

- *Obesity* – ↑ risk post-menopause
- *Physical activity* – 30% ↓ risk if taking regular physical activity
- *High-fat diet* – probably associated with ↑ risk
- *Alcohol* – ↑ risk by 7%/unit consumed/d.

Reproductive history

- *Early menarche or late menopause* – ↑ risk
- *Pregnancy* – ↑ parity → ↓ risk (32% ↓ risk in women reporting 3 births compared to women reporting 1); late age when first child is born ↑ risk
- *Breast feeding* – ↓ relative risk by 4.3% for each year of breast feeding
- *Combined oral contraceptive pill* – slight ↑ risk (relative risk 1.24 for current users) – excess risk disappears within 10y. of stopping
- *HRT* – risk ↑ by 6 cases/1000 after 5y. combined HRT use and 19 cases/1000 after 10y. use. Risk for combined oestrogen and progestogen preparations is greater than oestrogen-only preparations. HRT also ↓ sensitivity of mammography

Other past medical history

- *Past history of breast disease* – ductal or lobular carcinoma *in situ*, florid hyperplasia, and papilloma with fibrovascular core all ↑ risk
- *Ionising radiation* – exposure ↑ risk

Family history: Referral algorithm – Figure 2.5

- *1 first-degree relative with breast cancer (mother or sister)* – ↑ risk x2 – but 85% of women with breast cancer have no family history
- *Several family members with early-onset breast cancer* – refer for genetic screening – BRCA1 and BRCA2 genes account for 2–5% all breast cancers

🕚 Family relationships

- *First-degree relative* – mother, father, sister, brother, daughter, son
- *Second-degree relative* – grandparents, grandchildren, aunt, uncle, niece, nephew, half-sister, half-brother

Breast cancer screening: 📖 p.52

Figure 2.5 Referral of women with family history of breast cancer[N]

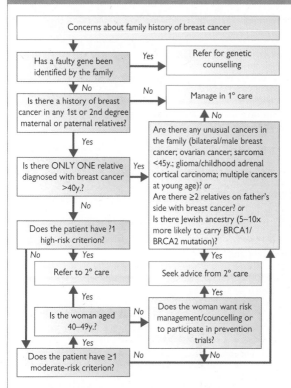

Concerns about family history of breast cancer

Has a faulty gene been identified by the family — Yes → Refer for genetic counselling

No

Is there a history of breast cancer in any 1st or 2nd degree maternal or paternal relatives? — No → Manage in 1° care

Yes

Is there ONLY ONE relative diagnosed with breast cancer >40y.? — Yes → Are there any unusual cancers in the family (bilateral/male breast cancer; ovarian cancer; sarcoma <45y.; glioma/childhood adrenal cortical carcinoma; multiple cancers at young age)? or Are there ≥2 relatives on father's side with breast cancer? or Is there Jewish ancestry (5–10x more likely to carry BRCA1/BRCA2 mutation)?

No

No

Does the patient have ?1 high-risk criterion? — Yes

Refer to 2° care — Yes → Seek advice from 2° care — Yes

Is the woman aged 40–49y.? — No → Does the woman want risk management/councelling or to participate in prevention trials?

Yes

Does the patient have ≥1 moderate-risk criterion? — No

High-risk criteria for Female breast cancer:

1x 1st degree relative + 1x 2nd degree relative diagnosed < average age of 50y.

2x 1st degree relatives diagnosed < average age of 50y.

1x 1st degree relative with bilateral breast cancer where first primary diagnosed at <50y.

≥3x 1st/2nd degree relatives

Male breast cancer:

1x 1st degree relative

Breast and ovarian cancer:

1x 1st/2nd degree relative with breast cancer + another with ovarian cancer (1 must be 1st degree relative)

Moderate-risk criteria for Female breast cancer:

1x 1st degree relative <40y.

1x 1st degree relative + 1x 2nd degree relative diagnosed > average age of 50y.

2x 1st degree relatives diagnosed > average age of 50y.

Prevention: Consider referral to secondary/tertiary care if family history of breast cancer (📖 p.57).

- Lifestyle measures – ↓ alcohol intake; ↓ weight; avoid exogenous sex hormones (e.g. HRT); breast feed.
- Chemoprophylaxis – tamoxifen ↓ risk of breast cancer by 40% in high-risk women but use is limited by side-effects (thromboembolism and endometrial carcinoma) – other drug trials are in progress.
- Prophylactic surgery – ↓ risk by 90% in very high-risk women.

Presentation: Often found at breast screening (📖 p.52). Clinical presentations include:

- breast lump (90%)
- breast pain (21% present with painful lump; pain alone <1%)
- nipple skin change (10%). Any red, scaly lesion or eczema around the nipple suggests *Paget's disease of the breast* – intraepidermal, intraductal cancer
- family history (6%)
- skin contour change (5%)
- nipple discharge (3%)
- rarely presents with distant metastases, e.g. bone pain
- in the elderly, may present with extensive local lesions.

Management

- Refer for urgent assessment (<2wk.) to a breast surgeon.
- Specialist investigation includes USS; mammography ± fine-needle aspiration or core biopsy.
- If diagnosis is confirmed further investigations include tumour markers, CT/MRI, liver USS and/or bone scan to stage disease and evaluate spread.

Treatment: Includes surgery (lumpectomy ± axillary clearance, mastectomy), radiotherapy and/or chemotherapy.

Adjuvant endocrine therapy: Oestrogen has an important role in the progression of breast cancer. Oestrogen and progesterone receptors determine the response to endocrine therapy.

- *Tamoxifen* – ↑ survival of patients with oestrogen receptor +ve tumours (60% tumours) of any age but rarely causes endometrial carcinoma – warn patients to report any untoward vaginal bleeding. Continue tamoxifen for ≥5y. – take advice from a specialist prior to stopping.
- *Anastrozole* (Arimidex®) – blocks synthesis of oestrogen. Superior efficacy when compared to tamoxifen for post-menopausal woman with hormone-sensitive early breast cancer and first-choice drug for post-menopausal woman with advanced breast cancer. Continue for ≥5y. – take advice from a specialist prior to stopping.
- *Trastuzumab* (Herceptin®) – monoclonal antibody directed against HER2, a receptor found in 1:5 breast cancers. Affects division and growth of breast cancer cells. Treatment option for woman with early HER2 +ve cancer at high risk of reccurrence and woman with advanced HER2 +ve breast cancer. Administered IV every 3wk. for 1y.

🚫 Optimum treatment regimes for breast cancer change regularly and there are regional variations. Many women will be asked to participate in clinical trials to answer important questions about optimum treatments.

Table 2.3 Classification of breast cancer stage

Virtually all breast cancers are adenocarcinoma (85% ductal; 15% lobular)

Stage	Features
In situ	Non-invasive
Stage I	≤2cm diameter No LNs affected No spread beyond breast
Stage II	2–5cm diameter and/or LNs in armpit affected No evidence of spread beyond armpit
Stage III	>5cm diameter LNs in armpit affected No evidence of spread beyond armpit
Stage IV	Any sized tumour LNs in armpit affected Spread to other parts of the body

ⓘ The T (Tumour) N (Node) M (Metastases) system of staging is in common use clinically in the UK

GP Notes: Sentinel lymph node biopsy

Prognosis and decisions surrounding adjuvant treatment are based on knowledge of the axillary node status. The only way to assess axillary lymph node involvement is to remove nodes surgically and look at them under the microscope. Axillary node clearence can result in lymphoedema and reduced arm function. Sentinel node biopsy is the removal of the key or sentinel lymph node in patients undergoing surgery for early breast cancer to accurately predict the state of nodal disease in the remaining axillary lymph nodes. Radical axillary surgery to clear the axillary nodes can then be reserved for the 20–40% with a +ve sentinel lymph node biopsy.

Further information

Adjuvant Online Decision-making tool for professionals assessing risks and benefits of additional therapy after surgery
🖳 www.adjuvantonline.com

Prognosis

- 72% of women diagnosed now will live 10y.; 64% live ≥20y.
- Recurrence is most likely <2y. after treatment – late recurrences do occur but the longer since diagnosis, the less the chance of recurrence.
- Prognosis for a given individual depends on age (patients aged 50–69y. have best prognosis), stage of disease (Figure 2.6), grade of tumour, and oestrogen receptor status (oestrogen receptor –ve tumours have poorer prognosis). Women who live in affluent areas have better survival rates than women in deprived areas.

Psychological impact of breast cancer: Depression, anxiety, marital and sexual problems are common. Be sensitive. Discuss possibilities of reconstructive surgery or breast prostheses as appropriate. Refer to the specialist breast care nurse for support and advice.

Lymphoedema: Due to obstruction of lymphatic drainage resulting in oedema with high protein content. In patients with breast cancer it usually affects one arm but may affect both arms and/or head and neck.

Risk factors

- ↑ with age
- Obesity
- Lack of physical exercise

Causes: Axillary involvement or treatment (axillary surgery, postoperative infection or radiotherapy) of breast cancer.

Presentation

- Swollen limb ± pitting – Figure 2.7
- Impaired limb mobility and function
- Discomfort/pain related to tissue swelling and/or shoulder strain
- Neuralgia pain – especially when axillary nodes are involved
- Psychological distress

Management: Untreated lymphoedema becomes increasingly resistant to treatment due to chronic inflammation and subcutaneous fibrosis.

Avoid injury: In at-risk patients (e.g. patients who have had breast cancer with axillary clearance) or those with lymphoedema, injury to the limb may precipitate or worsen lymphoedema. Avois sunburn and cuts (e.g wear gloves for gardening). Do not take blood from the limb or use it for IV access or vaccination.

Skin hygiene

- Keep the skin in good condition with moisturizers, e.g. aqueous cream.
- Treat fungal infections with topical agents, e.g. clotrimazole cream.
- Cellulitis is a common complication and causes rapid ↑ in swelling. Treat with oral antibiotics (e.g. penicillin 500mg qds). If ≥2 episodes of cellulites consider prophylactic antibiotics, e.g. penicillin V 250mg bd.

External support

- Intensive support can be provided with special compression bandages – refer to specialist physiotherapy or the palliative care team.
- Maintenance therapy with a lymphoedema sleeve is helpful – contact the palliative care team or breast care specialist nurse for information.

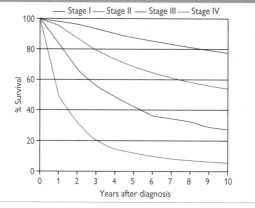

Figure 2.6 Prognosis of breast cancer according to stage at diagnosis

— Stage I — Stage II — Stage III — Stage IV

% Survival vs Years after diagnosis

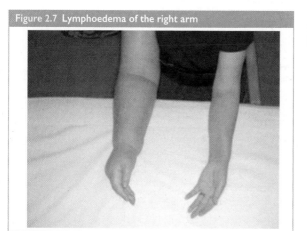

Figure 2.7 Lymphoedema of the right arm

Figure 2.6 is reproduced with permission from Cancer Research UK, News and Resources website (2007) ▣ www.cancerresearchuk.org/cancerstats

Figure 2.7 is reproduced with permission from Harlington Hospice, ▣ www.harlingtonhospice.org

Exercise: Advise gentle daily exercise of the affected limb, gradually increasing range of movement. ❶ Patients should wear their compression bandages or lymphoedema sleeve whilst doing their exercises.

Massage: Very gentle fingertip massage in the line of drainage of the lymphatics can help – refer to specialist physiotherapist for advice.

Diuretics: If the condition develops/deteriorates after corticosteroid or NSAID use, or if there is a venous component, consider trial of diuretics, e.g. furosemide 20mg od. Otherwise diuretics are of no benefit.

Further information

NICE ▢ www.nice.org.uk
- Improving outcomes in breast cancer (2002)
- Classification and care of women at high-risk of familial breast cancer in primary, secondary and tertiary care (2004)
- Breast cancer: diagnosis and treatment (due for publication in 2008)

Clinical evidence ▢ www.clinicalevidence.com
- Stebbing *et al.* Breast cancer (metastatic) (2006)
- Rodger *et al.* Breast cancer (non-metastatic) (2005)

Cancer Research UK Breast cancer survival statistics
▢ http://info.cancerresearchuk.org/cancerstats

Cochrane Badger *et al.* Physical therapies for reducing and controlling lymphoedema of the limb (2004)

GMS contract			
Cancer 1	The practice can produce a register of all cancer patients defined as a 'register of patients with a diagnosis of cancer excluding non-melanotic skin cancers from 1/4/2003'	5 points	
Cancer 3	% of patients with cancer diagnosed within the last 18mo. who have a patient review recorded as occurring within 6mo. of the practice receiving confirmation of the diagnosis	up to 6 points	40–90%
Palliative care 1	The practice has a complete register available of all patients in need of palliative care/support	3 points	
Palliative care 2	The practice has regular (at least 3-monthly) multidisciplinary case review meetings where all patients on the palliative care register are discussed	3 points	
Education 7	The practice has undertaken a minimum of 12 significant event reviews in the past 3y. which could include new cancer diagnoses	4 points	for 12 reviews

Advice for patients:

Patient experiences of diagnosis of breast cancer

'The fact is, I was so shocked because I wasn't expecting it whatsoever, that I didn't do anything. I just sat deadly still and I didn't know what to do. It was awful because no one was there and then they went out the room and they went into the office, and they left me on my own in that little room and that's when I burst into tears. That's when, that's when the reality hit me.'

'And people's reactions to it [cancer] were sort of: 'Ughhh!', you know. They don't like, I mean a lot of people just don't like, mentioning the word... And sometimes I felt some people avoided me because they didn't know what to say. So that was, that was hard to bear really, I think. I mean some people were great but some people, and I mean it wasn't that people didn't want to help, they just didn't know what to say. And so they just avoided it. And avoided me, which was difficult.'

Patient experience of worries over body image

'You know how most men have a favourite part of the anatomy – my husband's happens to be the breast. So I did think that that would be difficult for him and me. If I ever talk to him about it now all he'll say is that he would rather have me with one breast or no breast than not have me at all. But that's what he says to me. I don't think that is necessarily what he thinks.... But you still feel rejected in a way because you just feel that it can't be the same any more, no matter how much he says that it doesn't matter, because it must matter, it must make a difference.'

Breast cancer information and support

DIPEx Patient experience database ▯ www.dipex.org
Breakthrough Breast Cancer ☎ 08080 100 200
▯ www.breakthrough.org.uk
Breast Cancer Care ☎ 0808 800 6000
▯ www.breastcancercare.org.uk
Breast Cancer Campaign ▯ www.bcc-uk.org
Against Breast Cancer ▯ www.aabc.org.uk
Cancer Research UK ☎ 0800 226 237 ▯ www.cancerhelp.org.uk
Cancer Backup ☎ 0808 800 1234 (helpline)
▯ www.cancerbackup.org.uk

Lymphoedema information and support

Lymphoedema Support Network ☎ 020 7351 4480
▯ www.lymphoedema.org/lsn
UKLymph.com Online support network ▯ www.uklymph.com
Skin Care Campaign ▯ www.skincarecampaign.org
CancerHelp UK ☎ 0800 226 237 ▯ www.cancerhelp.org.uk
Royal Marsden Hospital ▯ www.royalmarsden.org.uk
Vascular Society ▯ www.vascularsociety.org.uk/patient/topics

Patient experiences are reproduced with permission from the DIPEx patient experience database ▯ www.dipex.org

Chapter 3

Gynaecological problems

Assessment of gynaecological problems 66
Congenital abnormalities 68
Puberty 70
The menstrual cycle 72
Premenstrual syndrome 74
Amenorrhoea 78
Menorrhagia 80
Dysmenorrhoea 84
Pelvic pain and dyspareunia 86
Endometriosis 90
Uterine problems 92
Prolapse 96
Ovarian cysts and tumours 98
Polycystic ovarian syndrome 104
Conditions of the cervix 106
Cervical cancer screening 110
Vaginal and vulval problems 114
Vaginal discharge 118
A–Z of sexually transmitted diseases 122
Sexual problems 132
Infertility 134
Urinary tract infection (UTI) 138
Urinary incontinence 142
The menopause 146
Hormone replacement therapy (HRT) 150
Osteoporosis 154

Assessment of gynaecological problems

Most women will have a gynaecological problem at some point in their lives. Women often find it embarrassing to talk about these problems and gynaecological examination is one of the most intimate examinations for a woman to undergo. Treat all women with sensitivity. *Try to:*

- Establish a constructive relationship with the patient to enable patient and doctor to communicate effectively, and to serve as the basis for any subsequent therapeutic relationship.
- Determine whether the patient has a problem and, if so, what that is.
- Assess the patient's emotions and attitudes towards the problem.
- Establish how it might be treated and involve her in the action plan.

History: Use open questions at the start, becoming directive when necessary – clarify, reflect, facilitate, listen. *Ask about:*

Presenting complaint: Chronological account, past history of similar symptoms (Figure 3.1)

Past medical history

- *Menstrual history* – last menstrual period (LMP), last normal period, age at menarche/menopause, cycle length, duration of bleeding, flow (number of tampons or pads/d., use of double protection, flooding, clots), bleeding between periods/post-menopausal bleeding, pain
- *Previous gynaecological disease*
- *Cervical smears* – date/result of last smear, previous abnormal smears
- *Obstetric history* – number of pregnacies/outcome/complications, history of infertility. *If pregnant* – estimated date of delivery/gestation, complications in earlier pregnancies/this pregnancy
- *Sexual history* – sexually active? Past history and risk of sexually transmitted infections, sexual problems, e.g. poor libido, dyspareunia
- *Other disease,* e.g. diabetes, thyroid disease, other endocrine disease; anorexia, irritable bowel syndrome, allergies
- *Past treatments,* e.g. surgery, radiotherapy/chemotherapy, current medication, medications previously tried, contraception, HRT

Family history: Ovarian cancer, breast cancer

Social history: Smoking, alcohol consumption, work (does the problem affect the job?), effect on relationships

Attitudes and beliefs: How does the patient see the problem? What does he/she think is wrong? How does he/she think other people view the situation? What does the patient want you to do about it?

Examination: Figure 3.1

Investigation: Figure 3.1

Action: Summarize the history back to the patient and give an opportunity for the patient to fill in any gaps. Draw up a problem list and outline a management plan with the patient. Further investigations and interventions are guided by the findings on history and examination – so a good history and examination is essential. Set a review date.

Figure 3.1 The gynaecological assessment

ASK
Chronological history of symptoms
- *Pain?* Type, location, radiation, relationship to cycle, exacerbating/relieving factors, pregnant?
- *Vaginal bleeding?* Absence/abnormal bleeding, relationship to menstrual cycle and/or sexual intercourse, pregnant?
- *Vaginal discharge?* Colour, smell, amount, itching, symptoms in partner, other symptoms, e.g. pain, rash
- *Urinary symptoms?* Frequency, nocturia, urgency, incontinence, haematuria, straining to void
- *Other symptoms?* Feeling of a 'lump coming down', vaginal dryness, pelvic mass/ abdominal swelling, weight loss, anorexia/nausea, pre-menstrual symptoms, headaches, galactorrhoea, body hair

Past medical history and drug history (including allergies)
Family and social history

EXAMINE
General: Pulse, BMI, weight ↓, fever/sweats
Breasts: If appropriate (p.42).
Abdomen: Tenderness, masses, organomegaly, ascites
Vaginal examination: Look at the vulva – check skin texture, lumps, excoriation, lichenification, whitening.
Speculum examination: Choose an appropriate size/type of speculum. Warm before use. Look at vaginal mucosa and note cervical abnormalities. Note vaginal discharge. Check for prolapse. Look for warts/herpes. If appropriate, check for retained tampon.
Bimanual examination: Feel for abnormalities of the vagina/cervix – roughness, hardness, lump; check uterine position, size, mobility, tenderness; feel adnexae bimanually for swelling/tenderness.
△ Only perform a vaginal examination if really needed. Ask if the patient would like a chaperone. If a chaperone is requested and not available, postpone the examination unless urgent.

TEST
Consider:
BP, temperature
Blood test: FBC, TFTs, LFTs, U&e, Cr, eGFR, FSH/LH, day 21 progesterone (if 28d cycle)
Microbiology: MSU, high/low vaginal swabs, endocervical swab
Cervical smear
Abdominal/pelvic ultrasound scan

Congenital abnormalities

Duplication: Duplication of the cervix and/or uterus, vaginal septum or bicornuate uterus (of varying degrees) is caused by failure of fusion of the paramesonephric ducts. Usually found incidentally. May cause problems with unstable lie in pregnancy and difficulty fitting an IUCD.

Imperforate hymen: May cause cryptomenorrhoea which presents as 1° amenorrhoea (📖 p.78). Refer for surgical release if suspected.

Congenital adrenal hyperplasia (CAH): Also known as *adreno-genital syndrome* or *adrenal virilism*. Autosomal recessive trait due to absence or deficiency of any of the enzymes needed for synthesis of cortisol. Each enzyme block causes a characteristic deficiency and >8 different syndromes have been described. The most common enzyme deficiencies are:

● *21-hydroxylase deficiency* (95%) – 1:5000 live births. Results in ↑ 17-alpha-hydroxyprogesterone and its metabolites – androstenedione and testosterone. Cortisol is also ↓ in 30%.
● *11-beta-hydroxylase deficiency* (5%) – 1:100,000 live births. Results in ↑ androstenedione and testosterone. Associated with hypertension.

Presentation: Ambiguity of the external genitalia. Less severe forms may go unnoticed until puberty. 2 patterns:
● androgens accumulate causing virilization of an affected female fetus
● androgen synthesis is impaired causing inadequate virilization of an affected male fetus (much rarer).

There may be a family history of CAH, ambiguous genitalia or neonatal death. Rarely presents with Addisonian crisis.

Management: Refer for specialist management. Treatment is usually with glucocorticoid ± mineralocorticoid replacement.

Testicular feminization: Also known as *androgen insensitivity syndrome (AIS)*. X-linked disorder affecting 1:62,000 male births. Complete or partial absence of testosterone receptors in target tissues results in the patient being genotypically male (46XY) but phenotypically female.

Presentation
● External genitalia are usually female (though if feminization is incomplete may be ambiguous) but the vagina is blind-ending and there is no uterus or ovaries.
● The testes fail to drop and are found in the groin (rarely abdomen).
● At puberty, breast development occurs and female contours form but there is little or no pubic or axillary hair.
● Adults present with primary amenorrhoea (📖 p.78).

Management: Patients have usually been treated as female since birth. It is very traumatic for patients (often teenage at the time of diagnosis) to be told they are male instead of female and unable to become pregnant or have children. Specialist support is always required. Undescended testes are removed at puberty as they have malignant potential. Oestrogens are given to complete 2° sexual development.

- Be honest – don't guess the gender of the child.
- Explain that there are rare conditions where girls may be virilized or boys undermasculinized, causing girls to look like boys and vice versa.
- Arrange paediatric assessment as soon as possible for further investigations, gender assignment and ongoing management.

Advice for patients: Information and support for children and parents

Climb Congenital Adrenal Hyperplasia UK Support Group
🖳 www.cah.org.uk
AIS Support Group (UK) 🖳 www.aissg.org

Female genital mutilation: Illegal in the UK but increasingly seen amongst immigrants from Africa, Asia and the Middle East. Many forms:

- Piercing and/or cauterization
- Circumcision – excision of the prepuce ± part/all of the clitoris
- Excision – removal of the clitoris ± part/all of the labia
- Infibulation – excision of external genitalia with stitching of the vulva to form a small opening to allow passage of urine and menstruation.

Consequences: Complications of the procedure (haemorrhage, infection, HIV transmission); non-consumation; infertility; problems with childbirth; recurrent UTIs; dysmenorrhoea; psychosexual problems.

Prevention: Educate at-risk populations about health consequences while maintaining cultural values.

⚠ **Circumcision of female infants:** It is not uncommon for infants to be taken abroad to be circumcized. If you suspect this might be going to happen to any patient of yours, inform social services and/or the police immediately.

Puberty

Puberty is defined as the time when the onset of sexual maturity occurs and the reproductive organs become functional. This is manifested in girls at 8–14y. by growth of the breasts and menstruation.

Assessment of abnormal puberty

History
- Previous growth and development
- Timing and sequence of changes of puberty (physical and emotional)
- Past medical history
- Family history: early or delayed puberty, genetic diseases
- If underweight and delayed puberty – diet and eating habits

Examination
- Plot height and weight on a growth chart – monitor growth velocity.
- Check genitalia and secondary sexual characteristics – document stage of puberty (Table 3.1).
- Check neurological examination – particularly optic fundi, visual fields and sense of smell (abnormalities associated with pituitary tumour).
- Look for evidence of thyroid dysfunction.

Further investigations: Usually carried out in secondary care.

Delayed puberty: No pubertal changes in a girl aged 13y. or failure of progression of puberty over 2y. Affects ~2% population. In all cases refer to paediatrics for further investigation.

Causes: Constitutional delay accounts for 90%. Other causes include:
- chromosomal abnormalities, e.g. Turner's syndrome
- GnRH deficiency, e.g. pituitary lesions, gonadal failure, thyroid disease
- hypothalamic suppression, e.g. anorexia or malnutrition, sportsmen, systemic illness (e.g. chronic renal failure, Crohn's disease).

Precocious puberty: Puberty before the normal age for the population. In the UK, this is <8y. for girls. $\male:\female \approx$ 5:1. In all cases refer for specialist investigation and advice on management. *Types:*

True: Course and pattern are normal, but early. *Causes:*
- Idiopathic (90%)
- Hypothalamic tumour
- Other CNS pathology

Pseudo: Pattern is abnormal – ≥1 element of puberty occurs (e.g. breast development), but other elements do not. *Causes:*
- Ovarian tumour
- Congenital adrenal hyperplasia
- Hepatoblastoma
- Adrenal virilizing tumours
- Cushing's syndrome

Primary amenorrhoea (without delayed puberty): No menstruation ≥16y. with normal growth/sexual development – 📖 p.78.

Contraception and the under 16s: 📖 p.195

Table 3.1	Stages of normal puberty in girls (Tanner stages)	
Stage	**Pubic hair**	**Other effects – female**
I	No different to abdominal hair	Papilla raised
II	Sparse longer, darker hairs close to genitalia	Breast buds form Fastest growth*
III	Hair is darker, curly and more widespread	Breast and areola are both more raised
IV	Adult type over less of body	Periods start Areola appears as distinct mound
V	Reaches onto inner thigh	Papilla projects with areola receding

Advice for patients: Information and support for teenagers

Childline 24h. confidential counselling ☎ 0800 1111
🖳 www.childline.org
Brook Advisory Service Contraceptive advice and counselling for teenagers ☎ 0800 0185 023 🖳 www.brook.org.uk
Sexwise For under-19s ☎ 0800 28 2930 🖳 www.ruthinking.co.uk
Teenage Health Freak 🖳 www.teenagehealthfreak.org

Figure 3.2 The normal female reproductive system

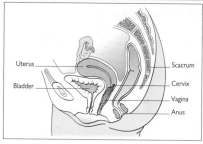

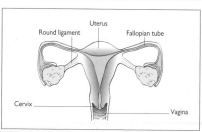

Figure 3.2 is reproduced with permission (copyright EMIS and PiP, 2007) from 🖳 www.patient. co.uk; where you can find comprehensive, free, up-to-date health information as provided by GPs to patients during consultations.

The menstrual cycle

A good working understanding of the menstrual cycle is essential to understand its endocrine disorders and their management. One menstrual cycle lasts from the start of one period until the day before the start of the next. The average length of a cycle is 28d., but anything from 24–35d. is common. The menstrual cycle is split into 4 (Figure 3.3).

Follicular or proliferative phase

Hormone changes: Levels of oestrogen and progesterone are low. There is ↓ negative feedback on the pituitary as a result so follicle stimulating hormone (FSH) levels ↑. FSH stimulates follicle development in the ovary. The developing follicles then produce oestrogen.

Changes within the reproductive organs
- *Ovaries* – Follicles develop. One follicle becomes dominant.
- *Uterus* – Lining thickens (proliferates).
- *Vagina* – Tends to be drier with thicker mucus.

Ovulation: Occurs ½ way through a cycle (~14d. after the start of the period). The dominant follicle ruptures and an egg is released into the fallopian tube. The follicle fills with blood after rupturing and there may be brief pain – *Mittelschmerz*. The egg travels along the fallopian tube into the uterus, and may be fertilized if the woman is sexually active and not using contraception.

Secretory or luteal phase

Hormone changes: After ovulation, the ruptured follicle forms the corpus luteum (yellow body), and secretes oestrogen and progesterone.

Changes within the reproductive organs
- *Ovaries* – Corpus luteum forms. If pregnancy does not occur the corpus luteum begins to degenerate ~4d. prior to menstruation.
- *Uterus* – Progesterone causes the lining of the uterus to alter so that it is ready to receive a fertilized egg. The endometrium becomes oedematous, more vascular and the glandular component becomes coiled and tortuous.
- *Vagina* – Mucus becomes thinner, more watery, and slippery. It becomes thicker again towards the next period as progesterone ↓.
- *Other changes* – Progesterone may cause 'water retention', breast tenderness and mood changes.

Periods (menstruation): With the regression of the corpus luteum, oestrogen and progesterone levels ↓. There is necrosis, bleeding and sloughing of the endometrium, resulting in a period or menstruation. Periods begin aged 11–16y. and continue until the menopause – usually between 45–55y. Bleeding can last from 1–8d. (average 5d.) and is generally heaviest in the first 2d. Blood loss each period is ~20–60ml (>80ml is associated with anaemia). Some period pain is common and normal.

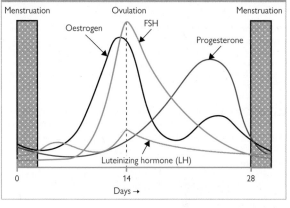

Figure 3.3 Hormone changes throughout the menstrual cycle

GP Notes: Postponing menstruation

- *Combined oral contraceptive (COC) pill* – started ≥1mo. before and continued throughout the time the withdrawal bleed should have occurred (2 packets back-to-back without a break). The withdrawal bleed will occur after the second packet is finished.
- *Combined oral contraceptive patch* – can be used for 6wk. without a patch-free break to postpone a period.
- *Norethisterone* – 5mg tds starting 3d. before the anticipated onset of menstruation. Menstruation will occur 2–3d. after stopping the norethisterone.

Premenstrual syndrome

Most women of reproductive age notice some symptoms/bodily changes in the days/weeks leading up to their periods. These changes resolve, or ↓ significantly, during the period. They are termed premenstrual tension (PMT), or premenstrual syndrome (PMS) if they occur on a regular basis and are severe enough to interfere with quality of life. >95% women have some symptoms but <1:5 seek help. Debilitating symptoms occur in 5%.

Cause: Underlying mechanism is not fully understood but is thought to be due to the hormonal changes that occur after ovulation affecting neurotransmitters in the brain. Premenstrual symptoms can also be precipitated by giving exogenous hormones such as the pill or HRT.

Symptoms: >100 symptoms described. Commonest are:
- psychological – nervous tension, mood swings and/or irritability (when severe termed *premenstrual dysphoric disorder* – PMDD)
- ↑ weight and abdominal bloating
- breast tenderness
- headache.

Management: Aims to alleviate symptoms. Usually symptoms return when treatment is stopped.
- Be sympathetic.
- Take a history of symptoms and ask the patient to keep a diary to establish cyclical nature of symptoms (☐ p.76).
- Many drug treatments have been advocated for PMS but there is no good evidence of efficacy for many.
- If mild/moderate symptoms – try lifestyle and/or dietary modification first (☐ p.77). Step up treatment according to severity and/or response.
- Consider drug therapy if symptoms are severe (e.g. PMDD) or do not respond to diet and lifestyle measures.
- Drug choice is based on symptoms.
- For all treatments try a 3–6mo. trial and follow up – the first treatment may not work.

ⓘ Bromocriptine, oestrogen patches, and gonadotrophin-releasing hormone analogues are usually only used by specialists for severe or resistant PMS/PMDD, because of side-effects.

Further information
RCOG PMS guideline currently being updated – will be available on 🖳 www.rcog.org.uk
MeReC bulletin 13(3) Tackling premenstrual syndrome (2003) Accessed via 🖳 www.npc.co.uk/merec_bulletins.htm

---

Advice for patients: Information and support for patients and their partners

National Association for Premenstrual Syndrome ☎ 0870 777 2177 🖳 www.pms.org.uk

Table 3.2 Treatment of premenstrual tension

Treatment	Effective?	Notes
Hormonal manipulation		
Progesterone/ progestogens[S]	✓	May induce PMT but systematic review shows a significant ↓ in symptoms.
Low-dose oestrogen[CE]/COC[CE]	✓	Do not give unopposed oestrogen if the uterus is intact. If progestogen causes PMT try local application instead, e.g. via IUS or topical gel (Crinone®).
GNRH analogues[R], danazol[R], bromocriptine[R]	✓	Use limited by side-effects. Usually reserved for specialist care. Bromocriptine and danazol help breast tenderness (📖 p.46).
Antidepressants		
SSRIs[C]	✓	↓ physical as well as psychological symptoms.
Anxiolytics/other antidepressants[CE]	✓/✗	Some evidence certain anxiolytics are effective but not usually used for PMS alone.
Other drugs		
Diuretics[CE]	✓	Spironolactone is effective for bloating/ breast tenderness. Many women prefer 'natural' diuretics, e.g. Waterfall®, though there is no evidence of effectiveness.
NSAIDs[CE]	✓	Effective for a range of symptoms but particularly helpful for premenstrual pain and to ↓ menstrual bleeding.
Surgery		
Hysterectomy ± oophorectomy	✓	Observational studies have found that hysterectomy + bilateral oophorectomy is curative.
Complementary therapies		
Oil of evening primrose[S]	✓/✗	Conflicting evidence – may help breast tenderness. May cause fits in patients with epilepsy.
Vitamin B₆[S]	✓	Most studies suggest effective – advise women to take 10mg/d. High doses (>100mg/d.) may cause reversible peripheral neuropathy.
Chaste tree berry (Vitex agnus-castus)[S]	✓	Evidence of effectiveness is generally positive – can cause menstrual irregularity.
Magnesium supplements[S]	✓/✗	Conflicting results.
Calcium supplements[S]	✓	↓ symptoms including breast tenderness and swelling, headaches, migraine and abdominal cramps.
Exercise[CE]	✓	High-intensity exercise improves symptoms > low-intensity exercise.
Cognitive therapy[CE]	✓	Evidence that effective though size of effect is unclear.
Relaxation[R]	✓/✗	Conflicting evidence – can do no harm.

	Jan	Feb	Mar	Apr	May	Jun	Jul	Aug	Sep	Oct	Nov	Dec
1												
2												
3												
4												
5												
6												
7												
8												
9												
10												
11												
12												
13												
14												
15												
16												
17												
18												
19												
20												
21												
22												
23												
24												
25												
26												
27												
28												
29												
30												
31												

Keeping a PMS chart

Keep the chart for at least 3 months. The chart will accurately reflect your symptoms and will show the days on which they occur, the days they are absent, the days of menstruation and the duration of the cycle. Choose a symbol for your 2 or 3 worst symptoms and use them to record the symptoms on the chart, e.g.

- H = Headache
- S = Sore breasts
- T = Tiredness

Record when you have a period with a P for period.

Advice for patients:

Things you can do to help yourself manage your PMS

Talk to people: Talk to people about your PMS and how it affects you. Friends, family and colleagues may be more supportive when you are suffering symptoms if they understand how you feel. It also often helps to discover that you're not the only one to suffer from premenstrual problems. In particular talk to you partner – over half of all relationships are affected by PMS and men often find symptoms difficult to deal with.

Menstrual diary: Keep a diary of your symptoms. This can help you understand more about how PMS affects you and plan ahead so that you can make allowances for your PMS. It can also help plan and monitor effects of treatment if you try self-help measures or decide to go to your GP for help with your symptoms.

Make allowances: If you can, try to arrange your life so that you have less to do on days your symptoms are likely to be worst.

Clothes: If you get bloated before a period, wear loose clothes on the days you are affected. Wear a supportive, comfortable bra if you suffer from sore breasts.

Look after you general health
- Make sure you are getting plenty of sleep.
- Try to take some regular exercise such as swimming, walking or yoga. Strengthening your tummy muscles can help ease discomfort due to premenstrual abdominal swelling.

Watch your diet
- Eat regularly and make sure your diet is low in fat and salt, and contains plenty of fresh fruit and vegetables.
- Some women find that eating small, frequent meals high in complex carbohydrates like bread, pasta, rice or potatoes can be helpful.
- If you suffer from bloating, cut down on your fluid intake or try eating foods with a natural diuretic effect, e.g. strawberries, water melon, aubergines, prunes, figs or parsley.
- Avoid sweet snacks between meals.
- Cut down on coffee, tea and alcohol.

Vitamin and mineral supplements and herbal remedies: Remedies which have been shown to have some effect include the following.
- Vitamin supplements – vitamin B_6 (pyridoxine) – but don't take more than 100mg each day. Vitamin E is often taken for breast tenderness but there is little evidence that it works.
- Mineral supplements – calcium and magnesium supplements may help.
- Agnus castus (chasteberry) fruit – one trial has shown this is effective but it is unclear how much you need to take for the best effect.
- Evening primrose oil – commonly used for PMS but no good evidence of effectiveness.

Further information
National Association for Premenstrual Syndrome ☎ 0870 777 2177
🖥 www.pms.org.uk

Amenorrhoea

Oligomenorrhoea: Infrequent periods. Manage as for amenorrhoea.

Primary amenorrhoea: No 2° sexual characteristics or menstruation by age 14y. with growth failure *or* no menstruation by age 16y. when growth and sexual development is normal. *Causes:*
- *Outflow abnormalities:* Mullerian agenesis, transverse vaginal septum, androgen insensitivity (testicular feminization – 📖 p.68), imperforate hymen.
- *Ovarian disorders:* PCOS; gonadal dysgenesis due to chromosomal abnormalities, e.g. Turner's syndrome – ⚠ gonads have malignant potential.
- *Pituitary disorders:* Prolactinoma.
- *Hypothalamic disorders:* Kallman's syndrome (gonadotropin deficiency and absent sense of smell – rare).

Secondary amenorrhoea: Absence of menses for ≥6mo. in a previously menstruating woman.

Causes: See Figure 3.4

History: Always consider the possibility of pregnancy.
- *Symptoms*
  - Galactorrhoea – 30% prolactinomas
  - Weight change
  - Hirsutism
  - Life crisis or upset, e.g. exams, bereavement
  - Level of exercise – gymnasts are frequently amenorrhoeic
  - Sweats and/or flushes
  - Cyclical pain.
- *Family history* of premature menopause or late menarche
- *Drug history*, particularly contraceptives, e.g. injectable progestogens
- *Past history* of chemo- or radiotherapy or gynaecological surgery.

Examination
- *Weight and height* – common if BMI <19kg/m^2
- *External genitalia* – structural abnormality, virilism
- *Vaginal examination* – including cervical smear if overdue
- *Pelvic examination* – ovarian masses, uterine size
- *General examination* – 2° sexual characteristics, hirsutism, ↓ weight, systemic disease
- *Visual fields and retinal examination*

⚠ Replace vaginal and pelvic examination with pelvic USS in young girls.

Investigation
- *Blood* – serum prolactin; TFTs; FSH/LH; karyotype if phenotypical abnormality; serum testosterone if LH high, hirsutism or virilism.
- *USS pelvis* – if structural abnormality or PCOS suspected.

Management: Treat the cause.

Contraception
- Injectable progestogens – periods usually return within a year.
- Other hormonal methods – look for another cause.

↓ Weight: Investigate and treat reasons (e.g. anorexia). Encourage weight ↑. If no response refer to gynaecology.

Physical exercise: Explain the reason for the amenorrhoea. Many refuse to cut their activity levels, so consider HRT/COC pill to protect bone density.

Stress: Reassure. Treat any psychiatric problems – periods should return spontaneously. Set a limit for return (e.g. another 3–4mo.). If periods do not return within that time consider referral as there may be another cause.

Endocrine
- Thyroid dysfunction – treat hyper- or hypothyroidism.
- Hypothalamic causes – after 6mo. there is ↑ risk of coronary heart disease and osteoporosis. Consider use of HRT or COC pill.
- Hyperprolactinaemia – refer to gynaecology or endocrinology.

Gynaecological
- Premature menopause – 📖 p.148
- PCOS – 📖 p.104

Cause not found: Refer to gynaecology.

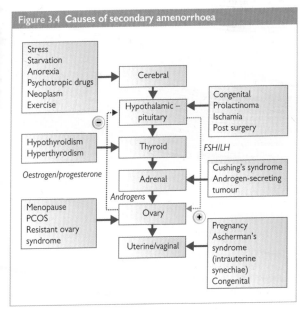

Figure 3.4 Causes of secondary amenorrhoea

Further information
Clayton, Monga & Baker. *Gynaecology by ten teachers.* Hodder Arnold (2006) ISBN: 0340816627

Menorrhagia

Menorrhagia (heavy periods) is defined as menstrual loss ≥80ml/mo. 10% meet this criterion but 1:3 feel their loss is excessive. Ask about number of tampons or pads used/d., use of double protection to prevent leaks, flooding and clots to gauge how heavy the bleeding is. Ask how periods affect life and activities. A menstrual diary may help (📖 p.83).

Assessment: Figure 3.5

Differential diagnosis: Physiological bleeding or dysfunctional uterine bleeding (50%). *Other causes:*

- Fibroids
- Congenital uterine abnormality e.g. bicornuate uterus
- Pelvic infection
- Endometriosis
- Endometrial/cervical polyps
- Presence of IUCD
- Endometrial carcinoma
- Bleeding tendency
- Hormone-producing tumours.

❗ Hyper- or hypothyroidism, diabetes mellitus, adrenal disease, prolactin disorders, kidney disease, liver disease and certain medications can also lead to menstrual disturbance.

Dysfunctional uterine bleeding: Excessive menstrual loss in the absence of any detectable abnormality. May be ovulatory or anovulatory.

Management: Figure 3.6 (📖 p.82)

Management of very heavy bleeding

- Resuscitate as necessary – admit if shocked – D&C in the acute situation can ↓ haemorrhage by 75–80%.
- Correct anaemia.
- Stop bleeding with progestogen, e.g. norethisterone 5mg tds for 10d. Effective in 24–48h. A lighter bleed will follow on stopping. Alternatively consider tranexamic acid (1g tds for 4d.) to ↓ bleeding.
- Refer for gynaecology assessment.

Reasons for treatment failure
- Very high blood loss *or* low pre-treatment blood loss
- Unsuspected uterine pathology
- Lack of compliance

Referral to gynaecology
- Symptoms suggestive of other pathology (Figure 3.5)
- Risk factors for endometrial carcinoma (Figure 3.5)
- Uterus >10/40, other pelvic mass or uterine tenderness
- Failed medical treatment

Secondary care management
- Assessment of endometrium: aspiration techniques or hysteroscopy
- Surgical treatment of menorrhagia: endometrial resection and ablation, myomectomy, hysterectomy ± oophorectomy

Further information
NICE Heavy menstrual bleeding (2007) 🖥 www.nice.org.uk

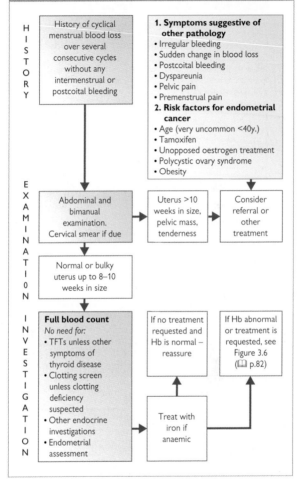

Figure 3.5 Assessment of menorrhagia in primary care

HISTORY

History of cyclical menstrual blood loss over several consecutive cycles without any intermenstrual or postcoital bleeding

1. Symptoms suggestive of other pathology
- Irregular bleeding
- Sudden change in blood loss
- Postcoital bleeding
- Dyspareunia
- Pelvic pain
- Premenstrual pain

2. Risk factors for endometrial cancer
- Age (very uncommon <40y.)
- Tamoxifen
- Unopposed oestrogen treatment
- Polycystic ovary syndrome
- Obesity

EXAMINATION

Abdominal and bimanual examination. Cervical smear if due

Uterus >10 weeks in size, pelvic mass, tenderness

Consider referral or other treatment

Normal or bulky uterus up to 8–10 weeks in size

INVESTIGATION

Full blood count
No need for:
- TFTs unless other symptoms of thyroid disease
- Clotting screen unless clotting deficiency suspected
- Other endocrine investigations
- Endometrial assessment

If no treatment requested and Hb is normal – reassure

If Hb abnormal or treatment is requested, see Figure 3.6 (📖 p.82)

Treat with iron if anaemic

Figure 3.6 Medical management of menorrhagia in primary care

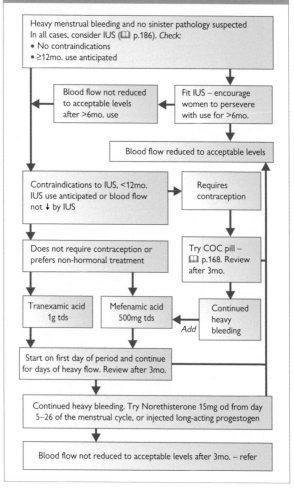

Heavy menstrual bleeding and no sinister pathology suspected
In all cases, consider IUS (📖 p.186). *Check:*
• No contraindications
• ≥12mo. use anticipated

Fit IUS – encourage women to persevere with use for >6mo.

Blood flow not reduced to acceptable levels after >6mo. use

Blood flow reduced to acceptable levels

Contraindications to IUS, <12mo. IUS use anticipated or blood flow not ↓ by IUS

Requires contraception

Does not require contraception or prefers non-hormonal treatment

Try COC pill – 📖 p.168. Review after 3mo.

Tranexamic acid 1g tds

Mefenamic acid 500mg tds

Continued heavy *Add* bleeding

Start on first day of period and continue for days of heavy flow. Review after 3mo.

Continued heavy bleeding. Try Norethisterone 15mg od from day 5–26 of the menstrual cycle, or injected long-acting progestogen

Blood flow not reduced to acceptable levels after 3mo. – refer

MENSTRUAL DIARY

Month ....

Day	1	2	3	4	5	6	7	8	9	10	11	12	13	14	15	16	17	18	19	20	21	22	23	24	25	26	27	28	29	30	31
Menstrual flow																															
Fill in if any pain																															

Month ....

Day	1	2	3	4	5	6	7	8	9	10	11	12	13	14	15	16	17	18	19	20	21	22	23	24	25	26	27	28	29	30	31
Menstrual flow																															
Fill in if any pain																															

Month ....

Day	1	2	3	4	5	6	7	8	9	10	11	12	13	14	15	16	17	18	19	20	21	22	23	24	25	26	27	28	29	30	31
Menstrual flow																															
Fill in if any pain																															

Menstrual flow
+++ **Heavy**: needing sanitary towels as well as tampons. Large clots and/or 'flooding' (blood staining clothing or bedding).
++ **Moderate**: regular changes of towels or tampons. No social inconvenience.
+ **Light**: needing some protection to prevent staining of underwear.
S **Spotting**: very light loss staining underwear.

Pain
+++ **Severe**: requiring painkillers. Not able to do normal activities.
++ **Moderate**: needing mild pain killers but can carry on normal activities.
+ **Mild**: but not needing painkillers.

83

Dysmenorrhoea

Dysmenorrhoea (painful periods) is an important problem. >½ pre-menopausal women have some degree of pelvic discomfort around the time of their period and up to 1:10 find period pain significantly interferes with their lifestyle. Adolescent girls with severe period pains do less well at school and older women who suffer from dysmenorrhoea take more time off work than other women.

Primary dysmenorrhoea: No underlying pelvic pathology. Tends to start 6–12mo. after menarche when ovulatory cycles are established. Due to uterine hypercontractility associated with ↑ prostaglandin production. Ischaemia of the uterine wall during a contraction causes pain.

Presentation
History
- Started when a teenager.
- Lower abdominal cramps ± back ache which occur in the first 1–2d. of each period.
- May be associated GI disturbance, e.g. diarrhoea/vomiting.

Examination
- *Young women (<20y.) with no other symptoms* – not necessary unless pathology suspected.
- *Older women or atypical history* – see secondary dysmennorhoea.

Treatment
- NSAID, e.g. mefenamic acid (500mg tds), naproxen (500mg initially then 250mg 6–8 hourly), ibuprofen (200–400mg tds) – effective in 80–90% – start when bleeding starts.
- COC pill – effective in 80–90%. Mechanism of action is unclear but may prevent prostaglandin production by the endometrium.

🟠 10–20% do not respond – consider a missed secondary cause.

Secondary dysmenorrhoea: Pain is due to underlying pathology.

Causes
- Endometriosis
- Adenomyosis
- Chronic pelvic infection
- IUCD
- Endometrial polyps
- Cervical stenosis
- Submucous fibroid
- History of pelvic/abdominal surgery
- Intrauterine adhesions following sugery or infection (Asherman's syndrome)
- Psychosexual problems.

Presentation
History
- Starts later than teenage years or may be a change in pattern, type or intensity of usual pain.
- Pain can last throughout the period and start just before.
- Often associated with deep dyspareunia and may be other associated symptoms, e.g. abnormal bleeding, vaginal discharge.

Examination: Perform an abdominal, vaginal speculum and bimanual pelvic examination. Look for tethered/fixed uterus, uterine tenderness, masses, and/or endocervical polyps.

Investigation
- Cervical smear – if overdue or clinical abnormality of cervix
- Endocervical swabs – including chalmydia swabs if infection is suspected
- Pelvic USS.

Management: Treat underlying cause if found, or else refer for further investigation (e.g. laparoscopy, hysterosalpingogram for identifying intrauterine adhesions).

Advice for patients: Frequently asked questions about period pains

What is period pain? Period pain is a crampy lower abdominal pain which commonly spreads to the lower back or upper thighs. It usually starts when your period starts though may start a day or two before. It goes away after 1–3 days. Some periods may be worse than others.

Are there any other symptoms? Many women do have other symptoms apart from pain. These include headaches, tiredness, nausea and diarrhoea.

Who gets period pains? Most women have some pain during periods but that pain is usually mild. 1 in 10 people have pain severe enough to affect their day-to-day activities. Painful periods are particularly common in teenagers and young adults and periods tend to become less painful as you get older. In most cases, there is no underlying cause of the pain. A few women do have an underlying cause of the pain. This is less common and more likely to occur in women in their 30s and 40s.

What can I do about my period pains? Some people find warmth helps (such as a hot bath or hot water bottle wrapped in a towel held against your lower abdomen). Simple painkillers such as paracetamol may also help. Otherwise try ibuprofen 200mg tablets from the pharmacist. Start taking 1 or 2 tablets 3 times a day after food when your pain starts or period starts – whichever comes first. Continue taking the ibuprofen regularly 3 times a day for 2–3 days. You can take paracetamol as well as ibuprofen.

When should I be worried about period pains? See your GP if:
- you develop period pains for the first time in your 30s or 40s
- you have other symptoms as well as period pain such as a change in your usual bleeding pattern, pain between periods, vaginal discharge, or pain or bleeding after sex or are concerned about sexually transmitted infection
- you are not able to control your period pains with over-the-counter medicines.

Pelvic pain and dyspareunia

History: Allow the woman to tell her story.
- Pain – site, onset (pregnant?), character, radiation, associated features, timing/pattern (relationship to menstrual cycle and/or sexual intercourse), exacerbating/relieving factors, severity
- Bowel/bladder symptoms
- Past history – ectopic pregnancy, pelvic infection or surgery, psychological symptoms.

Examination: Abdominal, pelvic and vaginal examination, including rectal examination if indicated and cervical smear if overdue. Normal pelvic and vaginal examination makes a gynaecological cause unlikely.

Investigation: *Consider:*
- Urine – pregnancy test, dipstick urine for RBCs, M,C&S
- Blood – FBC, CRP
- Radiology – pelvic USS if gynaecological cause is suspected, IVP, lumbar spine X-ray.

Causes of pelvic pain: Table 3.3

Management
- *Acute pelvic pain:* Admit unless cause is clear and ectopic pregnancy can be excluded.
- *Chronic pelvic pain:* Pain for ≥6mo. Affects 1:6 women.
  Decide whether the cause is gynaecological – patients usually have dyspareunia and pain may be cyclical. ⓘ May be due to a combination of factors.
  - If gynaecological cause is suspected and pelvic USS is normal, refer for laparoscopy.
  - If GI pain is likely, consider referral for colonoscopy.

Mittelschmerz: Mid-cycle pain which occurs around the time of ovulation. Reassure. No action needed.

Dysmenorrhoea: Painful periods – 📖 p.84.

Dyspareunia: Pain on intercourse. 10% women admit sexual intercourse usually causes discomfort. It may be *superficial* (felt around the introitus) or *deep* (felt deep inside). There is a psychological element in most cases (a vicious cycle of pain leading to fear of intercourse which exacerbates symptoms). Address both physical and psychological aspects.

Superficial dyspareunia: Examine if possible but do not insist. Treat cause (Table 3.4). If no specific treatment, try lidocaine gel. Most can be treated successfully especially if the patient has support from a sympathetic partner.

Deep dyspareunia: *Causes:*
- Endometriosis
- Pelvic inflammatory disease
- Retroverted uterus
- Ovarian cancer (rarely).

Management: Examine, treat any cause found, else refer for further investigation. If no cause is found or cause is untreatable, pain can be ↓ by limiting penetration. Often becomes a chronic problem.

Table 3.3 Causes of pelvic pain

Gynaecological		Non-gynaecological	
Acute	**Chronic**	**Acute**	**Chronic**
Ectopic pregnancy	Endometriosis	Appendicitis	Irritable bowel syndrome
Infection	Adhesions	Cystitis	
Endometriosis	Fibroids	Neurological	Musculoskeletal
Torsion of fibroid	Ovarian cyst	Colitis	Psychological*
Dysmenorrhoea	Venous congestion	Psychological	Bowel or bladder cancer
Ovarian cyst (torsion, bleeding or rupture)	Pelvic inflammatory disease		Neurological

🚯 Psychological causes of pelvic pain do occur but be careful not to dismiss organic symptoms as psychological. Psychological pain may be a consequence of and perpetuate physical pain. Diagnosis is one of exclusion.

Table 3.4 Causes of superficial dyspareunia

Vulval	Vaginal	Urethral
Vulvitis – atrophic, infective (candida, HSV)	Vaginismus (📖 p.132)	Urethritis
Dystrophy	Lack of lubrication	Urethral caruncle
Neoplasm	Vaginitis – atrophic, infective	Urethral diverticulum
Lichen sclerosis	Congenital – imperforate hymen, atresia	
	Post-surgery, e.g. painful episiotomy scar	
	Contracture – atrophy, post-surgery, post-radiotherapy	

87

Advice for patients: Information for patients with chronic pelvic pain

Royal College of Obstetricians and Gynaecologists Factsheet
🖥 www.rcog.org.uk

Endometriosis: 📖 p.90

Pelvic inflammatory disease (PID): May be asymptomatic. Peak age 15–25y. >10% develop tubal infertility after 1 episode; 50% after 3 episodes. Risk of ectopic pregnancy ↑ x10 after a single episode.

Acute PID[G]: Only 70% of those with acute PID clinically have diagnosis confirmed on laparoscopy. Most cases of PID are associated with sexually transmitted infections. In 20% no cause is found. Usual organisms are Chlamydia (50% – 📖 p.122) and/or Gonorrhoea (📖 p.122).

History
- Fever >38°C and malaise
- Acute pelvic pain and deep dyspareunia
- Dysuria
- Abnormal vaginal bleeding – heavier periods, intermenstrual and/or postcoital bleeding
- Purulent vaginal discharge.

Examination
- Pyrexia
- Vaginal discharge
- Cervical excitation
- Adnexal tenderness.

Investigations: Consider:
- *Swabs* – high vaginal swab and endocervical swab for M,C&S and chlamydia screening
- *Blood* – FBC – may show leucocytosis, ↑ ESR/CRP.

Management: Admit if very unwell or ectopic pregnancy or other acute surgical emergency cannot be excluded, otherwise:
- Advise rest and sexual abstinence; provide analgesia.
- Treat with ofloxacin 400mg bd and metronidazole 400mg bd for 14d. If the patient has an IUCD consider removal but only if symptoms are severe. If removed advise re alternative contraception and emergency contraception if sexual intercourse <7d. before.
- Arrange contact tracing via GUM clinic (📖 p.119).
- If no improvement after 48h. admit; if slow recovery consider referral for laparoscopy to exclude abscess formation.

Chronic PID: Due to inadequately treated acute PID. Presents with pelvic pain, dysmenorrhoea, dyspareunia (1:5) ± menorrhagia. *Examination:* lower abdominal/pelvic tenderness, cervical excitation ± adnexal mass.

Management: Screen for chlamydia and gonorrhoea (📖 p.122). A –ve result does not exclude diagnosis. If suspected, or chronic pelvic pain with no obvious cause, refer to gynaecology. Once diagnosis is confirmed, treatment options include long-term antibiotics or surgery.

Pelvic venous congestion: Chronic pelvic pain due to dilation and congestion of pelvic veins. Presents with chronic pelvic pain. Refer to exclude PID and endometriosis. Once confirmed, treatment is with progestogens, e.g. medroxyprogesterone 30mg od for 6mo., or GnRH analogues, e.g. goserelin 3.6mg monthly for 6mo. Symptoms often recur following treatment.

Advice for patients: Frequently asked questions about PID

What is pelvic inflammatory disease (PID)? Pelvic inflammatory disease is an infection of the uterus and/or fallopian tubes in women.

What causes PID? PID is caused by bacteria which usually travel to the uterus from the vagina or cervix (neck of the womb). The bacteria are usually passed on through sex. The most common cause is chlamydia and another common cause is gonorrhoea. These bacteria may not cause symptoms immediately so it is possible to develop PID weeks or even months after having sex with an infected person.

Who gets PID? The most commonly affected age group are women aged 15–24y. PID is a common disease and roughly 1 in 50 sexually active women develop it each year. Your risk goes up if you have a lot of sexual partners or if you have recently changed your sexual partner, if you have had an intrauterine contraceptive device (IUCD) in the past 3 weeks, or have had any recent operations involving your uterus such as a D&C or termination of pregnancy.

What symptoms does PID cause? The most common symptom is pelvic and/or lower abdominal pain. Other common symptoms include pain during sex, abnormal vaginal discharge and/or bleeding (such as heavier periods, or bleeding between periods or after sex), fever and low back pain. Some people do not get any symptoms at all or get very mild symptoms but can still get complications. The diagnosis is usually confirmed by taking swabs from your vagina and cervix.

What are the complications of PID? Early treatment with antibiotics for 2 weeks prevents complications but many women who only have mild symptoms, or have no symptoms at all, do not get treatment. Possible complications include chronic pain, infertility, ectopic pregnancy, other complications of pregnancy (e.g. miscarriage, premature birth and stillbirth), and Reiter's syndrome (arthritis and eye inflammation). If you have had PID and become pregnant, ask for an early scan to make sure the pregnancy is in the womb.

Does my partner need to be treated too? Yes, your latest sexual partner should be tested and treated, even if the tests are negative. Any other sexual partner you have had in the past 6 months should also be tested for infection.

How can I prevent PID? 1 in 5 women who have PID get a further infection within 2 years. Risk of infection goes up with the number of partners you have. Using condoms protects against infections which cause PID.

Further information for patients
Women's Health ☎ 0845 125 5254 🖳 www.womens-health.co.uk

89

Further information
RCOG Management of acute pelvic inflammatory disease (2003)
🖳 www.rcog.org.uk
British Association for Sexual Health and HIV (BASHH) Management of PID (2005) 🖳 www.bashh.org

Endometriosis

Presence of tissue histologically similar to endometrium outside the uterine cavity and myometrium. Most commonly found in the pelvis but can occur anywhere. Affects 10–15% of women presenting with gynaecological symptoms. Ovarian deposits may result in *chocolate cysts* or *endometriomas*.

Risk factors
- Age
- Family history
- Heavy periods
- Frequent cycles.

! Oral contraceptives and pregnancy are protective.

Theories of pathogenesis
- *Reflux and implantation:* Menstrual loss flows backwards through Fallopian tubes into the pelvis where it implants into the peritoneum and continues to grow under the influence of oestrogen.
- *Transformation/induction:* Peritoneal tissue transforms into endometrium either under the influence of ovarian steroids or as a result of factors released when menstrual loss refluxes into the peritoneum.
- *Mechanical transplantation:* Endometrium transplanted from one location to another (e.g. during surgery) will grow at that new site.
- *Vascular ± lymphatic spread:* Thought to explain distant deposits, e.g. lungs, brain.

Presentation
History
- Pelvic pain: cyclical ± non-cyclical, dyspareunia, dysmenorrhoea (spasmodic dysmenorrhoea is highly predictive of endometriosis)
- Menorrhagia
- Infertility.

Examination: Abdominal, speculum and bimanual pelvic examination, looking for:
- Pelvic tenderness
- Pelvic mass
- Fixation of the uterus
- Occasionally tender nodules can be felt on the utero-sacral ligaments.

Investigation: Refer to gynaecology for laparoscopy/transvaginal USS. Magnetic resonance imaging may also be useful.

! Laparoscopic findings of endometriosis are common and extent often does not correlate with severity of symptoms. Only treat if symptomatic.

Management
Infertility: Refer for specialist opinion – 📖 p.134.
- If tubal damage – reconstructive surgery or IVF.
- If no tubal damage – laparoscopic ablation may improve fertility.

Pain and bleeding

- Cyclical pain and/or heavy periods – NSAID, e.g. ibuprofen 400mg tds prn from 1st day of period.
- If a woman is not trying to conceive and there is no evidence of a pelvic mass, try a progestogen (e.g. norethisterone 10–15mg/d. for at least 4–6mo. starting on d.5 of cycle; if spotting occurs ↑ dose to 20–25mg/d. and ↓ once bleeding has stopped) or continuous COC (3 or 4 packets without a break then 7d. break).
- If symptoms are not controlled – refer.

Specialist treatments

- *Medical options:* include danazol, gestrinone and GnRH agonists (e.g. goserelin). Side-effects can be troublesome.
- *Surgical options:* include laparoscopy or laparotomy with ablation of lesions and division of adhesions; tubal surgery; hysterectomy. Laparoscopic ablation of mild endometriosis may improve fertility.

❶ For all forms of specialist treatment there is a 15–20% recurrence rate. If relapse in <6mo., treatment has failed and an alternative form of treatment should be tried. If relapse >6mo., consider the condition to have relapsed and repeat treatment.

Psychological support: Many women will have had pain for years. Often there is delay in diagnosis of the cause, and frequently they have been told it is psychosomatic. Be sympathetic and supportive and use a cooperative strategy for management.

Adenomyosis: Usually affects multiparous pre-menopausal women aged >35y. Caused by extension of endometrial tissue and stroma into the uterine myometrium. May co-exist with endometriosis (15%) but a separate entity.

Presentation: May be asymptomatic. Dysmenorrhoea (pain often peaks towards the end of menstruation), dyspareunia and menorrhagia. On examination, the uterus may be symmetrically enlarged and tender.

Management: No treatment needed if asymptomatic. Refer for further investigation of symptoms. MRI may confirm diagnosis but diagnosis is often only confirmed on histology after hysterectomy. Treatment is usually surgical with hysterectomy ± bilateral salpingo-oophorectomy. Medical treatment with GnRH analogues is a short-term option but symptoms return once withdrawn unless the woman has reached the menopause in the interim.

Further information

RCOG The investigation and management of endometriosis (2000) ⊞ www.rcog.org.uk

---

Advice for patients: Information and support for patients with endometriosis

National Endometriosis Society ☎ 020 7222 2781
⊞ www.endo.org.uk
Women's Health ⊞ www.womens-health.co.uk

Uterine problems

Congenital malformation: 📖 p.68

Uterine retroversion: 20% women have a retroverted, retroflexed uterus. May be difficult to palpate bimanually – push on the cervix to antevert. Rarely may fail to lift out of the pelvis during pregnancy, causing discomfort and urinary retention – refer (treated with catheterization).

Fibroids/uterine leiomyoma: Benign tumours of the smooth muscle of the myometrium affecting 1:5 women. Often multiple. Oestrogen dependent so regress post-menopause. Named by location:

- Pedunculated
- Intramural (centrally in myometrium)
- Cervical
- Subserosal (bulge into peritoneum)
- Submucosal (bulge into endometrium)
- Separate from uterus, especially in broad ligament from embryonal remnants.

Risk factors for clinically significant fibroids

- Nulliparity
- Obesity
- Family history of fibroids
- African racial group.

Symptoms: Usually asymptomatic. May cause:

- *Menorrhagia* – usually submucous fibroids distorting endometrial cavity
- *Pain* – torsion (pedunculated fibroid); degeneration. *Red degeneration* may occur in pregnancy (pain, fever and local tenderness until degeneration is complete)
- *Pelvic pressure/discomfort and/or backache*
- *Urinary symptoms* – may press on the bladder → ↑ frequency or a feeling of incomplete emptying or difficulty passing urine
- *Infertility* – may act as a 'natural IUCD'
- *Problems in pregnancy* – abnormal lie and ↑ risk of post-partum haemorrhage. Risk of miscarriage is not ↑

⚠ Calcification of fibroids may be an incidental finding on X-ray.

Signs: Bulky uterus ± pelvic mass felt abdominally.

Investigation: Pelvic USS is diagnostic. Check FBC if menorrhagia to exclude anaemia.

Management

- *Asymptomatic/ mild symptoms* – monitor growth by USS or bimanual pelvic examination after 6–12mo.
- *Medical* – COC pill may ↓ menstrual loss; GnRH analogues (maximum use 6mo. due to risk of osteopoenia) – cause fibroid shrinkage by up to 50% – used around menopause to avert surgery and pre-surgery to make surgery easier (controversial). Soon selective progesterone receptor modulators (e.g. asoprisnil) will be available in the UK. They ↓ fibroids by 30% without inducing a hypoestrogenic state.
- *Surgical* – myomectomy (removal of fibroids only); hysteroscopic resection (only suitable for submucosal fibroids); hysterectomy.
- *Uterine artery embolization* – radiological technique. A catheter is placed in each of the 2 uterine arteries and small particles injected to block the arterial branches that supply blood to the fibroids.

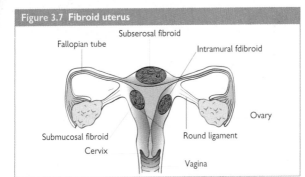

Figure 3.7 Fibroid uterus

Subserosal fibroid

Fallopian tube

Intramural fdibroid

Ovary

Round ligament

Submucosal fibroid

Cervix

Vagina

Post-menopausal bleeding: *All* women presenting with post-menopausal bleeding require referral for further investigation.

NICE guidance: A full pelvic examination, including speculum examination of the cervix, is recommended for all patients presenting with post-menopausal bleeding.

Refer urgently to a team specializing in gynaecological cancer:
- All patients with post-menopausal bleeding who are NOT taking HRT.
- Patients on HRT with persistent or unexplained post-menopausal bleeding after cessation of HRT for 6wk.
- All patients taking tamoxifen with post-menopausal bleeding.

❶ Endometrial thickness >4mm on USS needs further investigation.

Differential diagnosis: Most commonly due to atrophic change. *Other causes:* endometrial hyperplasia, endometrial polyps, endometrial malignancy (10% referred), cervical malignancy, uterine sarcoma.

Further information

SIGN Investigation of post-menopausal bleeding (2002),
🖳 www.sign.ac.uk

Pelvic or abdominal mass: Refer urgently for an ultrasound scan patients with a palpable abdominal or pelvic mass on examination that is not obviously uterine fibroids or not of gastrointestinal or urological origin. If the scan is suggestive of cancer, an urgent referral should be made. If urgent USS is not available, an urgent referral should be made without USS.

Advice for patients: Information for patients about fibroids

Women's Health 🖳 www.womens-health.co.uk

93

Figure 3.7 is reproduced with permission (copyright EMIS and PiP, 2007) from 🖳 www.patient. co.uk; where you can find comprehensive, free, up-to-date health information as provided by GPs to patients during consultations.

Endometritis: Acute infection of the endometrium. Uncommon amongst pre-menopausal women and usually occurs after surgery (including IUCD insertion) or childbirth.

Presentation: Fever, lower abdominal pain, uterine tenderness and/or purulent discharge (which may be bloodstained).

Investigation: High vaginal and endocervical swabs for M,C&S (including swab for chlamydia – 📖 p.122).

Management: Treat with antibiotics, e.g. doxycycline 100mg bd for 14d. + metronidazole 400mg bd for 1wk. or azithromycin 1g stat for chlamydia. *Pyometra* is a complication (uterine cavity fills with pus) – suspect if fails to clear. Refer to gynaecology urgently (associated with endometrial cancer).

Endometrial proliferation: Oestrogen causes endometrial proliferation, progesterone causes endometrial maturation, shedding follows withdrawal of oestrogen and progesterone (📖 p.72).

If oestrogen is given alone, the endometrium proliferates unchecked, resulting in irregular, heavy bleeding, polyps and ↑ incidence of endometrial carcinoma. *Causes:*
• Anovulatory cycles *or*
• Administration of unopposed oestrogen

Endometrial carcinoma: ~6000 women each year are diagnosed with endometrial cancer in the UK (4% of all female cancers). It is predominantly a disease of post-menopausal women with 93% of cases diagnosed in women >50y. (Peak age 61y.)

Risk factors
• Age
• Obesity
• Nulliparity
• Late menopause
• Diabetes mellitus
• Drugs – unopposed oestrogen, tamoxifen
• Granulosa cell ovarian tumour
• Family history of breast, ovary or colon cancer
• Previous pelvic irradiation.

Risk is ↓ with current or past use of the COC pill and/or progestogens.

Presentation: Post-menopausal bleeding (PMB) (>90%) – any woman presenting with a PMB has endometrial carcinoma until proven otherwise. Pre-menopausally tends to occur in overweight women and present with continual bleeding. Rarely detected on routine cervical smear.

Management: Refer any PMB to gynaecology for further investigation. Assessment comprises transvaginal USS to look at endometrial thickness ± endometrial sampling with pipelle or hysteroscopy.

Treatment: TAH and BSO ± radiotherapy, progestogen therapy and/or chemotherapy depending on stage and differentiation of the tumour. Staging and prognosis – Table 3.5.

Further information
NICE Referral guidelines for suspected cancer (2005) 🖳 www.nice.org.uk
Cancer Research UK Uterine (womb) cancer statistics
🖳 http://info.cancerresearchuk.org/cancerstats

GMS contract			
Cancer 1	The practice can produce a register of all cancer patients (excluding non-melanotic skin cancers) from 1/4/2003	5 points	
Cancer 3	% of cancer patients diagnosed ≤18mo. ago who have a patient review recorded as occurring <6mo. after the practice received confirmation of diagnosis	up to 6 points	40–90%
Education 7	The practice has undertaken a minimum of 12 significant event reviews in the past 3y. which could include new cancer diagnoses	4 points	for 12 reviews

Table 3.5 Stage and prognosis of endometrial cancer

Stage		Sub-stage	
I	Cancer confined to the corpus uteri	A	Tumour limited to endometrium
		B	Invasion to <50% of the myometrium
		C	Invasion to >50% of the myometrium
II	Cancer involves the corpus and the cervix but has not extended outside the uterus	A	Endocervical glandular involvement only
		B	Cervical stromal invasion
III	Cancer extends outside the uterus but is confined to the pelvis	A	Tumour invades the serosa and/or adnexa and/or positive peritoneal cytology
		B	Vaginal metastases
		C	Metastases to pelvic and/or para-aortic LNs
IV	Cancer involves the bladder or bowel mucosa or has metastasized to distant sites	A	Tumour invasion of bladder and/or bowel mucosa
		B	Distant metastases, including intra-abdominal and/or inguinal LNs

Grade:

G1: ≤5% of a non-squamous or non-morular growth pattern
G2: 6–50% of a non-squamous or non-morular growth pattern
G3: >50% of a non-squamous or non-morular solid growth pattern

Survival: Depends on age of the patient, stage and grade – overall 10y. survival is 75%

Stage I tumours – 5y. survival 85% (grade 1 stage IC – 81%; grade 3 stage IC – 42%)
Stage IV tumours – 5y. survival 25%

Advice for patients:

Information about hysterectomy
Hysterectomy Association ▢ www.hysterectomy-association.org.uk
Information about womb cancer
Cancer Research UK (Cancer Help) ▢ www.cancerhelp.org.uk

Prolapse

Pelvic organs sag into the vagina due to poor pelvic muscle tone and weakness of pelvic ligaments. Affects 12–30% of multiparous and 2% of nulliparous women.

Risk factors: Good obstetric practice ↓ risk. Risk is increased by:
- Childbirth
- Menopause
- Coughing and straining
- Congenital connective tissue disorders.

Terminology: Named according to the organs involved:
- **Cystocoele** – bladder bulges into the vagina
- **Urethrocoele** – urethra bulges into the vagina
- **Rectocoele** – rectum bulges into the vagina
- **Enterocoele** – loops of intestine bulge into the vagina
- **Uterine** – uterus descends into the vagina.

Uterine prolapse is further classified by degree (Figure 3.8). The most dependent portion of the prolapse is assessed whilst straining.

Presentation: Dragging sensation, feeling of 'something coming down' or a 'lump'. Symptoms are only present when upright, i.e. whilst awake, and get worse if standing for a long time, coughing or straining.

Associated symptoms: Stress incontinence (📖 p.142), difficulty of defaecation, recurrent cystitis, frequency of micturition, and/or dyspareunia depending on structures involved. In severe cases renal failure may occur due to ureteric kinking.

Examination: In left lateral position with Sims speculum, ask the patient to bear down and watch the vaginal walls. Exclude pelvic mass by bimanual examination.

Investigation: Dipstick urine and send MSU if suggestive of UTI.

Management: Choice of treatment depends on patient preference, general health, degree of prolapse, severity of symptoms and wish to preserve fertility and sexual activity. Options include:
- **Lifestyle measures:** Weight loss; smoking cessation.
- **General measures:** Treatment of co-existing conditions exacerbating prolapse, e.g. chronic cough due to COPD or asthma, constipation, menopause (📖 p.146)/atrophic vaginitis (📖 p.114).
- **Physiotherapy:** Pelvic floor exercises (📖 p.145). Refer to specialist physiotherapy if simple self-help techniques fail.
- **Ring pessary:** Useful for those too frail for surgery, women who have symptoms but don't want surgery or as a temporary measure whilst awaiting surgery. Change the pessary every 4–6mo. *Shelf pessaries* may be useful in women who can't retain a ring pessary – consider referral.
- **Surgery:** Refer to gynaecology if the woman is fit for surgery and:
  - symptoms are of sufficient severity to warrant operation *and/or*
  - incontinence *and/or*
  - recurrent UTI.

Surgical options include: Repair operations (anterior or posterior colporrhaphy), colpo/vaginal suspension, hysterectomy (vaginal or abdominal).

Figure 3.8 Degrees of uterine prolapse

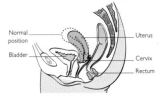

Normal position

Uterus

Bladder

Cervix

Rectum

1st degree prolapse – the cervix remains in the vagina

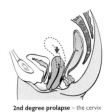

2nd degree prolapse – the cervix protrudes from vagina on coughing/straining

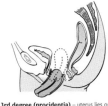

3rd degree (procidentia) – uterus lies outside the vagina and may ulcerate

GP Notes: Fitting a ring pessary

- Measure the approximate size required manually – the distance between posterior fornix and pubic bone can be measured roughly against the index finger.
- Soften the ring in hot water and lubricate it well.
- Insert the ring into the posterior fornix and tuck it above the pubic bone.
- Change the pessary every 4–6mo. Inspect the vagina for damage (e.g. ulceration) before inserting the new ring.

Potential problems

- *Discomfort* – ring may be too big or atrophic vaginitis.
- *Infection* – remove, clear infection, then try again.
- *Ulceration* – remove, allow to heal, consider alternatives or reinsert when fully healed.
- *Expulsion* – ring may be too small, pelvic musculature inadequate or retropubic rim unsuitable.

Advice for patients: Information about prolapse

Women's Health London ▢ www.womenshealthlondon.org.uk

Figure 3.8 is reproduced with permission (copyright EMIS and PiP, 2007) from ▢ www.patient.co.uk; where you can find comprehensive, free, up-to-date health information as provided by GPs to patients during consultations.

Ovarian cysts and tumours

Simple, physiological or functional cysts: Very common and often incidental finding on USS in *pre-menopausal* women. May cause pain due to tension within the cyst, rupture, torsion, or bleeding into the cyst.

- *Follicular cyst:* An ovarian follicle fails to rupture in the course of follicular development and ovulation. Unilocular and can reach a diameter of 10cm. Usually regresses during the subsequent cycle.
- *Luteal cyst:* Forms if there is excessive bleeding into the corpus luteum. May be tender, cause abdominal pain (sometimes acute abdomen) and delay the next period.

Management: As for ovarian tumour (below).

Ovarian hyperstimulation: Iatrogenic condition resulting from overstimulation of the ovaries in the course of infertility treatment.

- *Mild hyperstimulation:* >10% patients receiving gonadotrophin therapy. The ovaries enlarge and cysts form, resulting in abdominal pain and swelling ± vomiting/diarrhoea. Manage with rest and simple analgesia, e.g. ibuprofen or paracetamol prn.
- *Severe hyperstimulation:* 1% patients receiving gonadotrophin therapy. Abdominal pain/distention, vomiting/diarrhoea, ascites, pleural effusion, and/or venous thrombosis. Admit.

Polycystic ovarian syndrome: 📖 p.104

Ovarian tumours: May be solid or cystic. In women of reproductive age, >80% are benign. The remainder are borderline or malignant. In post-menopausal women, the proportion of malignant ovarian tumours rises to ~50%. Classified according to tissue of origin:

- Tumours of surface epithelium – 60% – Table 3.6
- Germ cell tumours – 15–25%
- Gonadal stromal tumours – 5–10%
- Metastatic (from breast, stomach, colon or genital tract) – 5–10%.

Presentation: Early tumours are often asymptomatic and may be an incidental finding on pelvic examination done for another reason (e.g. when doing a cervical smear) or on USS. Symptoms include:

- Non-specific – weight ↓/cachexia, constipation, early satiety, fatigue
- Abdominal pain – rapid expansion of tumour, rupture, torsion, infection or bleeding
- Abdominal distension/bloating – tumour or ascites
- Pressure effects, e.g. urinary retention/frequency, prolapse
- Menstrual disturbance
- Endocrine effects – due to hormone production by tumour.

Management: If suspected, refer for urgent USS.

- If USS is suggestive of ovarian cancer, check CA125 and refer urgently to gynaecology (to be seen in <2wk.).
- If pre-menopausal – refer any cysts with multilocular or solid elements, cysts >8cm diameter, or cysts <8cm which fail to regress in <6wk.
- If post-menopausal – refer any cyst/ovarian mass.

NICE guidance

Abdominal/pelvic masses: Refer urgently for an USS all patients with a palpable abdominal or pelvic mass on examination that is not obviously uterine fibroids or not of gastrointestinal or urological origin. If the scan is suggestive of cancer, an urgent referral should be made. If urgent ultrasound is not available, an urgent referral should be made.

Ovarian cancer: Ovarian cancer is difficult to diagnose. In patients with vague, non-specific, unexplained abdominal symptoms such as:

- bloating
- constipation
- abdominal pain
- back pain
- urinary symptoms

Carry out an abdominal palpation. Also consider a pelvic examination.

Table 3.6 Tumours of surface epithelium

Type of tumour	Subtype	10y. survival
Serous Peak age 30–40y.; 20–50% ovarian tumours; 30% bilateral	Benign serous cystadenoma – 60% serous tumours; 25% of all benign ovarian tumours	100%
	Borderline serous cystadenoma – 10% serous tumours	90–95%
	Malignant serous cystadenocarcinoma – 35–50% serous tumours; bilateral in 40–60%; 40–50% of all malignant ovarian tumours; 85% have spread outside the ovaries at the time of diagnosis; >50% are >15cm diameter at diagnosis	15%
Mucinous Can be very large; often multilocular; often contain viscid mucin – if burst can cause *pseudomyxoma peritonei* (mucin secreting cells are spread throughout the peritoneum)	Benign mucinous cystadenoma – Peak incidence aged 30–50y.; 80% mucinous tumours; bilateral in 5–10%; 20–25% of all benign ovarian tumours	100%
	Borderline mucinous cystadenoma – 10% mucinous tumours; bilateral in 10%	90–95%
	Malignant mucinous cystadenocarcinoma – Peak age 40–70y.; 10% mucinous tumours; bilateral in 15–30%; 5–10% of all 1° ovarian cancers; average diameter at diagnosis ≈16cm	34%

Endometrioid
Peak age 50–60y.; 30–50% bilateral; benign tumours are rare; malignant tumours account for 20–25% of all malignant ovarian neoplasms; 30% co-exist with endometrial cancer; 10% co-exist with endometriosis

Clear cell (mesonephroid)
5% bilateral; 5–10% of all malignant ovarian neoplasms; 25% co-exist with endometriosis; associated with hypercalcaemia

Brenner (transitional cell)
Rare – 2–3% all ovarian tumours; >90% are benign; if malignant have poor prognosis; <5% are bilateral; associated with mucinous cystadenoma and cystic teratoma in 1:10 cases

Undifferentiated carcinoma
<10% epithelial neoplasms; no histological features that characterize it

Epithelial ovarian cancer (EOC): 90% of ovarian cancers. ~7000 cases are diagnosed each year in the UK (2.5% of all cancers) and ovarian cancer accounts for 6% of ♀ deaths. Incidence is rising.

Risk factors
- **Age** – peak age 50–70y.; 85% ovarian cancers occur in ♀ >50y.
- **Family history** – mutations in BRCA1, BRCA2 and hereditary nonpolyposis colorectal cancer (HNPCC) genes are associated with ↑ risk of ovarian cancer, although only 10% of ovarian cancers occur in women carrying these mutations. Women who have inherited a gene mutation that puts them at high risk of ovarian cancer may consider having prophylactic surgery (bilateral oophorectomy). Regular screening (with USS and CA125) for the early signs of ovarian cancer is currently only available as part of a research study in the UK.
- **Nulliparity** – odds ratio 2.42 compared to women with ≥4 children.
- **Infertility** – odds ratio for women trying to conceive for >5y. = 2.67 compared to women trying to conceive for <1y. – this is probably *not* an effect of infertility drugs.
- **Obesity** may ↑ risk.

Protective factors
- **Pregnancy** – the more pregnancies, the lower the risk.
- **COC pill** – ↓ risk by ~60%. Protective effect is maintained >20y. after the COC pill has been discontinued.
- **Breast feeding** – may ↓ risk by 20%.
- **Tubal ligation** – ↓ risk by 30–70%.
- **Hysterectomy** – may ↓ risk.

Presentation and primary care management: See ovarian tumours – 📖 p.98. In the UK, ~80% of patients with ovarian cancer have had symptoms for <4wk. before seeing their GP.

Treatment: Specialist management is with laparotomy ± adjuvant treatment with chemotherapy dependent on stage of disease. Radiotherapy may be used for palliation. Staging and prognosis – Table 3.7.

Prevention: Ovarian cancer fulfils some of the criteria necessary for the introduction of population screening – it is an important health problem, and early detection is associated with improved outcomes. Although both USS and tumour markers (e.g. CA125) can detect a significant proportion of ovarian cancers pre-clinically, there is no evidence that early detection through screening ↓ mortality. To clarify this issue, 2 large-scale trials of screening are underway in the UK.

UK Familial Ovarian Cancer Screening Study – 5000 women aged >35y. with a significant family history of ovarian cancer. Screening involves annual CA125 measurement and USS.

UK Collaborative Trial of Ovarian Cancer Screening – 200,000 postmenopausal women. Screening tests used are annual CA125 and/or transvaginal USS. Due to be completed in 2010.

GMS contract			
Cancer 1	The practice can produce a register of all cancer patients defined as a 'register of patients with a diagnosis of cancer excluding non-melanotic skin cancers from 1/4/2003'	5 points	
Cancer 3	% of patients with cancer diagnosed within the last 18mo. who have a patient review recorded as occurring within 6mo. of the practice receiving confirmation of the diagnosis	up to 6 points	40–90%
Palliative care 1	The practice has a complete register available of all patients in need of palliative care/support	3 points	
Palliative care 2	The practice has regular (at least 3-monthly) multidisciplinary case review meetings where all patients on the palliative care register are discussed	3 points	
Education 7	The practice has undertaken a minimum of 12 significant event reviews in the past 3y. which could include new cancer diagnoses	4 points	for 12 reviews

Table 3.7 Stage and prognosis of ovarian cancer

Stage			Sub-stage	5y. survival
I	Tumour confined to the ovaries (20% new diagnoses)	A	Tumour limited to one ovary	73%
		B	Tumour limited to both ovaries	
		C	IA or IB with tumour on external surface of the ovary, ruptured capsule or malignant cells in ascites or peritoneal washings	
II	Tumour involving one/both ovaries with pelvic extension	A	Extension and/or implants in uterus and/or Fallopian tubes	34%
		B	Extension to other pelvic organs	
		C	IIA or IIB with malignant cells in ascites or peritoneal washings	
III	Tumour involving one/both ovaries with microscopically confirmed peritoneal metastases outside the pelvis and/or regional lymph node metastases	A	Microscopic peritoneal metastases outside the pelvis	27%
		B	Peritoneal metastases ≤2cm diameter outside the pelvis	
		C	Peritoneal metastases >2cm diameter outside the pelvis and/or pelvic, para-aortic or inguinal lymph node metastases	
IV	Distant metastases (40% new diagnoses)			16%

Germ-cell tumours: Arise from the germ cell elements of the ovary.

Presentation and primary care management: See ovarian tumours – 📖 p.98.

Types
- *Mature teratoma (or ovarian dermoid cyst):* Benign; 25% of all ovarian tumours; bilateral in 20%. Peak age at diagnosis is 20–30y. Frequently an incidental finding. May contain skin, hair, cartilage, bone, or other structures. Rarely secete thyroxine if thyroid tissue is present within the cyst and can cause hyperthyroidism. Usually removed surgically. Rarely malignant change can occur in older women.
- *Immature teratoma:* Malignant tumour. Rare – <1% of ovarian teratomas but 20% of malignant germ cell tumours. Presents in the first 2 decades of life. Usually unilateral. ↑ serum AFP (used as tumour marker). Treated with surgery and chemotherapy. 5y. survival 60–90%.
- *Dysgerminoma:* 30–40% malignant germ cell tumours (1–3% of ovarian cancers). Peak incidence in women in their teens and 20s. Unilateral in 85–90%. Highly sensitive to radio- and chemotherapy. Placental alkaline phosphatase (PLAP) is used as a tumour marker. 5y. survival rate ~95%
- *Endodermal sinus tumour (yolk sac tumour):* 20% malignant germ cell tumours. Unilateral in 95%. Tends to be fast growing and present with an acute abdomen. ↑ serum AFP (used as a tumour marker). 5y. survival 60–70%.
- *Rare tumours:* Embryonal carcinoma, choriocarcinoma and gonadoblastoma. Associated with ↑ AFP and/or ↑ β-HCG (both are used as tumour markers). All are treated with surgery and chemotherapy. Overall 5y. survival is ~60%.

ⓘ Mixed germ cell tumours account for ~10% of malignant germ cell tumours – usually contain dysgerminoma and endodermal sinus tumour.

Gonadal stromal tumours: Derived from the mesenchymal stroma of the gonad.

Presentation and primary care management: Usually present early with symptoms of hormone production. See ovarian tumours – 📖 p.98.

Types: All are rare. Treatment is surgical.
- *Granulosa cell tumours:* Most common. May be non-functional or secrete oestrogens. Associated with endometrial cancer in adults due to unopposed oestrogen secretion. Prognosis is good.
- *Thecomas:* >65% occur in post-menopausal women. Usually secrete oestrogen (rarely virilizing). Often, tumours have both granulosa and thecal elements – granulosa – theca cell tumours.
- *Fibromas:* Benign tumours consisting of fibrous tissue. Do not secrete anything. May occur in association with pleural effusion (Meig's syndrome) ± ascites. Mechanism is not understood.
- *Sertoli cell and Leydig cell tumours or Leydig cell (lipid cell tumours):* Very rare. Usually androgenic and/or virilizing.

Chocolate cysts/endometrioma: 📖 p.90.

Advice for patients:

Experiences of women with ovarian cancer

Symptoms

'Ovarian cancer is called the "silent killer" for a reason because, you know, I think women always have pains, and because I was reaching menopausal age I really kind of thought these pains were related to my ovaries drying up or, you know, your body going through the change, because you expect that … you tend to incorporate those pains and not necessarily think that they're linked to something that's, you know, worrying.'

'And I really hadn't felt ill, I'd lost a lot of weight prior to that, but I'd had a year of [stress] … and, so I'd put all my weight loss down to that. And that was the only real indication that I had that anything was wrong with me.'

Diagnosis

'In the beginning I told them they must be dreaming. It cannot happen to me, because in my family there's nobody who has ever had it. Even up to this day I believe it's a dream, and to me it's a dream, it's a bad, bad dream.'

'Well, the consultant showed me the scan of this little cauliflower thing and he told me what it was, and I felt quite calm actually. Just sat there, I suppose because it really didn't sink in, and he told me what would happen with me. I'd go in, have the operation, have both ovaries out and some lymph glands. And I drove home quite calm and it wasn't until I came in the street door that it suddenly hit me, and I just burst into tears.'

Adjusting after treatment

'I think I left hospital and I really was aware that despite being told that everything looks like it's going to be fine, they can't say a hundred percent, but it looked really good and the prognosis was great. I felt absolutely terrified and I knew that there was a huge kind of conflict between what I was being told and what I felt.'

Ovarian cancer information and support

Ovacome ☎ 020 7380 9589 🖳 www.ovacome.org.uk
DIPEx Patient experience database 🖳 www.dipex.org.uk
Cancer Research UK (Cancer Help) ☎ 0800 226 237
🖳 www.cancerhelp.org.uk
Cancer Backup ☎ 0808 800 1234 (helpline)
🖳 www.cancerbackup.org.uk

Patient experiences are reproduced with permission from 🖳 www.dipex.org.uk

103

Further information

NICE Referral guidelines for suspected cancer (2005) 🖳 www.nice.org.uk
Cancer Research UK Ovarian cancer statistics
🖳 http://info.cancerresearchuk.org/cancerstats
Clayton, Monga & Baker. *Gynaecology by ten teachers.* Hodder Arnold (2006) ISBN: 0340816627

Polycystic ovarian syndrome

Polycystic ovarian syndrome (PCOS) or *Stein – Leventhal syndrome* is a condition of unknown cause. Often there is a family history. Hormonal cycling is disrupted and ovaries are enlarged with multiple cysts. Up to 1:3 of pre-menopausal women have polycystic ovaries on ultrasound scan – 1:3 of those women have PCOS. Diagnosis requires presence of ≥2 of:

- oligomenorrhoea and/or anovulation
- hyperandrogenism – clinical and/or biochemical
- polycystic ovaries – defined as the presence of ≥12 follicles in each ovary measuring 2–9mm in diameter and/or ovarian volume >10cm^3.

Symptoms and signs Patients may be asymptomatic or suffer from any or all of the following:

- menstrual irregularity – oligomenorrhoea or amenorrhoea (affects ~67% of women with PCOS – more common in women with BMI ≥30kg/m^2), dysfunctional uterine bleeding
- anovulatory infertility
- central obesity
- acne
- hirsutism
- male pattern baldness.

Investigations

- **USS ovaries** – >12 cysts of 2–9mm in diameter (string of pearls sign)
- **Blood** – ideally take blood during the first week after menstruation:
  - normal FSH
  - ↑ LH (>10iu/l – LH:FSH ratio ↑ from 1:1 to 2–3:1)
  - ↑ testosterone (>2.5nmol/l – if >4.8nmol/l exclude other causes of androgen hypersecretion, e.g. tumour, Cushing's syndrome)
  - ↓ sex hormone binding globulin (SHBG).

Complications

- Insulin resistance/impaired glucose tolerance – 2x ↑ incidence of DM
- ↑ cardiovascular risk factors – central body fat distribution, obesity, ↑ BP, ↑ triglycerides, ↓ HDL cholesterol – 3x ↑ risk of stroke/TIA
- ↑ endometrial cancer risk.

Management

- In all cases, encourage weight ↓ and exercise.
- If oligomenorrhoeic, consider progestogens to induce a withdrawal bleed every 2–3mo. to ↓ risk of endometrial hyperplasia.
- Consider the COC pill to regulate menstruation (though may induce DM). COC pills with anti-androgen, e.g. Dianette®, may ↓ acne/hirsutism.
- Clomifene can be used to induce ovulation – 📖 p.136.
- Metformin (unlicensed) may be helpful for insulin sensitivity, menstrual disturbance and is also used for infertility to stimulate ovulation in overweight women with PCOS in whom clomifene has failed.
- Hirsutism – 📖 p.336.

Further information

RCOG Long-term consequences of polycystic ovary syndrome (2003) 🖥 www.rcog.org.uk

Advice for patients:

Frequently asked questions about PCOS

What is PCOS? Polycystic ovarian syndrome (PCOS) is a hormone imbalance that can cause irregular periods, unwanted hair growth, and acne. It affects up to 1 in 10 women. Not all people with PCOS realize they have it but symptoms usually start during the teenage years and can be anything from mild to severe.

What are the signs of PCOS? Some of the most common signs include:
- irregular periods – periods that come every few months, not at all, or too frequently
- extra hair on your face or other parts of your body, called 'hirsutism'
- acne
- weight gain and/or trouble losing weight.

What causes PCOS? PCOS is caused by an imbalance in the hormones (chemical messengers) in your brain and your ovaries which results in extra production of testosterone (or male hormone) from your ovaries. Many women also have higher than normal levels of insulin from the pancreas which may affect their blood glucose levels.

How is PCOS diagnosed? Your doctor will ask questions about your symptoms and examine you. If a diagnosis of PCOS is suspected, it can be confirmed with a blood test and ultrasound scan of your ovaries. Typically women with PCOS have lots of tiny cysts (like bubbles) in their ovaries. These are not harmful and do not need to be removed.

Why are my periods so irregular? Having PCOS means that your ovaries are not getting the right hormonal signals from your pituitary gland. Without these signals you will not ovulate (make eggs). Your periods may be irregular or you may not have a period at all.

Why do I get acne and/or extra hair on my body? Acne and extra hair on your face and body can happen if your body is making too much testosterone. All women make testosterone, but if you have PCOS, your ovaries make a little bit more testosterone than they are supposed to.

Will PCOS affect my ability to have children some day? Women with PCOS have a normal uterus and healthy eggs but many women with PCOS have trouble getting pregnant. Some have no trouble at all though. If you have trouble conceiving, see your doctor as there are now many treatments which can help.

What can I do about having PCOS? While you can't cure PCOS, you can treat it. A healthy lifestyle is very important, including healthy eating and daily exercise. There are also treatments which can help you manage irregular periods, hair growth, and acne.

Further information and support

Verity Support for women with PCOS 🖳 www.verity-pcos.org.uk
Well-being of women Leaflet on PCOS 🖳 www.wellbeing.org.uk
Women's Health 🖳 www.womens-health.co.uk

Conditions of the cervix

Cervical intraepithelial neoplasia (CIN): Invasive carcinoma of the cervix is preceded by pre-malignant lesions. The vast majority of these changes are detected in women <45y. with peak incidence in the 25–29y. age group. CIN is a histological diagnosis resulting from biopsy, usually following an abnormal smear.

Classification
- CIN 1 – Nuclear atypia confined to basal $^1/_3$ epithelium (mild/moderate dysplasia)
- CIN 2 – Nuclear atypia in basal $^2/_3$ epithelium
- CIN 3 – Nuclear abnormalities through the full thickness of the epithelium (severe dysplasia/carcinoma *in situ*).

Natural history: Unclear – and unethical to test. CIN 1 may revert to normality. Any stage can progress to cervical cancer – though more likely with CIN3.

Treatment: Depends on stage and ranges from local ablation (diathermy, laser diathermy, cold coagulation) through large loop excision of the transformation zone (LLETZ), and cone biopsy to hysterectomy. Excisional techniques are preferred as tissue is preserved for histology.

Cervical cancer: In the UK, 2800 women each year are diagnosed with cervical cancer (2% of all female cancers). There are 2 peaks of incidence – women in their late 30s and women in their 70s and 80s (Figure 3.9). 80% are squamous cell cancer – the remainder adenocarcinoma. Incidence is dropping probably due to the cervical cancer screening programme and changes in sexual practices.

Risk factors
- Social class
- Smoking
- Early age of 1st intercourse
- Early age of 1st pregnancy
- Multiple sexual partners
- HPV infection (types 16, 18, 31 & 33)
- History of dyskaryosis
- Method of contraception (↓ with barrier methods; ↑ if >5y. COC use)
- Immunosuppression, HIV.

Presentation
- Routine cervical screening – 📖 p.110
- Postcoital, intermenstrual or post-menopausal bleeding
- Offensive vaginal discharge
- Cervical ulceration/mass or cervix which bleeds easily.

Management: Refer urgently to gynaecology. Treatment is with surgery ± radiotherapy depending on the stage of the disease:
- *Stage 1:* microinvasive cancer (A)/cancer confined in the cervix (B). 5y. Survival 70–95%
- *Stage 2:* invasion into the upper 1/3 of the vagina (A) or parametria (B) but not to the pelvic side wall. 5y. survival 60–90%
- *Stage 3:* Extension to the lower 1/3 of the vagina (A) or pelvic side wall (B). 5y. survival 30–50%
- *Stage 4:* tumour involving bladder/rectum (A) or extrapelvic spread (B). 5y. survival 20–30%.

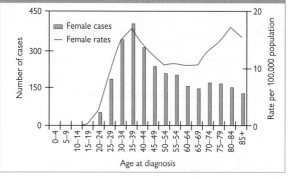

Figure 3.9 Numbers of new cases and age-specific incidence of cervical cancer in the UK (2002)

NICE guidance

Refer urgently (to be seen in <2wk.) to a team specializing in gynaecological cancer:

- Patients with clinical features of cervical cancer on examination. A smear test is NOT required before referral and a previous negative result should not delay referral.
- All patients with post-menopausal bleeding who are NOT taking HRT.
- Patients on HRT with persistent or unexplained post-menopausal bleeding after cessation of HRT for 6wk.
- All patients taking tamoxifen with post-menopausal bleeding.

Consider urgent referral: Patients with persistent intermenstrual bleeding and negative pelvic examination.

Refer urgently for an USS: Patients with a palpable abdominal or pelvic mass on examination that is not obviously uterine fibroids or not of gastrointestinal or urological origin. If the scan is suggestive of cancer, an urgent referral should be made. If urgent USS is not available, an urgent referral should be made.

Perform a full pelvic examination: Including speculum examination of the cervix, for patients with:

- alterations in the menstrual cycle
- intermenstrual bleeding
- postcoital bleeding
- post-menopausal bleeding
- vaginal discharge.

Further information

NICE Referral guidelines for suspected cancer (2005) ⊞ www.nice.org.uk
Cancer Research UK Cervical cancer statistics
⊞ http://info.cancerresearchuk.org/cancerstats

Figure 3.9 is reproduced with permission from Cancer Research UK, News and Resources website (2007), ⊞ www.cancerresearchuk.org/cancerstats

>65% of women present with stage 1 cancer so overall 5y. survival is 70%. <6% of cervical cancer deaths occur in women <35y. mainly because they tend to be diagnosed at an earlier stage.

Cervical erosion/ectropion: Physiological. An erosion or ectropion is the area of columnar epithelium visible within the vagina when the squamo-columnar junction moves down the cervix at times of high oestrogen exposure (e.g. pregnancy, COC pill, puberty). Only treat if:
- abnormal cervical smear *or*
- symptoms are causing problems, e.g. postcoital or intermenstrual bleeding, or excess discharge – refer to gynaecologist for cautery. If using the COC pill, consider switching to an alternative form of contraception.

Nabothian cysts: Mucus retention cysts on cervix. Usually asymptomatic and need no treatment. If causing troublesome discharge, refer for cautery.

Cervicitis: Presents with vaginal discharge. Speculum examination reveals mucopurulent discharge, and inflamed and friable cervix. Causes include Chlamydia (50%), gonococcus and HSV.

Management: Treat cause (📖 pp.122–9).

Cervical polyps: Develop from the endocervix and protrude into the vagina through the external os. Usually asymptomatic though there may be ↑ vaginal discharge and the lowest part of the polyp may ulcerate and bleed, causing intermenstrual, post-menopausal and/or postcoital bleeding. The vast majority are benign.

Treatment: Avulsion (send for histology). Cauterize base with silver nitrate stick if possible. Frequently recur. If post-menopausal, intermenstrual or postcoital bleeding, refer to gynaecology.

Cervical incompetence: Diagnosis is usually made on the basis of history of suggestive symptoms in past pregnancies – ≥1 late 2nd trimester or early 3rd trimester miscarriage (usually painless leaking of liquor or gradual painless dilation of the cervix). Refer all women with past history for early obstetric review.

Treatment: Cervical cerclage – a stitch is placed high up around the cervix to keep it closed, e.g. Shirodkar suture. The stitch is removed at ~37wk. and labour ensues rapidly if the diagnosis was correct.

GMS contract				
Cancer 1	The practice can produce a register of all cancer patients defined as a 'register of patients with a diagnosis of cancer excluding non-melanotic skin cancers from 1/4/2003'	5 points		
Cancer 3	% of patients with cancer diagnosed within the last 18mo. who have a patient review recorded as occurring within 6mo. of the practice receiving confirmation of the diagnosis	up to 6 points	40–90%	
Education 7	The practice has undertaken a minimum of 12 significant event reviews in the past 3y. which could include new cancer diagnoses	4 points	for 12 reviews	

Advice for patients: Patient experiences of discovering their cervical cancer

'I hadn't had a cervical smear for quite a while because like a lot of women I don't particularly like having them and it had just sort of lapsed. So I thought, well I'd better go and have one done, which I did at my local GP, and it came back with some abnormalities and surface abnormalities.

So they asked me to go to hospital to have a colposcopy, which I'd never had before, and that was really awful as I'm sure a lot of women would know. Sort of the full examination-lights, cameras, action and all the rest of it. And I found that quite traumatic. But I went to see the consultant at the hospital afterwards for the results and I went on my own. And the consultant said that they'd found not just abnormalities on the surface, but actual cancer cells deeper down in the neck of the womb.'

'I was angry and I felt it wasn't fair. Had I never ever been for a smear in my life I would have thought, well, tough, you've brought this on yourself and maybe if you'd been, you wouldn't be in this mess now. But when I'd been very diligent and it was just 18 months ago that it was totally clear – to suddenly have a tumour. I felt it was grossly unfair, I didn't want it.'

Cervical cancer information and support

DIPEx Patient experience database ⌨ www.dipex.org.uk
Cancer Research UK (Cancer Help) ☎ 0800 226 237
⌨ www.cancerhelp.org.uk
Cancer Backup ☎ 0808 800 1234 (helpline)
⌨ www.cancerbackup.org.uk

Patient experiences are reproduced with permission from ⌨ www.dipex.org.uk

Cervical cancer screening

Screening prevents ~1000–4000 deaths/y. in the UK from squamous cell cancer of the cervix (Figure 3.10). Cervical cancer almost exclusively occurs in women who are or have been sexually active.

Liquid-based cytology: In the UK, the traditional Papanicolou smear (Pap smear) is being replaced by liquid-based cytology. The sample is collected in a similar way but, rather than smearing the sample from the spatula onto a slide, the head of the spatula, where the cells are lodged, is broken off into a small glass vial containing preservative fluid, or rinsed directly into the preservative fluid. This method ↓ the number of inadequate smears taken as cervical cells can be examined even if the sample is contaminated with blood, pus or mucus.

Taking a smear: Ensure adequate training – poor smear taking misses 20% abnormalities. Courses are available – update skills every 3y. Give all women information about the test, condition being sought, possible results of screening and their implications.

Timing: Avoid menstruation if possible (note on the request form if unavoidable). Ideal time is mid-cycle. Routine bimanual examination is unnecessary – only do a pelvic examination if clinically indicated (e.g. painful/heavy periods).

Screening interval: A smear test is routinely offered to all women aged 25–64y. who are sexually active. There is no upper age limit for the 1st smear. Frequency of screening depends on age:
- 25–49y. – 3-yearly screening interval
- 50–64y. – 5-yearly screening interval
- 65y.+ – Only screen those who have not been screened since age 50y. or have had recent abnormal tests

Organization of the cervical screening programme: Practices undertaking cervical screening must:
- Provide information to eligible women to allow them to make an informed decision about taking part in the programme
- Perform the cervical screening test (and ensure staff are properly trained and equipped to perform the test)
- Arrange for women to be informed about the results of their tests
- Ensure that results are followed up appropriately *and*
- Maintain records of tests carried out, results and any clinical follow-up requirements.

The role of human papilloma virus testing: Infection with human papilloma virus (HPV) 16, 18, 31 and 33 is associated with CIN/cervical cancer. 99.7% of cervical cancers contain HPV DNA and women with HPV infection are 70x more likely to develop high-grade cervical abnormalities. A pilot of HPV testing is being conducted within the UK cervical screening programme. Women with borderline/mild dyskaryosis are tested for high-risk HPV (using the sample collected for cytology). If HPV is found, the woman is referred to colposcopy; if HPV is not found, the woman is invited for a repeat smear and further HPV test after 6mo.

GMS contract			
Cervical screening 1	% of patients aged 25–64y. (21–60y. in Scotland) whose notes confirm that a cervical smear has been performed in the last 5y.	up to 11 points	25–80%
Cervical screening 5	The practice has a system of informing all women of the results of cervical smears	2 points	
Cervical screening 6	The practice has a policy for auditing its cervical screening service and performs an audit of inadequate smears in relation to individual smear takers at least every 2y.	2 points	
Cervical screening 7	The practice has a protocol that is in line with national guidance and practice for the management of cervical screening, which includes staff training, management of patient call/recall, exception reporting and the regular monitoring of inadequate smear rates	7 points	

GMS practices are expected to perform cervical screening for all women aged 25–64y. (21–60y. in Scotland) registered with the practice as an additional service. Opting out → a 1.1% ↓ in the global sum payment.

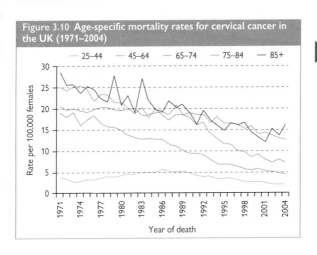

Figure 3.10 Age-specific mortality rates for cervical cancer in the UK (1971–2004)

Legend: — 25–44 — 45–64 — 65–74 — 75–84 — 85+

Y-axis: Rate per 100,000 females
X-axis: Year of death

Figure 3.10 is reproduced with permission from Cancer Research UK, News and Resources website (2007), 🖳 www.cancerresearchuk.org/cancerstats

Table 3.8 Interpretation of smear results and action

Result	What does it mean?	Action
Normal	No nuclear abnormalities	Place on routine recall
Inadequate (~9% conventional smears; ~2% with liquid-based cytology)	Insufficient material present or poorly spread/fixed. Vision of cells obscured by debris	Repeat the smear as soon as convenient After 3 consecutive inadequate results, refer for colposcopy
Borderline dyskaryosis (5–10% of smears are borderline or mild)	Some nuclear abnormalities but not clear whether these changes represent dyskaryosis	Repeat smear every 6mo. Most changes will have reverted to normal. After 3 consecutive normal smears, return to normal recall If abnormality persists 3 times, or worsens, refer for colposcopy If in a 10y. period there are 3 borderline or more severe results, refer for colposcopy
Mild dyskaryosis (5–10% of smears are borderline or mild)	Nuclear abnormalities indicative of low-grade CIN	Repeat smear every 6mo. Most changes will have reverted to normal. After 3 consecutive normal smears, return to normal recall If abnormality persists 2 times, refer for colposcopy If in a 10y. period there are 3 mild or more severe results, refer for colposcopy If CIN1 is confirmed on colposcopy, management options are to watch and wait (3 normal smears 6mo. apart are needed before return to normal recall) or treat*
Moderate dyskaryosis (1% of smears)	Nuclear abnormalities reflecting probable CIN2	Refer to colposcopy. If CIN is confirmed on colposcopy, treat*
Severe dyskaryosis or worse (0.6% of smears)	Nuclear abnormalities reflecting probable CIN3	Refer to colposcopy or (rarely) make referral to gynaecological oncologist if invasive carcinoma is suspected If CIN is confirmed on colposcopy, treat*

Other possible abnormalities seen on cervical smear
- Dyskaryotic glandular cells – refer for colposcopy.
- Atrophic – common in peri-/post-menopausal women. No action.
- Endometrial cells – may be normal if IUCD *in situ*, hormonal treatment or 1st half of 28d. cycle. Otherwise, discuss with laboratory. Refer if reported as abnormal.
- Inflammatory changes – common finding. Take chlamydial, endocervical and high vaginal swabs. Treat as necessary.
- Trichomonas, Candida or changes associated with HSV infection – treat trichomonas or candida. Discuss any new diagnosis of HSV with the patient.
- Actinomyces – associated with IUCDs – 📖 p.186.

* Following treatment, women with high grade disease (CIN2, CIN3 and cGIN) require a smear at 6mo. and 12mo. then annually for at least 9y. Women treated for low grade disease require a smear at 6mo., 12mo. and 24mo.

Advice for patients: Frequently asked questions about cervical screening

Should I have cervical screening if I'm pregnant or trying to get pregnant? Ideally women should not have cervical screening when pregnant or possibly pregnant. However, this will depend on your own individual circumstances. If you've had abnormal smears in the past, for example, or if you haven't accepted your past invitations for screening, then you should consult your doctor or practice nurse to ask for advice. If you have a normal smear history then it's better to wait until about 3 months after the delivery before you go for cervical screening.

When is the best time in the menstrual cycle to have cervical screening? Mid-cycle (usually between 10 and 16 days after your last period) is the best time because a clearer sample can be obtained around this time. But it's not a strict rule, so do take advice from your doctor or practice nurse if you can't make an appointment at that time.

Will cervical screening pick up any other infections? It might, but that's not really the aim of the programme which is to detect and treat early abnormalities which, if left untreated, could lead to cervical cancer. Incidental findings of infections may be reported. Your doctor will then act on them as needed.

I've had a hysterectomy – do I still need cervical screening? If your cervix is still present after your hysterectomy then you will still need cervical smears. Sometimes another sort of smear (a vault smear) is needed after hysterectomy even if you don't have a cervix. Normally, if you do not have a cervix, then you do not need cervical screening. The surgical team who performed the operation will decide what kind of follow-up is appropriate.

My cervical screening test showed borderline changes. Why do I have to wait 6 months for a repeat test – won't they get worse? The reason we repeat the test in 6 months is to give minor changes a chance to get better without any treatment, which is what usually happens. If the repeat test is normal, you will be asked to have two more tests in 6 and 12 months' time to check that the cells are still healthy. You can then go back to receiving routine invitations as before. If your repeat test still shows borderline changes (also called mild dyskaryosis), you may be referred for a colposcopy.

Further information for patients

Cervical screening – the facts 🖳 www.cancerscreening.org.uk
Womens Health – information on cervical screening and abnormal smears 🖳 www.womenshealthlondon.org.uk

Reproduced with permission in modified format from the NHS Cancer Screening Programmes 🖳 www.cancerscreening.org.uk

Further information
NHS Cervical Screening 🖳 www.cancerscreening.org.uk
Cancer Research UK Cervical Screening
🖳 http://info.cancerresearch.org.uk/cancerstats

Vaginal and vulval problems

Vaginal disorders

Vaginal discharge/infection: 📖 p.118

Atrophic vaginitis: Presents with vaginal soreness, dyspareunia and occasional spotting. On examination, the vagina looks pale and dry. Treat with topical oestrogens for up to 3mo. or consider other HRT.

❗ Refer any post-menopausal bleeding for further assessment – 📖 p.93.

Vaginal cysts: May arise from remnants of the mesonephric ducts (anterolaterally) or occasionally after healing following surgery or episiotomy (posterior, lower $^1/_3$). Usually no treatment is needed. If symptomatic or very large, refer for gynaecaology assessment ± removal.

Benign vaginal tumours: Benign leiomyomas or fibromyomas are common. Refer for surgical removal.

Vaginal intraepithelial neoplasia (VAIN): Multifocal. Occurs in upper $^1/_3$ of vagina. Usually occurs in association with CIN (📖 p.106). May be asymptomatic or present with postcoital staining or abnormal vaginal discharge. Treatment is by local ablation.

Vaginal cancer: Rare occurs in the 6th or 7th decade. 90% are squamous cell cancer – the rest are clear cell (associated with *in utero* exposure to stilboestrol), 2° tumours or sarcomas. Present with post-menopausal bleeding. Most are treated with radiotherapy though surgery is an option in the early stages. Refer all women with post-menopausal bleeding for gynaecological assessment – 📖 p.93.

Urethral caruncle: Due to prolapse of the posterior urethral wall. Occurs post-menopausally. Seen as a reddened area involving the posterior margin of the urethral opening. Usually asymptomatic though may bleed or cause dyspareunia. Treatment is with topical oestrogen. Surgical excision is only needed if symptoms do not resolve.

Vulval symptoms

Vulval lumps: Common and usually benign.

Non-gynaecological causes
- Sebaceous cyst
- Varicose veins
- Haematoma
- Malignant skin tumours (1° or 2°)
- Benign skin tumours (lipoma, fibroma, papilloma)
- Inguinal hernia.

Gyanecological causes
- Bartholin's gland cyst/abscess
- Genital warts (📖 p.130)
- Endometriosis
- Carcinoma of the vulva
- Mesonephric (Gartner's duct) or para-mesonephric cyst – usually near fornices.

Vulval itching (Pruritus vulvae): Common symptom. Take a history and examine the affected area. Treat the cause (Table 3.9). ❗ May be associated with diabetes mellitus. Check fasting blood glucose.

Figure 3.11 The anatomy of the vulva

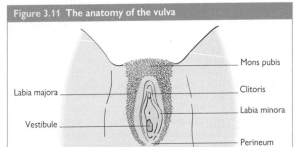

Mons pubis

Clitoris

Labia majora

Labia minora

Vestibule

Perineum

Anus

NICE guidance

Refer urgently (to be seen in <2wk.) to a team specializing in gynaecological cancer:
- Patients with an unexplained vulval lump
- Patients with vulval bleeding due to ulceration

For patients with vulval pruritus or pain: A period of 'treat, watch and wait' is reasonable. Active follow-up is recommended until symptoms resolve or a diagnosis is confirmed. If symptoms persist, refer to gynaecology. The referral may be urgent or non-urgent, depending on the symptoms and the degree of concern about cancer.

Further information

NICE Referral guidelines for suspected cancer (2005) 🖥 www.nice.org.uk

Table 3.9 Causes of vulval itching

Infection/infestation	Candida, herpes genitalis, genital warts, threadworms, pubic lice, scabies
Local irritants	Poor hygiene, contact dermatitis, vaginal discharge, urinary incontinence
Conditions specific to the vulva	Atrophic vulvitis (treat as for atrophic vaginitis), vulval dystrophy, vulval carcinoma
Other skin conditions	Eczema/contact dermatitis, intertrigo, psoriasis, lichen planus, urticaria
Generalized causes of pruritus	DM, thyroid disease, liver or renal disease, malignancy, iron-deficiency anaemia or polycythaemia, drug allergy, psychological causes

Vulvodynia: Feeling of burning, sometimes with stinging, rawness and pain. Cause unknown. Exclude other causes and then consider treatment with psychotherapy/counselling.

Genital ulcers: Take a history and examine. Consider:
- **Infective causes** – genital herpes, primary syphilis, *Behçet's syndrome* (triad of oral and genital lesions and inflammatory eye disease)
- **Non-infective causes** – vulval carcinoma, Crohn's disease

🛈 If vulval bleeding due to ulceration, refer to gynaecology urgently. If cause unknown and infective cause has been excluded, refer to gynaecology. If history of foreign travel/partner from abroad, refer to GUM.

Bartholin's gland swellings: Obstruction of the duct of a Bartholin's gland leads to cyst formation which presents as painless vulval swelling. If it becomes infected an abscess results, presenting as a painful, tender, red vulval lump. Cysts can be left to resolve spontaneously. Abscesses sometimes resolve with antibiotics (if early) or discharge themselves. If they do not resolve, acute admission for surgery (marsupialization) is indicated. The same procedure can be used to remove cysts.

Vulval dystrophy: Changes in the skin of the vulva. Usually presents with vulval itching and/or soreness. Classified histologically.

Hypoplastic (lichen sclerosus)
- Can occur at any age but peak age 45–60y. Most common of the vulval dystrophies.
- 25% have a family or personal history of autoimmune disease, e.g. vitiligo, thyroid disease and pernicious anaemia.
- Lesions occur on the vulva, inner thighs and/or perineum but do not extend into the vagina. 20% have white patches elsewhere on the body, but often these are asymptomatic.
- Initially presents with a reddened, sore, itchy area. Later the skin becomes fragile, thinned, and pale/white in appearance ± white patches (leukoplakia). Atrophy causes the skin to look whiter, and contours of the vulva slowly disappear. Narrowing of the introitus may cause superficial dyspareunia. Rarely fusion of the labia can cause urination difficulties.
- Associated with a small risk of malignant change (3–5%).

Management: If suspected, refer to gynaecology or dermatology for skin biopsy to confirm diagnosis. Treatment is with potent topical steroids for 3mo. then intermittently as needed thereafter. Advise women to wash the genital area with aqueous cream instead of soap and to avoid bath additives and biological washing powders. Refer back to gynaecology urgently if there is persistent ulceration or any new lesions appear.

Hyperplasic: Usually affects post-menopausal women. Characterized by thickened, hyperkeratotic lesions on the vulva ± excoriation. Lesions are often multiple and symmetrical. Refer to dermatology or gynaecology for biopsy to confirm diagnosis. Treatment is with topical steroids. <2% of lesions show malignant change.

🛈 Mixed patterns are common.

Vulval intraepithelial neoplasia (VIN): Previously known as *Bowen's disease* or carcinoma *in situ*. May be associated with other genital tract neoplasia (e.g. CIN – 📖 p.106).

Presentation: Abnormal looking skin of vulva (usually pinky-white and altered texture) ± white patches ± itch.

Diagnosis: There is some overlap between vulval dystrophy and VIN. Diagnosis is histological following skin biopsy:
- **VIN 1**   Epidermis is thickened. Atypia is confined to the basal $^1/_3$ of the epithelium.
- **VIN 2**   Nuclear atypia in the lower $^1/_2$ of the epithelium.
- **VIN 3**   Carcinoma *in situ* – nuclear atypia through the full thickness of the epithelium.

Management: Refer all patients with abnormal looking vulval skin (without candidal infection or other obvious cause) to gynaecology for skin biopsy and treatment. Treatment – depends on site, histology and extent – includes: observation with regular biopsies, surgery, cryocautery, laser vaporization, or topical chemotherapy.

Vulval carcinoma[G]: Rare. Mainly affects women in 8th decade. Most are squamous cell carcinoma; others – melanoma, basal cell carcinoma, Bartholin's gland carcinoma and adenocarcinomas. The majority occur on the labia and spread to local LNs. Present early with chronic pruritus vulvae ($>^2/_3$), vulval lump or ulcer. Refer for confirmation of diagnosis. Treatment is surgical. 5y. survival rate ≈ 95%.

Further information

British Association for Sexual Health and HIV (BASHH) National guidelines on the management of vulval conditions (2002) 🖥 www.bashh.org

British Association of Dermatologists Guidelines for the management of lichen sclerosus (2002) 🖥 www.bad.org.uk

RCOG Management of vulval cancer (2006) 🖥 www.rcog.org.uk

GMS contract			
Cancer 1	The practice can produce a register of all cancer patients defined as a 'register of patients with a diagnosis of cancer excluding non-melanotic skin cancers from 1/4/2003'	5 points	
Cancer 3	% of patients with cancer diagnosed within the last 18mo. who have a patient review recorded as occurring within 6mo. of the practice receiving confirmation of the diagnosis	up to 6 points	40–90%

Advice for patients:

National Lichen Sclerosus Support Group
🖥 www.lichensclerosus.org
Cancer Research UK (CancerHelp) ☎ 0800 226 237
🖥 www.cancerhelp.org.uk

Vaginal discharge

All women have some vaginal discharge. Physiological discharge is white, becoming yellow on contact with air. Amount varies considerably and is affected by menstrual cycle, sexual activity, use of COC pill, age, stress and pregnancy. 5 causes account for 95% cases presenting to GPs:

- Excessive normal secretions
- Bacterial vaginosis
- *Candida albicans*
- Cervicitis (gonococcal, chlamydial or herpetic)
- *Trichomonas vaginalis*.

ⓘ Discharge is only abnormal when it is different from a woman's normal discharge.

Rarer causes
- Cervical ectropion
- Chemical vaginitis – avoid perfumed or disinfectant bath additives
- Foreign body, e.g. retained tampon – remove and treat with metronidazole 400mg tds for 7d.
- IUCD
- Cervical polyp
- Fistula
- Necrotic tumour (rare).

History: Ask about:
- *Symptoms* – vaginal discharge (itchy, offensive, colour, duration), vulval soreness and irritation, lower abdominal pain, dyspareunia, heavy periods, intermenstrual bleeding, fever, vulval pain.
- *Sexual history* – recent sexual contact with new partner, multiple partners, presence of symptoms in partner, worries about sexually transmitted disease.
- *Medical history* – pregnancy, diabetes mellitus, recent antibiotics.
- *Attempts at self-medication*.

Examination: Abdominal, bimanual pelvic and vaginal speculum examination. Look for lower abdominal tenderness, tenderness on bimanual palpation, cervical erosion or contact bleeding, discharge, warts or ulcers.

Management: High vaginal swab for culture and endocervical swabs for gonorrhoea and chlamydia, opportunistic cervical smear. If herpes infection is suspected – viral swab (or if unavailable refer to GUM). Treat cause (below and 📖 pp.120–9). If unclear, refer to GUM or gynaecology.

Bacterial vaginosis (BV): Vaginal flora is changed from lactobacillus species to anaerobes. Not sexually transmitted. Affects 10–40% of pre-menopausal women – ~½ are asymptomatic. *Associated with:*
- ↑ risk of pre-term delivery (and ↓ risk if treated)
- Development of PID and endometritis following abortion or birth
- Infection post-hysterectomy.

Presentation:
- *History:* White–grey, fishy, offensive discharge; no vulval soreness.
- *Examination:* Discharge; cervix looks normal.

GPs are frequently presented with symptoms or signs found inciden-tally (e.g. when doing a cervical smear) that may indicate sexually transmitted disease (STD). The easiest (and often best) option is to refer suspected cases to genito-urinary medicine (GUM) clinics. Sometimes the patient is reluctant to go and 40% of referrals never attend, so it is still necessary for GPs to know how to prevent, diagnose and treat STDs themselves.

Contact tracing: Best done by GUM clinics. If a patient refuses to go then provide the patient with a letter to give to contacts stating the disease they have been in contact with, treatment given and suggesting contacts visit their local GUM clinic promptly.

Use of GUM clinics: In general, refer patients:
- who require contact tracing
- if counselling is needed, e.g. first-attack HSV, HIV
- if diagnosis is still unclear after investigation
- for confirmation of diagnosis, e.g. HSV
- if specialist treatment required, e.g. treatment of genital warts.

Advice for patients: Information about bacterial vaginosis (BV)

- BV is a very common condition of the vagina caused by an overgrowth of several bacteria. It is not just a simple infection.
- BV can affect any woman. It is not a sexually transmitted disease. Sexual partners of women with BV do not need any treatment.
- BV may not cause symptoms, but when it does the main symptom is white–grey vaginal discharge which often has a fishy smell. It does not usually cause itching or soreness. The smell may be most noticeable when having sex.
- BV is not caused by poor hygiene. In fact, excessive washing of the vagina may alter the normal balance of bacteria in the vagina, which may make BV more likely to develop.
- BV is usually diagnosed when a swab is taken to find out what is causing vaginal discharge.
- Once diagnosed, treatment is with antibiotics which your doctor will prescribe for you. This clears BV in 7 out of 10 cases. Not treating is an option if you are not pregnant as BV often clears without treatment. In pregnancy, BV can cause complications (such as premature labour or infections of the womb after birth), so treatment is always needed.
- BV recurs within 3 months in about ½ of women who have been successfully treated. If it does recur, a repeat course of antibiotics is usually successful. Avoid anything which might upset the natural balance of the vagina, like washing the area too often or putting detergents or perfumes in bath water, as this can make recurrences more likely.

119

Further information

British Association for Sexual Health and HIV National guidelines for consultations requiring sexual history taking (2005) 🖳 www.bashh.org

Investigation: Endocervical swab – M,C&S

Management: Without treatment, 50% remit spontaneously. Cure rates with all methods is ~85%. There is no benefit from treating the woman's partner. *Treatment:*

- Except in the 1st trimester of pregnancy, treat with metronidazole po (400mg bd for 7d.) or pv (5g bd for 5d.)
- In the 1st trimester of pregnancy, treat with clindamycin 2% cream 5g nocte pv for 1wk.
- Recurrent infection (1:3 recur) – metronidazole 400mg bd for 3d. at the start and end of menstruation *or* metronidazole 0.75% gel od for 10d. then twice weekly for 4–6 mo.

Candidiasis: Fungal infection. ~20% of patients are asymptomatic.

Predisposing factors

- Cushing's or Addison's disease
- DM
- Pregnancy
- Immunosuppression
- Steroid treatment
- Vaginal trauma
- Broad-spectrum antibiotics
- Radiotherapy/chemotherapy
- Tight-fitting synthetic underwear.

History: Pruritus vulvae, superficial dyspareunia, thick, creamy, non-offensive discharge.

Examination: Discharge (cottage cheese), sore vulva which may be cracked or fissured.

Investigation: Usually unnecessary. Confirm diagnosis if infection persists or recurs by sending a vaginal swab for M,C&S.

Management: Only treat if symptomatic.

- Try clotrimazole pessaries – cure rate ≈ 90%.
- An alternative is oral fluconazole – contraindicated in pregnancy or lactation – 83% cure rate.
- Sexual transmission is minimal and there is no benefit from treating the partner unless overt infection.
- Benefits of ingestion or topical application of live yoghurt are not clear, though it is probably not harmful.

Recurrent infection

- *If occurs pre-menstrually:* Consider prophylaxis with fluconazole 150mg on the 21st day of cycle or 500mg clotrimazole pessary on days 7 & 21.
- *If infection at other times:* Try a 2wk. course fluconazole 50mg od po or clotrimazole 100mg nocte pv. Advise loose underwear and avoidance of perfumes or disinfectants in bath.

Further information

British Association of Sexual Health and HIV (BASHH)
🖳 www.bashh.org
- Management of bacterial vaginosis (2001)
- Management of vulvovaginal candidiasis (2001)

Advice for patients: Frequently asked questions about thrush

What is thrush? Thrush is an infection caused by a yeast called *Candida albicans*. Small numbers of Candida live on the skin and around the vaginal area. These are usually harmless but occasionally, when conditions are right, will cause symptoms. Thrush is not usually a sexually transmitted infection.

What are the symptoms of vaginal thrush? Thrush causes a creamy, white vaginal discharge. This is often accompanied by soreness, itching and/or redness around the outside of the vagina.

Who gets thrush? Most women will have at least one episode of thrush at some point in their lifetime. In most cases it appears for no apparent reason. Some people are more likely to get thrush than others though. Thrush is more common in pregnancy, amongst women with a poor immune system (for example, due to steroids, chemotherapy or AIDS), amongst diabetic women or women who are taking antibiotics.

Do I need to see a doctor about thrush? Some women are prone to thrush and know what it feels like. They often buy treatment from the pharmacist and do not need to see a doctor. If you have never had thrush before, see a doctor or nurse to confirm the diagnosis and for advice on treatment. Tests are not always necessary if symptoms and signs are typical but the doctor or nurse may take a swab of the discharge to confirm the cause of infection if the diagnosis is not clear. Always see your GP if symptoms do not go away with treatment.

How is thrush treated? Thrush can be treated with creams and/or pessaries, or tablets. Both are available on prescription or directly from the pharmacist without a prescription. They are equally effective but don't use tablets if you are pregnant or breast feeding. Always read the label before using any treatment. Side-effects are uncommon. Treatment does not clear symptoms in 1 in 5 cases. See your doctor if this happens.

Why does thrush treatment sometimes not work? There are several reasons why treatment can fail. These include:
• not using the treatment properly
• another cause, other than thrush, for the vaginal discharge
• resistance of the thrush germs to the medicine used
• further, new thrush infection.

If treatment has not worked or you get recurrent infections (more than 4 attacks a year), then see your doctor.

Further information
Women's Health ⊟ www.womens-health.co.uk
Family Planning Association (FPA) ⊟ www.fpa.org.uk

121

A–Z of sexually transmitted diseases

Chlamydia: Major cause of pelvic pain and infertility in women.

Presentation in women
- **History:** >70% are asymptomatic. *Symptoms:* vaginal discharge (30%); postcoital or intermenstrual bleeding; pelvic inflammatory disease (10–30% – 📖 p.88).
- **Examination:** Mucopurulent cervicitis; hyperaemia and oedema of the cervix ± contact bleeding; tender adnexae; cervical excitation.
- **Investigation:** Send endocervical swab for ELISA ± MSU to confirm diagnosis. Urine samples are used for screening asymptomatic women.

Presentation in men: Usually asymptomatic. May have urethritis. Send urethral swab for ELISA ± MSU to confirm diagnosis.

Presentation in neonates: Conjunctivitis, pneumonia, pharyngitis, otitis media – $^1/_3$ affected mothers have affected babies.

Screening: Chlamydia is a preventable cause of infertility, ectopic pregnancy and pelvic inflammatory disease. Screening using first-catch urine testing ↓ prevalence and incidence of pelvic inflammatory diseases. The DoH is implementing a national screening programme, initially aimed at young people aged 16–24y. who access sexual health services, through a phased roll-out in England. Similar programmes are being considered in the rest of the UK.

Management
- Doxycycline 100mg bd for 1wk.; azithromycin 1g po as a single dose is an alternative which ensures compliance.
- During pregnancy/breast feeding use erythromycin 500mg qds 1wk.
- Affected neonates – seek specialist advice.

Gonorrhoea

Presentation in women: Infection may cause pelvic inflammatory disease, abscess of Bartholin gland, miscarriage, pre-term labour and babies may have neonatal ophthalmia (purulent discharge ± swelling of eyelid <4d. after birth – permanent visual damage can result). Send endocervical swab for M,C&S to confirm diagnosis. Taking rectal and urethral swabs ↑ sensitivity.

Presentation in men: 50% acute infections are asymptomatic. May present with urethritis, prostatitis, urethral stricture, skin lesions or septic arthritis. Send urethral ± rectal swabs for M,C&S to confirm diagnosis.

Management
- 1×400mg cefixime po. Alternative is amoxicillin 3g + probenecid 1g or ciprofloxacin 1×500mg po, or ofloxacin 1×400mg po. Do not use cirofloxacin or ofloxacin in pregnancy. Refer to local protocol.
- If pelvic inflammatory disease add co-amoxiclav 250–500mg tds (or erythromycin) for 10d.
- Reculture 3–7d. after treatment. Contact tracing is essential – refer to GUM clinic.
- *Affected neonates:* seek specialist advice.

Advice for patients:

Information about chlamydia

- Chlamydia is an infection caused by a bacterium called *Chlamydia trachomatis*. In women, infection usually affects the cervix and uterus (womb). Men may have these infections without any symptoms.
- Chlamydia is usually passed on through sex with an infected person. Risk of infection increases with number of changes of sexual partner. Wearing a condom during sex helps to prevent chlamydia and other sexually transmitted infections.
- Symptoms include vaginal discharge, pain or burning on passing urine, bleeding or spotting between periods (particularly after sex), and lower abdominal or pelvic pain, but 7 out of 10 women have no symptoms.
- Diagnosis is confirmed by taking swabs from the vagina and cervix.
- Chlamydia infections need treatment, even if you have no symptoms. Untreated they can go on to cause pelvic pain or infection, infertility and/or ectopic pregnancy. Without treatment you can also pass the infection on to other sexual partners.
- Treatment involves a course of antibiotics. Your current (or last) sexual partner and any other sexual partners within the last 6 months should also be tested for infection and treated with antibiotics. Avoid sex for 1 week after completion of treatment.

Information about gonorrhoea

- Gonorrhoea is an infection caused by another bacterium, gonococcus, and is also known as 'clap'. In women, infection usually affects the cervix and uterus (womb). Men may have no symptoms.
- Usually passed on through sex with an infected person. Risk of infection increases with number of sexual partners. Wearing a condom helps to prevent gonorrhoea and other sexually transmitted infections.
- Symptoms include vaginal discharge, pain or burning on passing urine, bleeding or spotting between periods (particularly bleeding after sex), and lower abdominal or pelvic pain. You may have no symptoms at all. Diagnosis is confirmed by taking swabs from the vagina and cervix.
- Gonorrhoea infections need treatment, even if you have no symptoms. Untreated it can go on to cause acute pelvic infection, pelvic pain, infertility and/or ectopic pregnancy. Without treatment you can also pass the infection on to other sexual partners.
- Treatment involves a course of antibiotics. Your current (or last) sexual partner and any other sexual partners within the last 6 months should also be tested for infection and treated with antibiotics.

Information sheets: Available from ▣ www.patient.co.uk, ▣ www.fpa.org.uk and ▣ www.ssha.info

Further information

Department of Health ▣ www.dh.gov.uk
- National Chlamydia Screening Programme
- National Strategy for Sexual Health and HIV (2001)

British Association of Sexual Health and HIV (BASHH) ▣ www.bashh.org
- Management of *Chlamydia trachomatis* genital tract infection (2006)
- Management of gonorrhoea in adults (2005)

Hepatitis B (HBV): Common. Endemic in much of Asia and the Far East. The virus has 3 major structural antigens: surface antigen (HBsAg), core antigen (HBcAg), and e antigen (HBeAg). Spread is via infected blood, sexual intercourse, from mother to newborn baby or via human bites. Incubation period is 6–23wk. (average 17wk.).

High-risk groups: See GMS contract box (opposite).

Presentation: May be asymptomatic or present with fever, malaise, fatigue, arthralgia, urticaria, pale stools, dark urine and/or jaundice.

Investigation: LFTs (hepatic jaundice – ↑ bilirubin, ↑ ALT/AST, ↑ alkaline phosphatase), hepatitis serology (Figure 3.12).

- HBsAg is present from 1–6mo. post-exposure. If present >6mo. after the acute episode, defines carrier status.
- HBeAg suggests high infectivity. Present from 6wk.–3mo. after acute illness.
- Anti-HBs antibodies appear >10mo. after infection and imply immunity.

Management: In all cases advise patients to avoid alcohol. Refer for specialist advice. Treatment is supportive for acute illness. Chronic hepatitis is treated with interferon and lamivudine with varying success.

Prognosis: ~85% recover fully; 10% develop carrier status; 5–10% develop chronic hepatitis – may lead to cirrhosis and/or liver carcinoma. Fulminant hepatitis and death are rare (<1%).

Prevention: Advise patients re 'safe sex'. Immunize high-risk groups. Give passive immunization with human immunoglobulin to non-immune high-risk contacts of infected patients.

Hepatitis C (HCV): Common – a major cause of post-transfusion hepatitis. Prior to 1989 known as non-A, non-B hepatitis. Spread is usually via contact with infected blood, though can occur from mother to baby. Hepatitis C is NOT easily spread through sexual contact. In 10% no source of infection is found. Incubation is 2–25wk. (average 8wk.).

Risk factors: Blood transfusions; health-care workers; IV drug abusers; haemodialysis patients; infants born to infected mothers; multiple sexual partners.

Presentation and management: As for HBV. Anti-HCV antibody is detectable 3–4mo. post-infection. Refer for expert advice. Avoid alcohol. ½ develop chronic infection; 5% cirrhosis and 15% of those hepatoma.

Further information

British Association for Sexual Health and HIV National guidelines on the management of viral hepatidides (2005) ▣ www.bashh.org
Health Protection Agency (HPA) ▣ www.hpa.org.uk
UK Clinical Virology Network ▣ www.clinical-virology.org
Department of Health The Green Book ▣ www.dh.gov.uk

Advice for patients: Information for patients

British Liver Trust ☎ 01425 463080 ▣ www.britishlivertrust.org.uk

GMS contract

Hepatitis B vaccination: Can be provided to high-risk groups as an *additional service*. Opting out of giving vaccinations to the under 5s results in a 1% ↓ in global sum and opting out of giving other essential vaccinations results in a 2% ↓ in global sum. High-risk groups include:

- Injecting drug users
- Individuals who change sexual partner frequently
- Families adopting children from high/intermediate-risk countries
- Close family contacts of a case/carrier
- Patients receiving regular blood/ blood products and their carers
- Patients with chronic renal failure
- Patients with chronic liver disease
- Prison inmates

- People at risk due to their occupation, e.g. health-care workers
- Staff/residents of residential accommodation for individuals with mental handicap
- Patients travelling to high/intermediate-risk areas
- Foster parents
- Babies born to mothers who are chronic carriers of hepatitis B or who have had acute hepatitis B during pregnancy (📖 p.257)

Figure 3.12 Hepatitis B serology

(a) Acute hepatitis B infection with recovery

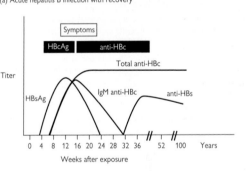

(b) Acute hepatitis B infection with progression to carrier state

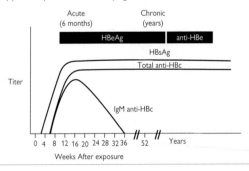

Permission to reproduce Figure 3.12 sought from the US Centres for Disease Control and Prevention 🖳 www.cdc.gov

Genital herpes: HSV is transmitted by direct contact with lesions. Lesions may appear anywhere on the skin or mucosa but are most frequent around the mouth, on the lips, conjunctiva, cornea, and genitalia.

History and examination: May be asymptomatic. If symptomatic, history and examination are diagnostic in 90% cases. Presents with multiple painful genital ulcers on a red background ± inguinal lymph nodes <1wk. after sexual contact. Lesions crust over then heal. Untreated lasts 3–4wk. *Complications:* Urinary retention, aseptic meningitis.

Management
- Refer to GUM if diagnosis is uncertain and for contact tracing.
- Treat with aciclovir if presents within the first few days of symptoms starting (↓ duration, symptoms and complications), analgesia, ice packs and salt baths.
- Advice – barrier methods of contraception (risk of transmission in monogamous relationships – 10%/y.).
- If pregnant, obtain specialist advice.

Neonatal infection: Presents at age 5–21d. with vesicular lesions around the presenting part or rarely systemic infection. Usually babies of women with no history of genital HSV. Refer as a paediatric emergency.

Recurrent infection: Reactivation of latent virus. Less severe than 1° infection. Neonatal transmission rates are low (<3%) – elective Caesarean section for those with active recurrences at term is controversial. Consider suppressive therapy if >5 attacks/y., e.g. aciclovir 400mg bd. Usually initiated under consultant supervision.

Human immunodeficiency virus (HIV): HIV is a retrovirus infecting T-helper cells bearing the CD4 receptor. Worldwide, the HIV epidemic continues, but prophylaxis and treatment is improving prognosis in developed countries where treatment is available.

Transmission
- Sexual (60–70%). Heterosexual intercourse –50% cases
- IV drug abuse (3%)
- Infected blood products
- Mother → child (90% HIV infections in children)
- Accidental exposure (e.g. needle-stick injuries – 📖 p.129)

Clinical disease
Primary HIV: Symptoms in ≈ ½ infected patients – glandular-fever like syndrome of diffuse maculo-papular rash, fever, fatigue and lymphadenopathy. Rarely acute neurological symptoms (aseptic meningitis, transverse myelitis, encephalitis). FBC may show atypical lymphocytes.

Early HIV: Follows seroconversion. Plasma viral load ↓ to a plateau. Level of the plateau is prognostic – 'fast progressors' have high and 'slow progressors' have low plateau levels. Most patients are asymptomatic. *Symptoms:* night sweats or generalized lymphadenopathy.

Advice for patients:

Self-help for recurrent genital herpes

After the first infection of genital herpes, the virus settles in a nearby nerve and stays there for the rest of your life. For most of the time, the virus is inactive and causes no symptoms. From time to time, in 1 in 5 people, the virus becomes 'active' and causes a further attack.

What are the symptoms of recurrent genital herpes?

- Often before anything is visible, you may feel a tingling or itching of the genital area.
- Within a day, blisters appear. These may weep and be sore.
- Over a few days the blisters scab over; the scab falls off after about a week, leaving no scar.

What triggers the virus to become active again?

Common triggers include:

- illness – such as colds, coughs and flu
- menstruation – common around the time of periods
- stress or being 'run down' for any reason
- sex with inadequate lubrication.

Are there any treatments for genital herpes? Yes.

- Pain can be eased by painkillers which you can buy at the chemist or supermarket such as paracetamol or ibuprofen. Ice packs made from wrapping ice cubes in a face flannel can also be soothing. If it hurts to pass urine, urinating whilst sitting in a warm bath can help or try application of local anaesthetic cream before passing urine.
- Antiviral tablets such as aciclovir help some people with severe symptoms, especially if used as soon as possible after symptoms start. You can get these tablets on prescription. If you get frequent attacks, talk to your doctor about taking tablets to prevent the attacks.

Can I pass on herpes to other people?

Yes. When you have blisters of genital herpes you should avoid sex until all the symptoms have gone. If you do have sex, use a condom. When you don't have blisters or sores, you are usually not infectious and it is unlikely you will pass the infection on, but wearing a condom reduces the risk further and protects against other sexually transmitted diseases too. If you have ever had genital herpes and are pregnant, tell your midwife as you can pass the infection on to your baby if the herpes is active at the time of delivery.

Further information

Herpes Association ☎ 0845 123 2305 🖥 www.herpes.org.uk
Family Planning Association (FPA) 🖥 www.fpa.org.uk

127

Further information

British Association for Sexual Health and HIV National guidelines for the management of genital herpes (2001) 🖥 www.bashh.org
Health Protection Agency (HPA) 🖥 www.hpa.org.uk
UK Clinical Virology Network 🖥 www.clinical-virology.org

Advanced HIV: Accompanied by immunosuppression or AIDS (if CD4 count <200cells/mm^3). Patients are at risk from opportunistic infection (e.g. pneumococcal infection, TB, CMV, *Pneumocystis carinii*, toxoplasmosis and cryptosporidial diarrhoea) and AIDS-associated malignancies (e.g. Kaposi's sarcoma, lymphoma).

Death: Due to multiple causes, including chronic incurable systemic infections, malignancies, neurological disease, wasting and malnutrition, and multisystem failure.

Management: Specialist treatment is essential.
- *Antiviral drugs:* A combination of antiviral drugs is usual. Adherence to therapy is essential to avoid resistance. Treatment failure requires switching or increasing therapy.
- *Prophylaxis against opportunistic infection:* Prophylactic antibiotics are used to prevent *Pneumocystis carinii*, toxoplasmosis and *Mycobacterium avium* for patients with low CD4 counts.
- *Psychological support:* Due to the stigma attached to HIV infection, patients and carers often lack the support offered by the community for most other serious illness.

Pubic lice: Pubic (or crab) lice are similar to head lice and may be sexually transmitted. All hairy areas (including eyelashes, eyebrows, pubic and axillary hair) can be affected. Carbaryl (unlicensed), phenothrin and malathion are all effective. Apply an aqueous solution to all parts of the body and rinse off after 12h. Repeat after 7d.

Scabies: The scabies mite (*Sarcoptes scabei*) is ~½mm long and spread by direct physical contact. Average infection consists of 12 mites. Symptoms appear 4–6wk. after infection.

Presentation: Intense itching. Examination reveals burrows (irregular, tortuous and slightly scaly, <1cm long. Itching results in excoriations. Untreated infection becomes chronic.

Management: Treat with scabicide, e.g. permethrin 5% cream. Apply to the whole body except head and neck (except child <2y. when head and neck should be included). Reapplication may be needed after 1wk. All close contacts need treatment. Advise patients to launder all worn clothing and bedding after application. Itching may persist for some time after elimination of infection – use oral antihistamines for symptomatic relief. Treat any 2° infection with topical or systemic antibiotics.

Syphilis: Caused by *Treponema pallidum*. Rare in the UK but incidence is increasing. *Incubation:* 9–90d. In all cases refer for specialist care. Contact tracing is essential. *4 stages:*
- *Primary syphilis:* Chancre at the site of contact
- *Secondary syphilis:* 4–8wk. after chancre – systemic symptoms: fever, malaise, generalized lymphadenopathy, anal papules (conylomata lata), rash (trunk, palms, soles), buccal snail-track ulcers, alopecia
- *Tertiary syphilis:* 2–20y. after initial infection – gummas (granulomas) in connective tissue
- *Quarternary syphilis:* Cardiovascular or neurological complications. *Investigation:* blood for VDRL or TPHA.

- Promotion of safe sex.
- Refer to A&E for prophylaxis if inadvertent exposure through needle-stick injury or similar.
- Consider prophylaxis if sexual contact with an infected (or high-risk if status unknown) individual <72h. before presentation – take advice from GUM clinic.
- ↓ IV drug abuse and ↓ needle sharing.
- Screening blood donors – seroconversion can take up to 3mo. so still small risk of transmission.
- Prevention of transmission from mother to child – risk can be ↓ to <5% by treatment with zidovudine given to the mother antenatally, during delivery, and to the neonate for 1st 6wk., elective Caesarean section and advising against breast feeding.
- Trials of HIV vaccines are in advanced stages.

Advice for patients:

Information and support for patients with HIV and carers
NAM Aidsmap ☎ 0207 840 0050 🖳 www.aidsmap.com
National AIDS Helpline ☎ 0800 567 123 (24h. helpline)
Terrence Higgins Trust ☎ 0845 1221 200 🖳 www.tht.org.uk

Information for patients with pubic lice, scabies or syphilis
Family Planning Association (FPA) 🖳 www.fpa.org.uk

Further information
Medical Foundation for AIDs and Sexual Health HIV in primary care (2004 and revision 2005) 🖳 www.Medfash.org.uk
Department of Health 🖳 www.dh.gov.uk
- Winning ways: reducing healthcare-associated infection in England (2004)
- National Strategy for Sexual Health and HIV (2001)
British HIV Association HIV treatment guidelines (2006)
🖳 www.bhiva.org
British Association of Sexual Health and HIV (BASHH)
🖳 www.bashh.org
- National guidelines on HIV testing (2006)
- Guideline for the use of post-exposure prophylaxis for HIV following sexual exposure (2006)
- National guidelines on the management of *Phthirus* pubis infestation (2001)
- National guidelines on the management of scabies (2001)
- Management of early syphilis (2002)
- Management of late syphilis (2002)

Trichomonas vaginalis (TV)

Presentation in women

History: 5% are asymptomatic. *Symptoms:*
- Vaginal discharge (25%) – copious, mucopurulent, yellow, smelly discharge – may be frothy
- Vaginal soreness
- Dysuria

Examination: Discharge, vaginal inflammation, typical strawberry cervix.

Investigation: Send endocervical swab for M,C&S. May also be detected on cervical smear.

Presentation in men: Almost always asymptomatic. May have dysuria. Take urethral swab for M,C&S.

Management

- Metronidazole po (400mg bd for 7d.) or pv (5g bd for 5d.); clindamycin is a suitable alternative in the 1st trimester of pregnancy.
- Consider referral to GUM clinic for contact tracing.
- Resistant TV – try a combination of po and pr metronidazole (keep total dose <4g/d. due to risk of neurotoxicity); for women, treat during menstruation when TV load is at its lowest.

Genital warts Caused by human papilloma virus (HPV). Usually sexually transmitted and >25% have concomitant STDs. Disease may be clinical (found on examination) or subclinical (changes associated with infection detected on smear). In women, CIN (🕮 p.106) is related to infection with HPV infection.

History and examination

Women: Often asymptomatic but may be associated with itching or vaginal discharge. Warts are usually seen on vulva or introitus. Warts enlarge during pregnancy.

Men: Warts are usually found on the penis or peri-anally.

Management

Clinical warts: Treatment does not eradicate the virus but removes lesions. Usually carried out in GUM clinics. Podophyllin paint 25% is applied weekly, left on 4h. and washed off – cure rates 50–60%. Paint must be applied by a doctor or nurse, protecting adjacent skin. *Alternative:* surgical treatment, e.g cryotherapy.

Subclinical warts: No treatment. Barrier contraception is needed for at least 3mo. after the warts are gone. Contact tracing is essential.

Further information

British Association of Sexual Health and HIV (BASHH)
🖥 www.bashh.org
- Management of *Trichomonas vaginalis* infection (2001)
- Management of HPV infection (2002)

Prevention of STIs: NICE recommends:

- Identification of high risk patients opportunistically in general practice e.g. at new patient checks, when attending for travel advice
- One-to-one structured discussions with individuals at high risk of STIs lasting 15–20min., and structured on the basis of behaviour change theories. They should address factors that can help ↓ risktaking.

High risk groups include: men who have had sex with other men; people who have come from/visited areas of high HIV prevalence; substance/alcohol misuse; early onset of sexual activity; unprotected sex and frequent change of/multiple partners

Young people from vulnerable groups: (e.g. from disadvantaged backgrounds; in/leaving local authority care; low educational attainment) should be offered one-to-one sessions educating them about sexual health and contraception

HPV vaccination: HPV vaccines are aimed at preventing infection with strains causing cervical cancer. Currently vaccines target strains 16 and 18 which account for ~70% of HPV-related cancer cases ± strains 6 and 11. The first vaccine has now been licensed in the UK and vaccination will be targetted at girls before the age at which they become sexually active (~11y.). Cervical screening will still be necessary as the vaccine does not protect against all strains causing cervical cancer.

Further information

NICE Preventing sexually transmitted infections and reducing under 18 conceptions (2007) 🖳 www.nice.org.uk

131

Advice for patients:

Information about trichomonas and genital warts
Family Planning Association (FPA) 🖳 www.fpa.org.uk

General information about sexual health
Family Planning Association (FPA) 🖳 www.fpa.org.uk
Department of Health Sexual Health Line ☎ 0800 567 123 (24h.); Sexwise (for under 19s) ☎ 0800 28 29 30

GMS contract

Specialized care of patients who need sexual health services may be provided by practices as a *national enhanced service*. Practices providing this service receive an annual payment plus a fee per patient per year.

Sexual problems

Sexual problems may have a physical or psychological basis but *all* develop a psychological aspect in time. Both partners have a problem in ~30% cases. Be supportive – your response will determine whether the patient receives appropriate help.

Assessment: Figure 3.13

Lack of sexual interest: Usually needs specialist help. Often there are underlying psychological difficulties which may relate specifically to sex, e.g. previous child abuse, or a general psychological disorder. Women frequently lose interest around the menopause or after operations (especially mastectomy or hysterectomy) or if their partner's performance repeatedly leads to frustration (e.g. impotence). Both sexes lose interest if depressed or after traumatic events.

Vaginismus: Usually apparent at vaginal examination – severe spasm of the vaginal muscles and adduction of thighs. May be detected incidentally when undertaking routine procedures, e.g. cervical smear Try to find the root cause. *Common causes:*
- Fear of the unknown
- Past history of rape, abuse or severe emotional trauma
- Defence mechanism against growing up

Management: Desensitize simple cases by encouraging the woman to examine herself, and also encourage the partner to be confident enough to insert a finger into the vagina. If no success, refer.

Orgasmic problems in women: *Consider:*

Physical reasons
- Drugs – major tranquillizers, antidepressants
- Neurological disease
- Pelvic surgery – recognized complication of hysterectomy

Psychological reasons
- *Women who have never achieved an orgasm* may have psychological reasons. Give 'permission' for the woman to investigate her body's own responses further by masturbation or vibrator. When she has learnt how to relax, encourage her to tell her partner and incorporate caressing into their usual lovemaking.
- *Women who have lost the ability to achieve orgasm* may need counselling, especially about current relationship or loss of self-image.

Dyspareunia: 📖 p.86

Further information about specialist doctors/therapists
British Association for Sexual and Relationship Therapy
☎ 020 8543 2707 🖥 www.basrt.org.uk
Institute of Psychosexual Medicine 🖥 www.ipm.org.uk

Figure 3.13 Assessment of sexual problems in general practice

History of sexual problem

What is the problem?
If new, when did it start?
Why consult now?
What outcome does the patient want?
Is the patient complaining or is her partner?

Sexual history

Details of sex education
Attitude towards sex
Past history of sexual problems (or lack of problems)

Always consider psychological aspects:

Poor self-image
Anger or resentment – relationship or financial difficulties, children, parents, work stress
Ignorance or misunderstanding
Shame, embarrassment or guilt–view that sexuality is 'bad', sexual abuse
Anxiety/fear about sex – fear of closeness, vulnerability, letting go and failure

Past medical history
• Chronic disease
• Psychiatric problems
• Current medication

Social history and recent life events

133

Examination

Genitalia for abnormalities or tenderness – helpful but don't insist – it may scare the patient away

---

Advice for patients: Further information

Brown P. Faulder C. *Treat yourself to sex*. Penguin (1989) ISBN 0140110186

Infertility

Failure to conceive after 1y. regular unprotected sexual intercourse in the absence of known reproductive pathology. Affects ~1 in 4 couples.

Pregnancy rates: The normal rate of pregnancy in the first year is 20–25% per cycle. 84% of couples in the general population will conceive after 1y. of unprotected intercourse (17 in every 20 couples); 92% will have conceived after 2y. (19 of every 20 couples); after 3y., the pregnancy rate is still ~25%/y.

Causes
- Ovulatory dysfunction – ~30%
- Pelvic disease – ~20%
- Male factor – ~20%
- Unknown – ~30%

Initial approach: Most couples tend to present at about 1y. Where possible, see the couple together. This shows mutual commitment and initiates ongoing, couple-centred management.

Couple: Ask about:
- Length of time trying to conceive
- Frequency of and/or difficulties with sexual intercourse, e.g. psychosexual problems, physical disability – includes excessive travelling which may limit optimal coital timing and indirectly affect fertility.

Women: Ask about:
- Previous pregnancies – children, miscarriages, same/different partner
- Menstrual cycle – length of cycle (normal cycle is 21–35d. duration), changes in cervical mucus through the cycle, ovulatory discomfort
- Past gynaecological history – cervical smears, previous pelvic surgery, sexually transmitted disease/pelvic inflammatory disease, PCOS
- Past medical history – systemic or debilitating disease, e.g. thyroid dysfunction, DM, inflammatory bowel disease, anorexia nervosa
- Drug history – chemotherapy, phenothiazines, cannabis, NSAIDs
- Lifestyle – occupation (exposure to pesticides?), smoking, alcohol, excessive exercise, stress.

Men: Ask about:
- Previous children, same/different partner
- Past history of mumps, other testicular disease, sexually transmitted disease
- Any systemic or debilitating diseases
- Drug history – sulfasalazine, nitrofurantoin, tetracyclines, cimetidine, ketoconazole, colchicines, allopurinol, A-blockers, tricyclic antidepressants, MAOI, phenothiazines, propranolol, chemotherapy, anabolic steroids, cannabis, cocaine
- Social history – occupation (exposure to pesticides, X-rays, solvents, paints, chemicals from smelting or welding), smoking, alcohol, excess exercise, stress, social or occupational factors which might cause testicular hyperthermia.

Box 3.1 Adverse factors

Maternal	Paternal
• Age (fertility falls off significantly from mid-30s onwards)	• BMI >29
	• Smoking
• BMI <19 or >29	• Excess alcohol
• Smoking (lowers fertility by ~$1/3$)	
• Excess caffeine (> equivalent 2 cups coffee/d.)	

GP Notes:

Menstrual history: A menstrual diary can be very helpful to show cycle regularity (cycles of 28d. ± 2d. are strongly suggestive of ovulation) and assist with interpretation of serum progesterone result (📖 p.83).

ℹ️ Ensure you and the patient both understand how to interpret cycle length – count from the first day of a period.

Advice for patients
- Advise regular sex 2–3x/wk.
- Avoid use of ovulation predictor kits and basal body charts.
- Give lifestyle advice – weight, smoking cessation, alcohol consumption.
- Provide written information wherever possible at all stages of investigation and treatment.

Pre-conceptual considerations: Check rubella status of women; advise women to take folic acid supplement (📖 p.200).

Counselling: Never underestimate the psychological effects of infertility and its treatment – consider early referral for specialist counselling. Access through national support groups and at local specialist fertility centres. Useful contacts:
- British Infertility Counselling Association 🖥️ www.bica.net
- British Fertility Society 🖥️ www.britishfertilitysociety.org.uk

Advice for patients: Advice and information for patients

Women's Health 🖥️ www.womens-health.co.uk
National Fertility Association (ISSUE) ☎ 09050 280 300
🖥️ www.issue.co.uk
National Infertility Support Network (CHILD) ☎ 01424 732361
🖥️ www.child.org.uk
Human Fertilisation and Embryology Authority (HFEA)
☎ 020 7377 5077 🖥️ www.hfea.gov.uk

Further information
RCOG Fertility: assessment and treatment of people with fertility problems (2004) 🖥️ www.rcog.org.uk

Examination: Consider pelvic/genital examination.

GP investigations: Perform investigations if no pregnancy after a year of trying to conceive – sooner if aged >35y.

Female
- Rubella status
- Chlamydia serology – indicator of possible tubal disease
- Mid-luteal progesterone – check on day 21 of the menstrual cycle for a woman with a 28d. cycle – adjust timing if longer/shorter cycle. Can only be accurately interpreted after the next period as aims to 'catch' the progesterone peak 7d. before the next period. Normal value (>30nmol/l) signifies ovulation
- FSH/LH – check if cycles are irregular (check on day 1–5 of the menstrual cycle)
- Thyroid function tests – if symptoms/signs of thyroid disease
- Prolactin – if galactorrhoea or any suggestion of pituitary tumour.

Male: Sperm problems affect ~1:5 couples with infertility problems. Sperm quality changes with time, so semen analysis is important even if the male already has children. It also shows equal commitment to fertility treatment. Try to use the same laboratory as the local infertility clinic. Sperm production takes ~70d. and is affected by febrile illness and major physiological/psychological stress. If first test is abnormal, advise loose trousers and underwear and repeat after 3mo. – or as soon as possible if grossly abnormal. ❶ Abnormal sperm do not fertilize ova.

Referral: Local protocols may vary – find out what local policy is. Generally refer after 18mo. of failure to conceive despite regular intercourse. Refer sooner if abnormal history, examination or investigations, e.g.
- *Female*: age >35y.; amenorrhoea/oligomenorrhoea; previous pelvic inflammatory or sexually transmitted disease
- *Male*: previous genital pathology or urogenital surgery; varicocoele; significant systemic illness

Initial investigations in secondary care
- *Female*: tubal patency test – hysterosalpingogram or laparoscopy and dye transit.
- *Male*: review of results from GP and further endocrine and other tests as appropriate.

Possible treatments GPs may need to continue to prescribe
- Clomifene – ovarian stimulation, treatment for some cases of oligospermia
- Tamoxifen – may be prescribed to women intolerant of clomifene
- Metformin – used as an adjunct to clomifene in overweight ladies with polycystic ovarian syndrome who fail to respond to clomifene alone
- Gonadotrophins, dopamine agonists (e.g. bromocriptine).

Complementary therapies: Frequently used – no firm evidence of effectiveness. Low-grade evidence that vitamin/mineral supplements (vitamins C, D, & E, zinc, selenium and folate) improve mild abnormalities in semen analysis.

Test	Normal value
Volume	≥2ml
Viability	≥50% viable
pH	≥7.2
Sperm concentration	≥20×10^6/ml
Morphology	≥30% with normal forms
Motility	≥50% (grades a and b) with forward progression within 60min. of ejaculation
MAR test	<50% of motile sperm with adherent particles

Table 3.10 Normal values of semen variables

Instructions for producing a semen sample for analysis

- No sex for 2d. beforehand and preferably no more than 7d. since last sex (may affect motility).
- Masturbate into labelled sterile pot without use of condoms or jellies.
- Keep the sample warm (e.g inside pocket), and deliver to the laboratory within 2h. Hand directly over to a member of laboratory staff if possible.

Advice for patients: Frequently asked questions about infertility

When is the best time in the menstrual cycle to try? Regular sex 2–3 times weekly throughout the cycle is the best strategy as cycle length and timing of ovulation can vary in women from month to month. Ovulation predictor tests and testing of basal body temperature are not generally recommended as they increase the stress of trying to conceive.

When is my most fertile time? Sperm last up to 5 days and sometimes up to 7 days. Eggs last only 12–24 hours. The most fertile time is therefore any time from 7 days before ovulation to 1 day after ovulation.

What are the chances of me conceiving at my age? Fertility falls off significantly from the mid-30s onwards. 94% of women aged 35y. and 77% aged 38y. will have conceived after 3y. of trying to become pregnant.

How is endometriosis linked with difficulty getting pregnant? Moderate or severe endometriosis can cause pelvic distortion due to scarring, or scarring or deformity of the ovary affecting ovulation. It is not clear how minor endometriosis affects fertility. Treatment may be offered at the time of laparoscopy to enhance fertility, though this only has a short-term effect.

No problem has been found – so why can't I conceive? 30% couples have unexplained infertility. This may be due to very minor endometriosis not detected at laparoscopy or due to other factors relevant to conception but not tested for, such as cervical mucus hostility, failure of fertilization or implantation.

Urinary tract infection (UTI)

UTI is one of the most common conditions seen in general practice, accounting for up to 6% consultations (1 case/average surgery). ♀>>♂. 20% of women at any time have asymptomatic bacteriuria and 20–40% of women will have a UTI in their lifetime. *Infecting organisms: E.coli* (>70%), *Proteus* sp., *Pseudomonas* sp., *Streptococci, Staphylococci.*

Risk factors

- Prior infection
- DM
- Pregnancy
- Stones
- Dehydration
- GU instrumentation
- Catheterization
- Sexual intercourse
- Diaphragm use
- ↓ oestrogen (menopause)
- Urinary stasis (e.g. obstruction)
- Genito-urinary (GU) malformations
- Delayed micturition (e.g. on long journeys).

Presentations

- *Cystitis:* Frequency, dysuria, urgency, strangury, low abdominal pain, incontinence of urine, acute retention of urine, cloudy or offensive urine, and/or haematuria.
- *Pyelonephritis:* Loin pain, fever, rigors, malaise, vomiting, and/or haematuria.

Initial investigation: If uncomplicated UTI in an otherwise healthy woman, test urine with a leucocyte esterase and nitrate dipstick. If +ve, treat for UTI.

Reasons to send MSU for M,C&S:

- Unresolved infection after antibiotics
- Recurrent UTI
- Catheterized woman with symptomatic UTI
- Pregnant woman – 📖 p.259
- Suspected pyelonephritis
- Haematuria – microscopic or macroscopic – always investigate further.

🛈 MSUs should be taken prior to starting antibiotics and sent to the laboratory fresh.

Further investigation: Consider further investigation with blood tests (U&E, Cr, eGFR) and/or radiology (renal tract USS, KUB, IVP) if:
- recurrent UTI in a woman
- pyelonephritis
- unusual infecting organism
- unclear diagnosis, e.g. persisting symptoms but negative MSU.

Management

Pregnant women: 📖 p.259

Catheterized patients: 90% develop bacteriuria <4wk. after insertion of a catheter. Always confirm suspected UTI with MSU – only treat if symptomatic or *Proteus* species grown. Infections can be difficult to eliminate. There is no good evidence bladder instillations help.

Haematuria: May be frank (visible) or microscopic.

Causes
- *Gynaecological* – menstruation, post-menopausal bleeding, bleeding in pregnancy, cervical bleeding, atrophic vaginitis
- *Kidney* – infection, stones, tumour, glomerulonephritis
- *Ureter* – stones, tumour (rare)
- *Bladder* – UTI, stones, tumour, chronic inflammation
- *Urethra* – inflammation

Refer urgently to urology (to be seen in <2wk.)[N]
- Patients of any age with painless macroscopic haematuria
- Patients aged ≥40y. who present with recurrent or persistent UTI associated with haematuria
- Patients aged ≥50y. who are found to have unexplained microscopic haematuria

For patients with symptoms suggestive of UTI who also have macroscopic haematuria, diagnose and treat the infection before considering referral. If infection is not confirmed, refer urgently to urology.

🛈 Rapid access one-stop clinics are now operated in most areas.

Refer non-urgently[N]: Patients <50y. with microscopic haematuria.
- If proteinuria or ↑ serum creatinine or ↓ eGFR – refer to a renal physician.
- If no proteinuria and serum creatinine and eGFR are normal – refer to urology.

Sterile pyuria: Presence of white cells (>10/mm³) in the urine in the absence of UTI.

Causes
- Inadequately treated UTI
- Appendicitis
- Calculi
- Prostatitis
- Bladder tumour
- Renal TB
- Papillary necrosis
- UTI with failure to culture organism
- Interstitial nephritis or cystitis
- Polycystic kidney
- Chemical cystitis, e.g. due to radiotherapy

Management: Initially repeat with clean-catch MSU. If finding persists, refer to urology.

Further information
NICE Referral guidelines for suspected cancer (2005)
🖳 www.nice.org.uk

All other patients
- ↑ *fluid intake* (>3l/24h.).
- *Alkalinize urine* (e.g. potassium citrate solution) to ease symptoms.
- *Oral antibiotics:* Trimethoprim 200mg bd is a good first choice – 80% organisms are sensitive. Use a 3d. course for women with uncomplicated UTI. Use a 2wk. course for patients with GU malformations or immunosuppression, relapse (same organism) or recurrent UTI (different organism). Use a 14d. course of a quinolone (e.g. ciprofloxacin 250–500mg bd) for patents with pyelonephritis.
- *Admission to hospital:* Rarely required if dehydrated or extremely systemically unwell.
- *Referral to urology:* If any abnormalities are detected on further investigation or unable to resolve symptoms.

Prevention of recurrent cystitis: Reinfection after successful treatment of infection (90%) or relapse after inadequate treatment.
- *General advice:* Advise patients to urinate frequently; ↑ fluid intake; double void (i.e. go again after 5–10 min.) and void after intercourse. Efficacy of cranberry juice is controversial.
- *Prophylactic antibiotics:* Consider prescribing either postcoitally (e.g. nitrofurantoin 50mg stat) or continuously (trimethoprim 100mg nocte or nitrofurantoin 50mg nocte).
- *HRT:* Topical oestrogen ↓ recurrent UTI in post-menopausal women[R].
- *Vaccines:* Results of large-scale trials are awaited.

Urethral syndrome: Symptoms of cystitis with –ve MSU. Unknown cause. Associated with cold, stress, nylon underwear, COC pill and intercourse. Advise patients to drink plenty of fluids and wear cotton underwear. Consider changing/stopping COC pill, or trying topical oestrogen if post-menopausal. Tetracyclines (e.g. doxycycline 100mg bd for 14d.) or azithromycin (500mg od for 6d.)[R] are helpful in some patients. If not settling, refer to urology. Urethral dilation/massage may be helpful.

Interstitial cystitis: Predominantly affects middle-aged women. Can cause fibrosis of the bladder wall. Main symptoms – frequency, urgency and suprapubic pain especially when the bladder is full. Often misdiagnosed as recurrent UTI. MSU – no bacteriuria. Refer to urologist for confirmation. There is no satisfactory treatment though antispasmodics, amitriptyline and bladder stretching under anaesthetic may help some patients.

Advice for patients: Frequently asked questions about cystitis

What is cystitis? Cystitis means inflammation of the bladder. It is usually caused by a urine infection. Typical symptoms are pain when you pass urine, and passing urine frequently. You may also have pain in your lower abdomen, blood in your urine, and fever (high temperature).

What causes cystitis? Most urine infections are due to bacteria (germs) that come from your own bowel. About half of women have at least one bout of cystitis in their life. For many it is a 'one-off'. It is a recurring problem for some women.

How do I know it is cystitis? Some conditions cause symptoms that may be mistaken for cystitis. For example, thrush. Also, soaps, deodorants, bubble baths, etc., may irritate your genital area and cause mild pain when you pass urine. Your doctor or nurse may do a simple 'dipstick' test on a urine sample to check for cystitis. This detects bacteria in urine. It is fairly reliable and usually no further test is needed. Sometimes a urine sample is sent to the 'lab' to find out which bacterium is causing the infection.

What is the treatment for cystitis? Usually antibiotics are prescribed for cystitis. A 3-day course is a common treatment. Symptoms usually improve within a day or so. See a doctor if symptoms are not gone, or nearly gone, after 3 days. Some bacteria are resistant to some antibiotics. If symptoms persist it is usual to send a urine sample to the laboratory. This finds which bacterium is causing the infection and which antibiotics will kill it. A change of antibiotic is needed in some cases to clear the infection.

What can I do to help myself? It is a good idea to drink plenty and avoid becoming dehydrated.

Potassium citrate or sodium citrate changes the acidity of the urine. It may help to ease the symptom of 'burning urine' but does not cure the infection. You can buy it at pharmacies without a prescription and it is available in solutions or flavoured sachets.

Paracetamol or ibuprofen ease pain or discomfort, and lower a high temperature.

Not taking any treatment is an option if you are not pregnant. Your immune system can often clear the infection. In about half of cases, the symptoms and infection go within 3 days without treatment. However, if you are pregnant, you should be treated with antibiotics to prevent possible complications.

See a doctor if you have recurring bouts of cystitis to discuss ways of preventing them.

Reproduced in modified format with permission from ▣ www.patient.co.uk

Urinary incontinence

Involuntary loss of urine which is objectively demonstrable and a social or hygienic problem. 14% women aged 30–70y. admit incontinence but this is probably an underestimate – roughly 1:3 with incontinence consult at outset, 1:3 consult later, 1:3 suffer in silence. Opportunistic questioning can identify sufferers.

Assessment

History

- Frequency of complaint
- Whether occurs with standing/coughing/sneezing
- Urgency/dysuria/frequency of micturition
- Volume passed
- Degree of incapacity
- Past obstetric/medical history
- Medication
- Mobility/accessibility of toilets.

Examination

- *Abdominal including rectal examination* – enlarged bladder, masses, loaded colon, faecal impaction, anal tone
- *Pelvic* – prolapse, atrophy, neurological deficit, retention of urine and pelvic masses

Investigation:

- *Intake/output diary* – evaluates problem and benchmark for progress – record drinks and passage of urine over a week
- *Urine* – glucose, RBCs, MC&S
- *Blood* – consider U&E, Cr, eGFR and/or FBG to exclude renal impairment or DM
- Specialist investigations include measurement of urinary flow rate, cystometry, IVP, USS, cystourethroscopy, and ambulatory monitoring

Drugs that exacerbate/cause incontinence: Diuretics, antihistamines, anxiolytics, α–blockers, sedatives and hypnotics, anticholinergic drugs, tricyclic antidepressants.

GP management: ❶ 30% have a mixed pattern.

General measures

- Manipulate fluid intake – amount, type (avoid tea, coffee, alcohol), timing
- Alter medication, e.g. timing of diuretics
- Treat UTI and chronic respiratory conditions which cause cough
- Avoid constipation
- Promote weight ↓
- Consider HRT (topical or systemic) for oestrogen deficiency

Stress incontinence

- *Symptoms* – small losses of urine without warning throughout the day related to coughing/exercise
- *Causes* – congenital; childbirth; deterioration of pelvic floor muscles/nerves
- *Treatment* – pelvic floor exercises (📖 p.145) continued >3mo. help 60% (can be taught by physiotherapists/continence advisors) – may be assisted by vaginal cones and/or electrical stimulation. Mechanical devices (e.g. Conveen continence guard®) help 75%

Table 3.11 Referral for incontinence problems

Specialist continence advisor (or district nurse)	Urodynamic studies	Gynaecology/urology opinion
Advice on aids and appliances Advice on primary care management Patient support	If type of incontinence is uncertain Atypical features of incontinence After unsuccessful surgery If a neurological problem is suspected	GP management has failed Severe symptoms Concomitant gynaecological problems (e.g. prolapse) Concomitant urological problems (e.g. chronic retention) Failed incontinence surgery Vesico-vaginal fistula Haematuria

GP Notes:

Incontinence aids and appliances

Pads: There are many different types. DNs or continence advisors are best aware of those available via the NHS locally. They are not prescribable on FP10 and are supplied by local NHS trusts on a 'daily allowance' basis. This varies across the country.

Bed covers: Absorb 1–4l of urine. Good laundry facilities are needed. If left wet can cause skin breakdown. Available via NHS trusts.

Catheters: Can be prescribed on NHS prescription. Approved appliances are listed in part IXA of the UK Drug Tariff.

Indwelling catheters: Only long-term Foley catheters are suitable for use in primary care. They last 3–12wk. Supply collecting bags to attach to the catheter. Only use catheters in patients with:
- urinary retention or neurogenic bladder dysfunction
- severe pressure sores
- inoperable obstructions that prevent the bladder emptying
- terminal illness
- inadequate carer support who are housebound.

Intermittent self-catheterization: Patient inserts a catheter into her bladder 4–5x/d. to drain urine. ↓ problems of infection and blockage. Useful for neurological bladder dysfunction. *Types:*
- *Reusable silver or stainless steel*
- *Reusable PVC* – wash and reuse for 1 wk. Usually supply 5/mo.
- *Single use* – need 125–150/mo. Expensive. Only use on consultant advice.

Further information

Prescription Pricing Authority Electronic drug tariff
🖳 www.ppa.org.uk

Urge incontinence: Detrusor instability or hyperreflexia cause the bladder to contract unintentionally.

- *Symptoms:* Frequency, overwhelming desire to void (often precipitated by stressful event), large loss, nocturia.
- *Causes:* Idiopathic, neurological problems (stroke, multiple sclerosis, DM, spinal cord injury, dementia, Parkinson's disease), local irritation (bladder stones, infection), surgery.
- *Treatment:* Try bladder training programmes – resist the urge to pass urine for increasing periods. Start with an achievable interval based on diary evidence and ↑ slowly. Drugs are helpful, e.g. oxybutynin 2. 5–5mg bd/tds, tolterodine 1–2mg bd, imipramine 50–75mg nocte (nocturnal symptoms). Spontaneously remits/relapses so reassess every 3–4mo.

Overflow: Uncommon amongst women.

- *Symptoms:* Constant dribbling loss day and night.
- *Causes:* Urethral stricture, faecal impaction, neurological (lower motor neurone lesions), side-effect of medication.
- *Treatment:* Treat the underlying cause if possible. Otherwise refer for specialist advice.

Urinary fistula: Communication between the bladder and the outside – normally through the vagina. Results in constant dribbling loss day and night. Refer to gynaecology/urology. *Causes:* Congenital, malignancy, complication of surgery.

Functional incontinence: No urological problem. Caused by other factors, e.g. inaccessible toilets/immobility, behavioural problems, cognitive deficit. Treat the cause.

Further information

Association for Continence Advice Advice for healthcare professionals ☎ 020 8692 4680 ▢ www.aca.uk.com

---

Advice for patients: Information and support for incontinence

Continence Foundation ☎ 0845 345 0165
▢ www.continence-foundation.org.uk

Advice for patients: Pelvic floor exercises

The pelvic floor is a large sling (or hammock) of muscles stretching from side to side across the floor of the pelvis. It is attached to your pubic bone in front, and to the coccyx (the tail end of the spine) behind. It forms your 'undercarriage'. The openings from your bladder (urethra), your bowels (rectum) and your womb (vagina) all pass through your pelvic floor.

What does the pelvic floor do?

- It supports your pelvic organs and abdominal contents, especially when you are standing or exerting yourself.
- It supports the bladder to help it stay closed. When the muscles are not working effectively you may suffer from leaking ('urinary incontinence') and/or urgent or frequent need to pass urine.
- It is used to control wind and when 'holding on' with your bowels.
- It has an important sexual function, helping to increase sexual awareness both for yourself and your partner.

How do I do pelvic floor exercises?

Exercise 1: Tighten the muscles around your back passage, vagina and front passage and lift up inside as if trying to stop passing wind and urine at the same time. It is very easy to bring other, irrelevant muscles into play, so try to isolate your pelvic floor as much as possible by:

- not pulling in your tummy
- not squeezing your legs together or tightening your buttocks and
- not holding your breath.

In this way most of the effort should be coming from the pelvic floor. Try holding the pelvic floor tight as long and as hard as you can. Build up to a maximum of 10 seconds. Rest for 4 seconds and then repeat the contraction as many times as you can up to a maximum of 10 times.

Exercise 2: It is important to be able to work these muscles quickly to help them react to sudden stresses from coughing, laughing or exercise that put pressure on the bladder. So you need to practise some quick contractions, drawing in the pelvic floor and holding for just 1 second before releasing the muscles. Do these in a steady manner. Aim for a strong muscle tightening with each contraction up to a maximum of 10 times.

How often should I do pelvic floor exercises?

Aim to do one set of slow contractions (exercise 1) followed by one set of quick contractions (exercise 2) 6 times each day. Get into the habit of doing the exercises by linking them to everyday activities – for example, do them after emptying your bladder or whenever you turn on a tap – or keep a simple exercise diary to help you remember. Practise the exercises when you are lying, sitting and especially standing.

Pelvic floor exercises should give optimum results with regular exercise within 3 to 6 months, but you should continue them for life. Ask your GP or the practice nurse for advice if you see little or no change in your symptoms after trying these exercises on your own for 3 months.

The pelvic floor exercises above are reproduced with permission from the Continence Foundation ☑ www.cancerscreening.nhs.uk/cervical/faqs.html

The menopause

From the Greek *'men'* (month) and *'pausis'* (halt). Menopause occurs when menstruation stops. Average age in the UK ≈ 50y. Smoking brings it forwards by ~2y. Impact on a woman's life varies and depends on cultural, health and social factors.

Diagnosis: >12mo. amenorrhoea with no other cause in ♀ >50y. *or* >24mo. amenorrhoea in ♀ <50y. The *climacteric* refers to the time as the ovaries fail, when production of oestrogen ↓ over a number of years.

What are the symptoms of the menopause?

Periods

- *Changes in menstrual pattern* – Common in the years before the menopause – typically cycle shortens after 40y. by up to 7–10d. Cycle then lengthens – periods may occur at 2–3mo. intervals until stopping.
- *Dysfunctional uterine bleeding* – Common leading up to the menopause but investigate post-menopausal, very heavy, painful, irregular, intermenstrual or postcoital bleeding.
- *Late menstruation (>54y.)* – Requires investigation due to ↑ risk of malignancy.

Flushes and sweats: 80% have flushes – 20% seek help. Often associated with palpitations.

Management:

Lifestyle changes: Exercise (↓ flushes by ~50%), deep breathing exercises, cool ambient temperature, wearing natural fibres, e.g. cotton, stress ↓, avoiding trigger foods/drinks (e.g. spicy foods, caffeine, alcohol).

Drug treatments

- HRT – Flushes are controlled successfully with oestrogen in the form of HRT (📖 p.150) in most women.
- SSRIs/SNRIs (e.g. fluoxetine 20mg od – unlicensed) ↓ flushes in >50%
- Norethisterone (5mg od) and megestrol acetate (40mg od) ↓ flushes in >80%. Megestrol acetate may cause vaginal bleeding on withdrawal.
- Clonidine – no more effective than placebo.

Complementary therapies

- Natural progesterone derived from yams has attracted interest – trials of effectiveness are awaited.
- Black cohosh seems to ease hot flushes in some women – long-term effects are unknown.
- Red clover may be of benefit – effectiveness studies have mixed results. Unsuitable for women taking warfarin.
- Foods containing phyto-oestrogens (e.g. soy foods) may be of benefit. Unlikely to be harmful.
- Dong quai, evening primrose oil, vitamin E and ginseng are no better than placebo.
- Avoid kava as it has been linked to cases of serious liver damage.

Psychological symptoms: Controversial. Some studies report depression and anxiety are more common, others find no association. Depression is multifactorial – consider social, physical and cultural factors before resorting to HRT as a solution.

Advice for patients:

Frequently asked questions about the menopause

What is the menopause? The menopause occurs when your periods stop. It is also called the 'change of life'. It happens because, as you get older, your ovaries make less oestrogen (the main female hormone). The average age of the menopause in the UK is 51.

Will I have problems when I go through the menopause? The menopause is a natural event. You may have no problems at all but it is more common to develop some symptoms due to the low level of oestrogen.

What are hot flushes and sweats? Hot flushes affect 3 in every 4 women. A typical hot flush lasts a few minutes and causes flushing of your face, neck, and chest. You may also perspire (sweat) during a hot flush. Some women become giddy, weak, faint, or feel sick during a hot flush. The number of hot flushes can vary from every now and then to many times a day. Hot flushes tend to start just before the menopause, and typically persist for 2–3 years.

Sweats commonly occur when you are in bed at night. In some cases they are so severe that sleep is disturbed and you need to change your bedding and night clothes.

Taking plenty of exercise, keeping cool, wearing loose clothes, and avoiding things that trigger the flushes such as alcohol, stress, spicy foods or caffeine may help. Eating foods containing plant oestrogens can also help. These foods include: certain fruits/vegetables (apples, plums, cherries, rhubarb, carrots, potatoes, peas, and all types of beans including lentils and soya); herbs/spices (cinnamon, parsley, sage, aniseed, fennel seeds); cereals (oats, rye, barley, rice); yeast and beer.

Will my appearance change? Skin and hair changes are common. The skin becomes drier, thinner, and more likely to itch. You may have less underarm and pubic hair and/or more facial hair. Dryness of vaginal tissues can cause soreness and make sex painful – you can buy lubricating jelly from the chemist. If this does not help, talk to your doctor.

Will I develop osteoporosis? Osteoporosis (brittle or thin bones) may, but does not always, develop after the menopause. If you have osteoporosis you may break a hip or wrist quite easily after a fall or minor injury. Protect your bones by doing plenty of weight-bearing exercise and making sure your diet contains plenty of calcium (milk, cheese, white bread and fortified soya milk are good sources) and vitamin D. Vitamin D and calcium supplements can be bought from the chemist.

Are there any other symptoms I might get? Other symptoms such as headaches, tiredness, palpitations, being irritable, difficulty sleeping, depression, anxiety, aches and pains, loss of libido (sex drive), and feelings of not coping as well as before are common.

Further information and support for patients
British Menopause Society 🖳 www.the-bms.org
The Menopause Amarant Trust ☎01293 413000
🖳 www.amarantmenopausetrust.org.uk

Sexual dysfunction: Vaginal dryness and atrophy are common. Manage with systemic or topical oestrogen. Loss of libido post-menopause (especially after surgical removal of the ovaries) responds to administration of androgens, e.g. testosterone implants, in combination with HRT until libido is re-established.

Urinary problems: Common — incontinence, nocturia and urgency. Stress incontinence does not respond to HRT but topical oestrogen may improve outcome of surgery. Recurrent UTIs in older women ↓ with use of topical vaginal oestrogen.

Ischaemic heart disease: Risk is ↑ ×2 after the menopause but there is no evidence to support use of HRT for 1° or 2° prevention of IHD.

Osteoporosis: Consider HRT to prevent osteoporosis in premature menopause (📖 p.154). In older women, HRT is now *not* recommended as first-line treatment of osteoporosis unless there are other reasons for prescribing the HRT.

Could the symptoms be due to another cause? *Exclude:*
- Physical illness, e.g. thyroid disease, anaemia, DM, chronic renal disease
- Side-effects of medication, e.g. Ca^{2+} antagonists cause flushing
- Social problems or psychiatric illness — depression screening questionnaires can be helpful.

Is the diagnosis in doubt? *Check FSH/LH:*
- Following hysterectomy with conservation of ovaries
- If amenorrhoea age <45y. *or*
- If having regular bleeds due to cyclical HRT/COC pill. Check at the beginning of a packet (oestrogen phase) or end of the pill-free week respectively. The COC/HRT can ↓ FSH/LH. To make a more accurate assessment, stop the preparation and check FSH levels 6 and 12 wk. after stopping. A FSH >30IU/l and amenorrhoea suggests the woman is post-menopausal.

⚠ It is unnecessary to check FSH/LH in other groups. FSH/LH levels may be normal in the peri-menopause.

Premature menopause: Menopause in a woman <40y. old. Associated with ↑ all-cause mortality and ↑ risk of osteoporosis and cardiovascular disease. *Causes:*
- Idiopathic
- Radiotherapy and/or chemotherapy
- Surgery — bilateral oophorectomy → instant menopause; hysterectomy without oophorectomy can also induce premature ovarian failure
- Infection — TB and mumps
- Chromosome abnormalities — particularly the X chromosome
- Autoimmune endocrine disease, e.g. DM, hypothyroidism, Addison's
- FSH receptor abnormalities
- Disruption of oestrogen synthesis.

Management: Usually HRT is recommended until the average age of menopause, i.e. 50y.

HRT: 📖 p.150

Fertility ↓ with age. A woman is post-menopausal and therefore not fertile 2y. after her last menstrual period if she is <50y. and 1y. after her last menstrual period if she is >50y. Contraception can be discontinued >55y.

ⓘ There is no definitive measure of loss of fertility. An FSH level >35 iu/l is suggestive of post-menopause. The confidence with which it can be interpreted ↑ with age, length of time the woman has experienced menopausal symptoms and duration of amenorrhoea.

Methods of contraception

Combined oral contraceptive (COC): Non-smokers without risk factors for ischaemic heart disease or breast cancer can use the COC until 50y. Consider switching to lower dose pills (20mcg oestrogen) and pills with lipid-friendly progestogen (e.g. gestodene or desogestrel). The COC pill can help menopausal symptoms and has a positive effect on menstrual symptoms and bone density. ↑ FSH at the end of the pill-free week is suggestive of menopause.

Progestogen-only pill (POP): Can be continued to 55y. Can be used as the progestogen component of HRT – but 3 POPs a day are needed for endometrial protection (unlicensed use and no data for Cerazette®). Does not interfere with FSH levels.

Injectable progestogen: Can be used up to 50y. in women without risk of osteoporosis (though the CSM advises benefits of using injectable medroxyprogesterone acetate for >2y. should be evaluated against risks of ↓ bone density). Helps menstrual disturbance. Masks the menopause.

Progestogen implant: Cannot be used as part of HRT regime. Masks the menopause.

Mirena: Helps menorrhagia and licensed for endometrial protection so can be used as part of an HRT regime. Masks the menopause.

IUCD: Does not mask the menopause. Copper intrauterine devices fitted in women >40y. may remain in the uterus until post-menopause.

149

Advice for patients: Advice and support for women with premature menopause

Daisy Network 🖳 www.daisynetwork.org.uk

Further information

RCP (Edinburgh) Consensus conference on hormone replacement therapy: final consensus statement (October 2003)
🖳 www.rcpe.ac.uk/education/standards/consensus/hrt_03.php

Hormone replacement therapy (HRT)

The concept of the menopause as a deficiency state needing replacement therapy with HRT emerged over recent years but recent research has highlighted ↑ breast cancer risks of HRT and suggested there is no rationale for using HRT to prevent cardiovascular disease. Thus long-term use of HRT is not indicated for healthy women without symptoms.

Short-term use of HRT is still recommended for the relief of menopausal symptoms. Carefully balance risks against benefits for each individual *.

Contraindications

- Cancer of the breast or endometrium
- Thromboembolic disease (including AF)
- Liver disease where liver function tests have failed to return to normal. In women with past history of liver disease, gallstones or taking liver enzyme-inducing drugs, consider transdermal therapy.

Particular indications

- Early menopause – consider alternatives if prescribing for osteoporosis prevention alone – continue until age 50y.
- Hysterectomy before menopause even if ovaries are conserved – ≈1:4 have early menopause
- Relief of symptoms related to oestrogen deficiency peri- and post-menopausally, e.g. flushes/sweats
- 2nd line treatment of osteoporosis – 📖 p.158.

Choice of preparation: *BNF 6.4.1.1.* Start with low dose and provide a 3mo. supply initially.

- For women without a uterus – give oestrogen alone unless past history of endometriosis. Endometrial foci may remain despite hysterectomy so consider addition of a progestogen.
- For women with an intact uterus – progestogen is required for the last 12–14d. of the cycle to prevent endometrial proliferation. Alternatively a preparation which provides continuous administration of an oestrogen and progestogen can be used.
- Tablets, patches, gels and implants are available.
- Continuous combined preparations or tibolone are not suitable for use in the peri-menopause or <12mo. after the last menstrual period.

Tibolone (Livial ®): Oestrogenic, progestogenic and weak androgenic action. Use in the same way as continuous combined HRT. Induce withdrawal bleed with progestogen if transferring from another form of HRT.

Topical vaginal preparations: Pessaries, vaginal tablets, creams and rings. Deliver oestrogen locally to vaginal tissues to alleviate vaginal dryness and atrophic vaginitis. No progestogen is needed though use is limited to 3–6mo. if the uterus is present. Consider prescribing a progestogen if given for longer periods or higher doses are used. Investigate any abnormal bleeding.

* See: Consensus conference on hormone replacement therapy: final consensus statement (October 2003) 🖥 www.rcpe.ac.uk/esd/consensus/hrt_03.html

History
- Has the woman had a hysterectomy?
- If not, ask about bleeding pattern. Investigate any abnormal bleeding prior to starting HRT.
- Ask about FH of breast cancer.
- Explore risk factors for osteoporosis, DVT and CHD.
- Drug history – ask about previous experience of HRT. Women taking thyroxine who start HRT may need to ↑ their dose of levothyroxine – check TFTs. Steroids may also be less effective. Anti-epileptics ↑ elimination of oestrogen.
- Ask the woman why she wants to start HRT and about her expectations of treatment.

Examination: Check:
- BP
- Weight
- Breasts – check no lumps, demonstrate breast self-examination techniques
- Check smear is up to date
- Consider examination for prolapse/vaginal abnormalities if symptoms

Explain the pros and cons of HRT: Support with written information; allow women time to consider their options.

Contraceptive requirement: HRT does not provide contraception. For women of <50y. the COC pill may provide contraception and alleviate menopausal symptoms (📖 p.168).

Health promotion: Support with general health education about smoking cessation, diet, exercise, alcohol consumption, the breast cancer screening programme etc.

151

Table 3.12 Risks and benefits of HRT

🛈 HRT does not prevent coronary heart disease or protect against ↓ in cognitive function and should not be prescribed for these purposes.

Risks	Short-term benefits	Long-term benefits
↑ Breast cancer (RR 1.43[Ψ]) ↑ DVT (RR 1.45[*]) ↑ Stroke (RR 1.15[*]) ↑ Gallbladder disease ↑ Ovarian cancer if using oestrogen-only HRT for >5y. No ↓ risk of CHD – may ↑ risk in the first year of use	Alleviation of menopausal symptoms, eg flushes/sweats/vaginal dryness ↓ recurrent UTIs	↓ Osteoporosis ↓ Colorectal cancer

[Ψ] Relative risk in women aged 50–64y. using combined HRT for 5y.
[*] Relative risk in women aged 60–69y. taking combined HRT for 5y.

Review side-effects after 3mo.: Check BP and weight. ↑ dose if symptoms are not controlled.

Common side-effects
- *Oestrogen related* – fluid retention, breast enlargement and tenderness, nausea, headaches
- *Progestogen related* – headache, ↑ weight , bloating and depression (↓ by changing to a preparation with a less androgenic progestogen, e.g. dydrogesterone or medroxyprogesterone).

Bleeding
- *Cyclical HRT* – may be erratic for the 1st 2–3mo. but should occur after the progestogen supplement in subsequent months.
- *Continuous combined preparations* – may cause spotting for up to 12mo. If bleeding continues >12mo., investigate to exclude endometrial abnormality and consider changing to a cyclical preparation.

Further follow-up: Annually or as needed if any problems. Check BP, weight, breasts, symptoms and bleeding pattern.

Stopping HRT: Review HRT use every 6–12mo. and reassess risks and benefits. HRT is usually needed for <5y. for vasomotor symptom control. When stopping, withdrawal flushes may be severe and distressing – stop in cold weather and half the dose for 1mo. first.

Reasons to stop immediately: HRT should be stopped, pending investigation and treatment, if any of the following occur:
- Sudden severe chest pain – even if not radiating to left arm
- Sudden breathlessness or cough with bloodstained sputum
- Unexplained severe pain in calf of one leg
- Severe stomach pain
- Serious neurological effects, e.g. severe headache, motor or sensory deficit, first epileptic seizure
- Hepatitis, jaundice, liver enlargement
- BP >160mmHg systolic and/or >100mmHg diastolic
- Detection of a risk factor, e.g. DVT, stroke
- Prolonged immobility after surgery or leg injury.

🛈 Major surgery is a predisposing factor for DVT – stop HRT 4–6wk. prior to surgery if possible. Restart after full mobilization.

Further information

RCP (Edinburgh) Consensus conference on hormone replacement therapy: final consensus statement (2003)
🖥 www.rcpe.ac.uk/education/standards/consensus/hrt_03.php
Clayton, Monga & Baker. *Gynaecology by ten teachers.* Hodder Arnold (2006) ISBN: 0340816627

Advice for patients: Further information and support for women

British Menopause Society 🖥 www.the-bms.org
Menopause Amarant Trust ☎ 01293 413000
🖥 www.amarantmenopausetrust.org.uk

Advice for patients: Frequently asked questions about HRT

What is hormone replacement therapy (HRT)? HRT replaces the oestrogen that your ovaries no longer make after the menopause. It is available as tablets, skin-patches, gels, nasal spray, or implants which are put under the skin. For women who have not had a hysterectomy, the oestrogen is given with another hormone, progesterone. If you don't take a progesterone with oestrogen and have not had a hysterectomy, there is an increase in the risk of cancer of the womb.

If you only have symptoms in the vaginal area, another option is to use a vaginal cream, pessary, or vaginal ring which contains oestrogen.

How do I take HRT? The way you take HRT depends on the preparation you are prescribed. HRT is available as tablets, gels, nasal sprays, patches, or implants. Talk to your doctor or practice nurse about which preparation is right for you.

What are the benefits of HRT? HRT tends to stop hot flushes and night sweats within a few weeks. It will also reverse vaginal dryness or soreness within the first 3 months of treatment (though occasionally takes longer). Its effects on other menopausal symptoms such as tiredness or irritability are less clear. With long-term use over a period of years, HRT protects against osteoporosis (thin bones) and bowel cancer.

What are the risks of HRT? Women taking HRT have an increased risk of deep vein thrombosis (or a clot in the deep veins of the leg), stroke and breast cancer. The increased risk of breast cancer only occurs in women over 50 taking HRT. It is small for the first 1–2 years of using HRT, and then gradually increases the longer you use it. If you use HRT and then stop taking it, your risk of developing breast cancer falls back to the normal risk within a few years of stopping treatment.

See a doctor urgently if you develop a red, swollen or painful leg, have sharp pains in your chest, or have any numbness or weakness of your arms, legs or face or problems with your speech or swallowing. You can greatly reduce your risk of developing heart disease and stroke by not smoking, taking regular exercise, and eating a healthy diet.

What are the side-effects of taking HRT? Side-effects with HRT are uncommon. Always read the leaflet that comes with the packet which gives a full list of possible side-effects. Side-effects include nausea (feeling sick), breast discomfort and leg cramps – all these tend to wear off in the first few months. Other side-effects include skin irritation with skin patches, dry eyes, and headaches or migraine. If side-effects are a problem, discuss changing the type or brand of your HRT with your doctor.

How long should I take HRT for? As a general rule, women taking HRT to ease menopausal symptoms need treatment for 1–3 years. If you are under 50 or are taking HRT as a treatment for osteoporosis, you may need to take HRT longer – discuss the risks and benefits with your doctor.

Osteoporosis

Lifetime risk of osteoporotic fracture is 40% in women and 13% in men. The main morbidity and financial costs of osteoporotic fracture relate to hip fracture where incidence ↑ steeply >70y. Treatment aims to prevent fracture.

Definition: Osteoporosis is defined as bone mineral density >2.5 standard deviations (SD) below the young adult mean (T score of –2.5). There is ↑ relative risk of fracture x2–3 for each SD ↓ in BMD.

🚺 Osteopoenia cannot be reliably diagnosed on X–ray, though vertebral fractures may be seen.

Bone mineral density (BMD) measurement: Hip and lumbar spine BMD measurement by dual energy X-ray absorptionometry (DEXA) scan can quantify risk of osteoporotic fracture (Figure 3.14).

Check BMD if
- <75y. and previous fragility fracture
- On long-term steroids and <65y.
- If other risk factors for osteoporosis (see below)
- Suggested osteopoenia on X-ray.

Follow local referral guidelines until national guidance is available (NICE will publish guidance on primary prevention of osteoporosis in 2007).

The report from the DEXA scan should contain information on fracture risk, management and time interval for rechecking BMD. Generally treatment with a bisphosphonate is started if the T score is ≤–2.5.

Age as a risk factor for osteoporosis: Risk of osteoporosis and associated fractures ↑ with age as bone mass declines (Figure 3.15).

Major age-independent risk factors for osteoporosis
- Glucocorticoid use (📖 p.156)
- Previous fragility fracture (📖 p.156)
- Low BMI (<19kg/m^2)
- FH of maternal hip fracture aged <75y.
- Untreated premature menopause, prolonged amenorrhoea
- Conditions associated with prolonged immobility
- Medical disorder independently associated with bone loss, e.g. inflammatory bowel or coeliac disease, chronic liver disease, hyperthyroidism, ankylosing spondylitis, chronic renal failure, type 1 DM, rheumatoid arthritis

---

Advice for patients: Information and support

Arthritis Research Campaign ☎ 0870 850 5000 🖥 www.arc.org.uk
National Osteoporosis Society ☎ 0845 450 0230 🖥 www.nos.org.uk

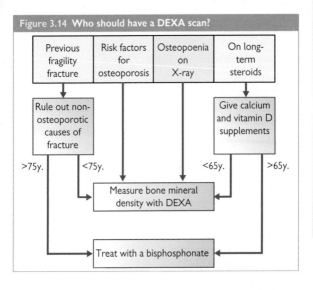

Figure 3.14 Who should have a DEXA scan?

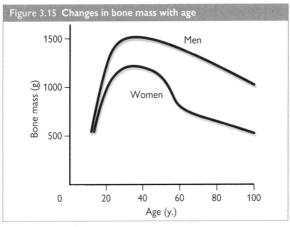

Figure 3.15 Changes in bone mass with age

Glucocorticoid use: Steroid use is a risk factor for osteoporosis.
- Minimize steroid dose.
- Advise *all* patients taking any dose of oral steroids to take calcium/vitamin D supplements[G].

In addition: For patients taking oral/high-dose inhaled steroids for >3mo.:
- Add a bisphosphonate for patients >65y. *or*
- Refer patients <65y. for DEXA scan and add a bisphosphonate if T score is ≤−1.5.

Previous fragility fracture: Fracture sustained falling from ≤ standing height – includes vertebral collapse (may not be a fall). Previous fracture is a risk for future fracture. Common fractures:
- *Hip* – associated with ↑ mortality
- *Wrist* – Colles'
- *Spine* – osteoporotic vertebral collapse causes pain, ↓ height and kyphosis. Pain can take 3–6mo. to settle and requires strong analgesia. Calcitonin is useful for pain relief for 3mo. after vertebral fracture if other analgesics are ineffective.

Investigation
- DEXA scan if <75y.
- Exclude other causes of pathological fracture, e.g. malignancy, osteomalacia, hyperparathyroidism. Check FBC, ESR, TSH, Cr, bone and liver function tests – all should be normal.
- Consider checking serum paraproteins/urine, Bence-Jones protein, bone scan and FSH/LH (if hormonal status unclear).

Management[N]
- If ≥75y., treat without DEXA once all non-osteoporotic causes of fracture have been ruled out.
- If 65–74y., treat if DEXA confirms osteoporosis (T score ≤−2.5)
- Treat if <65y. and very low BMD (T score ≤−3) *or* if T score ≤−2.5 and the patient has ≥1 additional age-independent risk factor (📖 p.154).

Lifestyle advice: Provide to all at-risk patients.
- *Adequate nutrition:* Approximate amounts of calcium in common foods are listed in Table 3.13.
  - Maintain body weight so BMI >19kg/m^2.
  - Give Ca^{2+} and/or vitamin D supplements to post-menopausal women with dietary deficiency[C].
  - Supplement with Ca^{2+} (0. 5–1g/d.) and vitamin D (800 iu/d.) if on long-term steroids[C], >80y., housebound or institutionalized[C].
- *Regular exercise:* Weight-bearing activity >30min/d. ↓ fracture rate[S].
- *Stop smoking[£]* pre-menopause → 25% ↓ fracture rate post-menopause.
- ↓ *alcohol consumption* to <14u/wk..

Table 3.13 Approximate calcium content of common foods

Food	Serving	Calcium (mg)
Whole milk	0.2l ($^1/_3$ pint)	220
Semi-skimmed milk	0.2l ($^1/_3$ pint)	230
Hard cheese	30g (1oz)	190
Cottage cheese	115g (4oz)	80
Low-fat yoghurt	150g (5oz)	225
Sardines (including bones)	60g (2oz)	310
Brown or white bread	3 large slices	100
Wholemeal bread	3 large slices	55
Baked beans	115g (4oz)	60
Boiled cabbage	115g (4oz)	40

An adult requires ~700mg of calcium/day to maintain healthy bones.

GP Notes: Measures to ↓ risk of falls and damage from falling

Falls are one of the biggest risk factors for fracture. Tendency to fall ↑ with age.

- Modify identified hazards or risk factors.
- Assess and correct vision, if possible.
- Correct postural hypotension – alter medication; consider compression stockings – but many elderly people cannot apply stockings tight enough to be of any use themselves.
- Treat other medical conditions, e.g. refer to cardiology if arrhythmia.
- Review medication and discontinue/alter inappropriate medication.
- Remove environmental hazards – arrange bath at a day centre, refer to OT to identify and correct hazards in the home, e.g. remove loose carpets, wheeled trolley for use indoors, commode or urine bottle for night-time use, moving the bed downstairs, etc.
- Liaise with other members of the primary health care team and social services to provide additional support if needed; refer to local council for 'carephone' or alarm system to call for help if any further falls.
- Refer to rehabilitation/physiotherapy to improve confidence after falls and for weight-bearing exercise (focusing on strength and flexibility) and balance training (↓ risk of falls).
- Use of hip protectors ↓ fracture risk in patients at high risk but compliance is a problem[c].

Treatment options

Bisphosphonates: e.g. alendronate 10mg od or 70mg once weekly; ibandronic acid 150mg/mo. ↓ bone loss and fracture rate[C]. Mainstay of treatment and prevention of osteoporosis.

Strontium ranelate: e.g. Protelos® 2g od in water. ↑ formation and ↓ resorption of bone. Use for post-menopausal osteoporosis, particularly when bisphosphonates are contraindicated or not tolerated. ↓ hip/vertebral fracture risk by 36–41%.

Selective oestrogen receptor modulator (SERM): e.g. raloxifene 60mg od – use if bisphosphonates are contraindicated/not tolerated or there is an unsatisfactory response (further fracture and/or ↓ in BMD after ≥1y. treatment) with bisphosphonates.

HRT: 📖 p.150. Postpones post-menopausal bone loss and ↓ fractures[C]. Optimum duration of use is uncertain (>5–7y.) but benefit disappears within 5y. of stopping. ↑ breast cancer and cardiovascular risk limits use[R].

> **CSM guidance (2003)**
> - **Premature menopause:** HRT is recommended for the prevention of osteoporosis until women reach 51y.
> - **>51y.:** HRT should **not** be considered 1st line therapy for long-term prevention of osteoporosis. HRT remains an option where other therapies are contraindicated, cannot be tolerated, or if there is a lack of response; risks and benefits should be carefully assessed.

Teriparatide: Most powerful treatment for osteoporosis currently available. Consider referral for consultant initiation if other treatment options are exhausted. Given by daily injection.

Referral: Routinely refer to endocrinology or menopause clinic (as appropriate) if:
- premature menopause (<40y.)
- unexplained cause of osteoporosis
- osteoporosis in a man, or
- problems with management.

Further information

NICE 🖥 www.nice.org.uk
- Osteoporosis – secondary prevention (2005)
- Osteoporosis – assessment of fracture risk and prevention in high-risk individuals – due for publication in 2007

National Osteoporosis Society Primary care strategy for osteoporosis and falls (2002) 🖥 www.nos.org.uk
Royal College of Physicians Osteoporosis: clinical guidelines for prevention and treatment (2003) 🖥 www.rcplondon.ac.uk
CSM guidance Further advice on safety of HRT (12/2003) 🖥 www.mhra.gov.uk
Million Women Study Collaborators Lancet (2003) 362 419–27
Women's Health Initiative Study 🖥 www.whi.org

Advice for patients: Frequently asked questions about osteoporosis

What is osteoporosis? Everybody loses bone as they get older. The amount of bone lost varies from person to person. Some people lose so much bone that their bones become fragile and break more easily. Those people have osteoporosis. Osteoporosis is far more common in women than men and usually comes on after the menopause.

Who is at risk of developing osteoporosis? Everyone is at risk of developing osteoporosis as they get older. Some factors make you more at risk. These include having an early menopause or having a period of time when your periods stopped due to an eating disorder, heavy exercise or illness; having a family history of osteoporosis; having a medical history of certain conditions such as an overactive thyroid; or taking steroid tablets for other medical conditions.

Your lifestyle can also put you at risk. You can lower your risk of having thin bones by eating foods which contain calcium and vitamin D or taking supplements, taking plenty of exercise, stopping smoking and cutting down on your alcohol intake.

How is osteoporosis diagnosed? Special X-ray machines do a dual energy X-ray absorptiometry (DEXA) scan which can check your bone density (thickness) and confirm osteoporosis. However, osteoporosis is often first diagnosed when you break a bone.

What are the symptoms and problems of osteoporosis? Osteoporosis usually develops slowly over several years without any symptoms. The major problem associated with osteoporosis is the increased risk of breaking a bone, even after a minor fall. A fractured bone in an older person can be serious. For example, about half the people who have a hip fracture are unable to live independently afterwards.

What are the treatments for osteoporosis? There are a number of medicines which can be prescribed to prevent your osteoporosis getting worse. The most commonly used drugs are the bisphosphonates which include alendronate, risedronate and etidronate.

You can also take measures to help prevent you from falling. This can reduce the chance of you breaking a bone. Check your home for hazards such as loose rugs, slippery floors, and objects you could trip on, and be careful outside in bad conditions, for example if it is wet or icy. If your medicine makes you drowsy, talk to your doctor to see if it can be changed and keep active. If you have had a fall, see your doctor as a 'falls assessment' may help prevent further falls.

Information and support for patients

Arthritis Research Campaign ☎ 0870 850 5000 🖳 www.arc.org.uk
National Osteoporosis Society ☎ 0845 450 0230 🖳 www.nos.org.uk

Chapter 4

Contraception

Summary of contraceptive methods 162
Emergency contraception 166
Combined oral contraceptives 168
Progestogen-only contraceptives 180
Intrauterine devices (IUDs) 186
Other methods of contraception 192
Consultation with teenagers 194
Termination of pregnancy (TOP) 196

🛈 Information in this section is based on WHO evidence-based recommendations for contraceptive use, the Faculty of Family Planning and Reproductive Health Care (FFPRHC)'s adaptation of the WHO guidelines for UK use and product data sheets. Recommendations sometimes go outside licensed uses and this is indicated in the text.

Summary of contraceptive methods

80% of women receive contraceptive advice and treatment through their GP. A sexually active woman has an 85% chance of becoming pregnant in <1y. without contraception and ~1:3 pregnancies are unplanned. Inadequate advice and choice results in women being dissatisfied with their method of contraception and not using methods correctly.

Choice of method: There is no ideal method of contraception. Choice of contraceptive method involves matching the method that best fits to the individual woman. Consider:
- The woman's personal preference
- Age
- Lifestyle
- Risk of sexually transmitted disease
- Gynaecological/obstetric history
  - Previous experience with contraception
  - Family/religious views about contraception
  - Future plans for pregnancy – does contraception need to be permanent, long- or short-term?
  - Past pregnancies?
  - Is the woman currently breast feeding?
- Intercurrent illness – epilepsy, DM, obesity, breast cancer, cardiovascular disease, migraine, history of thromboembolism, liver disease, other illness, current medication (enzyme-inducing drugs?)
- Family history – breast cancer, thromboembolism, heart disease/stroke
- Effectiveness of the preferred method
- Possible risks and side-effects.

Sexually transmitted diseases (STDs): When discussing contraception with women always discuss the risk of transmission of STDs, especially if contemplating using a non-barrier method. Advise high-risk groups (young, multiple sexual partners, past history of STD) to use barrier methods in addition to hormonal methods.

> **GP Notes: WHO medical eligibility criteria for contraceptive use**
>
> Useful way to clarify when contraceptive methods should/should not be used.
> - WHO 1 – No restriction for the use of the contraceptive method
> - WHO 2 – Advantages generally outway the disadvantages
> - WHO 3 – Theoretical/proven risks outweigh advantages
> - WHO 4 – Unacceptable health risk

Further information

World Health Organization (WHO) 🖳 www.who.int
- Selected practice recommendations for contraceptive use (2004)
- Medical eligibility criteria for contraceptive use (2004).

FFPRHC UK selected practice recommendations for contraceptive use (2002) 🖳 www.ffprhc.org.uk

Table 4.1 Summary of contraceptive methods

Method of contraception	% unintended pregnancies in the first year *	Advantages	Disadvantages
Sterilization (σ)	0.05 (1:2000)	No contra-indications Single procedure	Difficult to reverse Post-op. complications
Sterilization (φ)	0.5 (1:200)	No contra-indications Single procedure	Requires general anaesthetic and rarely results in laparotomy Post-op. complications Difficult to reverse ↑ risk ectopic pregnancy
Implanon (single capsule upper arm)	0.05	Lasts 3y. Immediately reversible	Needs training to insert and remove Can cause irregular bleeding Progestogenic side-effects
Progestogen-containing IUS (e.g. Mirena®)	0.1	No need for compliance Lasts 5y. ↓ bleeding, ↓ dysmenorrhoea, ↓ ectopic pregnancy risk Provides endometrial protection	May cause erratic bleeding Progestogenic side-effects
Combined oral contraceptive (COC)	0.3 (8)	Regular cycle Lighter periods ↓ dysmennorhoea Woman has cycle control	Compliance Side-effects *Health risks:* thromboembolism, breast cancer
Progestogen-only pill (POP)	0.3 (8)	Few side-effects and contraindications	Compliance Irregular bleeding Progestogenic side-effects
IUCD	0.6 (0.8)	No systemic effect Little compliance needed	Heavy periods Does not protect against PID or ectopic pregnancy
Injectable progestogen (e.g. Depot Provera)	0.3 (3)	Avoids pill taking ↓ bleeding and can help PMS ↓ risk of ectopic pregnancy, endometrial cancer	Menstrual irregularity Weight gain Unpredictable return of fertility ↑ risk osteoporosis
Barrier methods – diaphragm, condoms, female sheath	2 (32)	Barrier to transmission of STDs	User-dependent Allergy
Natural methods	1 (27)	No contraindications or side-effects	Teaching required High failure rate

* Failure rates stated are with perfect use. Rates in brackets are with typical use.

Contraceptive services: Provided by practices as an additional service, i.e. most practices are expected to provide this service and payment is included in the global sum. If a practice 'opts out' the global sum is ↓ by 2.4%.

Requirements: Practices providing contraceptive services should make these services available to all their patients who request them. This should include:

- Advice and information about the full range of contraceptive methods
- Advice and information about sexual health and sexually transmitted diseases
- Where appropriate, medical examination of patients requesting contraceptive advice
- Provision of contraceptives (excluding fitting of intrauterine devices/systems and implantation of contraceptive implants – both these can be provided as an enhanced service)
- Advice and information about emergency contraception and, where appropriate, provision of emergency hormonal contraception
- Advice and referral in cases of unwanted or unplanned pregnancy, including advice about free pregnancy testing within the practice area
- Referral as necessary to specialist sexual health services, including referral for testing for sexually transmitted diseases.

🛈 Where the practice or individual doctor/nurse seeing the patient has a conscientious objection to either emergency contraception or termination of pregnancy, prompt referral must be arranged to another provider of primary medical services who does not have such conscientious objections.

Fitting intrauterine devices: Intrauterine devices (including Mirena®) may be fitted as a *national enhanced service*. A payment is available for fitting the intrauterine device and a further payment is made for annual review.

Quality and outcomes framework points

CON 1	The team has a written policy for responding to requests for emergency contraception	1 point
CON 2	The team has a policy for providing preconceptual advice	1 point

Advice for patients: Further information for patients

Family Planning Association ☎ 0845 310 1334 🖥 www.fpa.org.uk

Exclude pregnancy: Take a menstrual and sexual history. You can be reasonably certain a woman is not pregnant if:
- she states that she has not had unprotected sexual intercourse since her last normal menstrual cycle
- has correctly and consistently been using a reliable method of contraception
- is within 7d. of the start of a normal menses
- is <4wk. post-partum
- is <7d. post-abortion or miscarriage
- is fully breast feeding, amenorrhoeic and <6mo. post-partum.

If in doubt, support your assessment with a pregnancy test which should be at least 3 weeks since the last unprotected sexual intercourse.

Provide information: Provide verbal and written information that will enable the woman to choose a method and use it effectively. This information should take into consideration the woman's individual needs and include:
- contraceptive efficacy
- duration of use
- risks and possible side-effects
- non-contraceptive benefits
- the procedure for initiation and removal/discontinuation
- when to seek help while using the method.

🕛 Prescriptions for contraceptives are free of charge for all women.

Contraception for teenagers: 📖 p.195

Contraception for women >35y.: 📖 p.149

Contraception after TOP or miscarriage: 📖 p.196

Post-partum contraception: 📖 p.275.

Further information
Guillebaud J. *Contraception: your questions answered*, 4th edn. Churchill Livingstone (2003) ISBN: 0443073430.
Family Planning Association (FPA) ☎ 0845 310 1334
🖥 www.fpa.org.uk
Faculty of Family Planning & Reproductive Health Care
🖥 www.ffprhc.org.uk
World Health Organization (WHO)
🖥 www.who.int/topics/contraception/en
NICE 🖥 www.nice.org.uk

Emergency contraception

History: Ask:
- when the woman's last menstrual period started and usual cycle length
- when she had unprotected intercourse and whether there were other episodes of unprotected intercourse during this cycle
- what other medication she is taking – including contraceptive pills
- whether she has any chronic or current medical conditions.

Hormonal emergency contraception: *BNF 7.3.1.* Use levonorgestrel 1.5mg – available OTC and on prescription. Single dose taken <72h. (3d.) after unprotected intercourse – the sooner it is taken, the greater the efficacy:
- 0–24h. – 95% efficacy
- 25–48h. – 85% efficacy
- 49–72h. – 58% efficacy

ⓘ Levonorgestrel is effective up to 120h. post-intercourse (unlicensed >3d.) but effectiveness ↓ the longer the delay.

Contraindications: Acute active porhyria, severe liver disease, allergy.

Possible pitfalls
- *Vomiting <3h. after taking levonorgestrel:* Give a replacement dose. If an anti-emetic is required, prescribe domperidone.
- *Enzyme inducing drugs:* e.g. anti-epileptics, St John's wort – efficacy may be ↓. Consider a copper IUCD or ↑ dose of levonorgestrel to 3mg (1.5mg immediately and 1.5mg 12h. later – unlicensed).

Copper-containing intrauterine device: Insertion of an intra-uterine device (IUD) is more effective than hormonal emergency contraception and prevents nearly 100% of pregnancies.

- Copper IUDs (*not* Mirena®) can be inserted for emergency contraception ≤120h. (5d.) after unprotected intercourse.
- Test for sexually transmitted diseases with endocervical swabs – if at risk, cover insertion with antibiotics, e.g. azithromycin 1g stat.
- If intercourse has occurred >5d. previously, the IUD can still be inserted up to 5d. after the earliest likely calculated ovulation (i.e. within the minimum period before implantation).
- There is a small ↑ in pelvic infections in the 20d. following insertion of an IUD.

Follow-up: 3–4wk. after prescribing emergency contraception or inserting an IUD – sooner if heavy vaginal bleeding or pelvic pain. Include:
- Checking the patient is not pregnant – may need a pregnancy test
- Talking about regular methods of contraception which would prevent pregnancy and the need for emergency contraception in future
- Screening for sexually transmitted diseases, if needed
- If the patient is pregnant, discussing options for pregnancy.

ⓘ There is no evidence treatment with levonorgestrel harms the fetus.

Further information
Department of Health CMO update 35 (2003) ▯ www.dh.gov.uk
FFPRHC Emergency contraception (2006) ▯ www.ffprhc.org.uk

Table 4.2 Emergency contraception for failure of contraception

Situation	Indication for emergency contraception
Combined oral contraceptive (21 active pills)	If ≥3 30–35mcg ethinyl estradiol or ≥2 20mcg ethinylestradiol pills have been missed, vomiting/severe diarrhoea or broad-spectrum antibiotic in the first week of pill-taking (i.e. days 1–7) and unprotected intercourse in the pill-free week or week 1
Progestogen-only pills (POP)	If ≥1 POPs have been missed or taken >3h. late (>12h. late for Cerazette®) and unprotected intercourse has occurred in the 2d. following this
Intrauterine contraception	If complete or partial expulsion is identified or mid-cycle removal of an IUD/IUS has been necessary and unprotected intercourse has occurred in the last 7d
Progestogen-only injectables	If the contraceptive injection is late (>14wk. from the previous injection for medroxyprogesterone acetate and >10wk. for norethisterone enantate) and unprotected sexual intercourse
Barrier method	Failure of a barrier method
Liver enzyme-inducing drugs	Patients taking the COC, POP or with a progestogen implant should use additional contraception if taking liver enzyme-inducing drugs. Use emergency contraception if barrier methods fail or there is unprotected intercourse during, or in the 28d. following, use of liver enzyme-inducing drugs

Advice for patients: Emergency hormonal contraception

- Contact your doctor if you vomit within 3 hours of taking your emergency contraceptive pill as it will not have had time to work. Your doctor can then give you a replacement pill.
- Use a barrier method of contraception until your next period.
- Your next period may be early or late. You may also get some spotting before you have your next period.
- If you get any lower abdominal pain or heavy bleeding or are worried in any other way, then talk to your doctor.
- Go back to your doctor in 3–4 weeks if you have not had a period or your period was abnormally light, brief or heavy.
- If the emergency contraceptive pill does not work, there is no evidence that it harms the baby.

If you do not use a regular contraceptive and are having unprotected intercourse, using emergency contraception is not a reliable way of preventing pregnancy. Talk to your doctor or local family planning clinic about methods of regular contraception which would be suitable for you, and ways to prevent sexually transmitted diseases.

GMS contract		
CON 1	The team has a written policy for responding to requests for emergency contraception	1 point

Combined oral contraceptives

Oral contraceptives containing an oestrogen and progestogen are known as combined oral contraceptives (COCs). 2 forms of the COC are now available – the combined pill and combined patch (Evra®).

Advantages of the combined oral contraceptive

- Reliable
- Easily and rapidly reversible
- ↓ menstrual symptoms – menorrhagia, dysmenorrhoea and pre-menstrual syndrome
- ↓ benign breast disease, benign ovarian cysts, pelvic inflammatory disease, ovarian & endometrial cancer, possible ↓ risk of osteoporosis

Risk of taking the COC is greater than benefit (WHO 3/4) if

- Aged >35y. and a smoker *or* age >50y. and non-smoker
- BMI >39kg/m^2 (if >30kg/m^2 ↑ risk DVT/PE – consider alternatives)
- BP is consistently >140mmHg systolic and/or 90mmHg diastolic
- Past medical history of cardiovascular disease (ischaemic heart disease, stroke/TIA or peripheral vascular disease)
- Past medical history of venous thromboembolism or >1 risk factor for venous thromboelbolism (see opposite)
- ≥2 risk factors for arterial disease (see opposite)
- Complicated valvular heart disease (pulmonary hypertension, risk of atrial fibrillation, history of subacute bacterial endocarditis)
- Focal migraine (Figure 4.1, 📖 p.170)
- Diabetes mellitus – if vascular complications or present for >20y.
- Liver disease – disorders of hepatic excretion (e.g. Dubin-Johnson or Rotor syndrome), acute hepatitis until LFTs are normal, liver adenoma, gallstones
- Female malignancy – breast cancer, genital cancer
- Hormone-related problems in pregnancy, e.g. hydatidiform mole, pruritus, cholestasis, pemphigoid gestationis, otosclerosis
- Fully breast feeding <6 months post-partum
- Porphyria.

🛈 Investigate any undiagnosed vaginal bleeding before starting the COC.

Before starting the COC

- Take a history – medical, sexual and reproductive health, medications and lifestyle. Use COC with caution if history of severe depression, inflammatory bowel disease or sickle cell disease. If hyperprolactinaemia, seek specialist advice.
- Check BP.
- Consider a routine thrombophilia screen if FH of deep vein thrombosis or pulmonary embolism in a 1st degree relative aged <45y. or multiple family members, and/or check cholesterol/triglycerides if FH of arterial disease in a 1st degree relative <45y. or multiple family members.
- Discuss side-effects and risks of the COC.
- Give directions on administration.
- Health education – discuss sexually transmitted diseases, cervical smears, smoking cessation, control of weight.

Table 4.3 Risks and benefits of the COC pill

Disease	Rates/100,000 women	Relative risk with COC use
Coronary artery disease	1500	Non-smoker – no ↑ Smoker – >20x ↑ risk
Stroke	100	2x ↑ in ischaemic stroke – no ↑ in haemorrhagic stroke Smoker (>15 cigarettes/d.) – 7x ↑ risk iaschaemic stroke
Venous thrombo-embolism	5	3x ↑ with norethisterone/levonorgestrel-containing COCs 5x ↑ with gestodene/desogestrel-containing COCs
Breast cancer	2000 (up to age 50y.)	Any small ↑ in risk disappears <10y. after stopping the COC pill
Cervical cancer	11	Small ↑ after 5y. use Risk ↑ x2 after 10y. use
Ovarian cancer	22	Halving of risk lasting ≥10y.
Endometrial cancer	15	Halving of risk lasting ≥10y.

Venous thromboembolism: Use COC with caution and avoid gestodene/desogestrel COCs if 1 risk factor is present. Avoid if >1:
- *Family history of venous thromboembolism* in 1st degree relative <45y.* or known prothrombotic coagulation abnormality, e.g. factor V Leiden or antiphospholipid antibodies
- *Obesity* – BMI >30kg/m^2 – avoid if BMI >39kg/m^2
- *Long-term immobilization* – avoid if bedbound or leg in a cast
- *Varicose veins* – avoid during sclerosing treatment or where definite history of thrombosis

Arterial disease: Use COC with caution if 1 risk factor is present. Avoid if >1:
- *Family history of arterial disease* in 1st degree relative <45y. – avoid if patient has hypercholesterolaemia/hypertriglyceridaemia
- *Diabetes mellitus* – avoid if complications present or present >20y
- *Hypertension* – BP >140/90mmHg – avoid if >160/100mmHg
- *Smoking* – avoid if smoking ≥40 cigarettes/d
- *Age* – >35y. – avoid if >50y. or if >35y. and smokes
- *Obesity* – avoid if BMI >39kg/m^2
- *Migraine* – Figure 4.1, 📖 p.170

* Refer to haematology for thrombophilia screen. Even if normal, risk of thromboembolism may be ↑.

Further information
FFPRHC First prescription of the combined oral contraception (2003) 🖥 www.ffprhc.org.uk

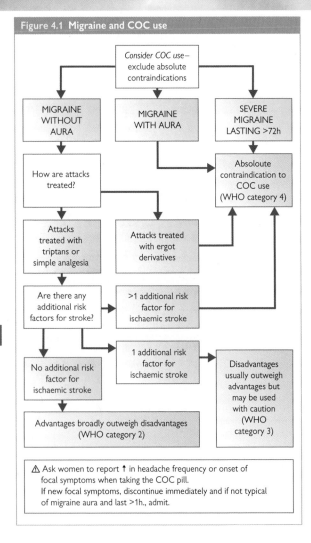

Figure 4.1 Migraine and COC use

Consider COC use—
exclude absolute
contraindications

MIGRAINE WITHOUT AURA

MIGRAINE WITH AURA

SEVERE MIGRAINE LASTING >72h

How are attacks treated?

Absoloute contraindication to COC use (WHO category 4)

Attacks treated with triptans or simple analgesia

Attacks treated with ergot derivatives

Are there any additional risk factors for stroke?

>1 additional risk factor for ischaemic stroke

No additional risk factor for ischaemic stroke

1 additional risk factor for ischaemic stroke

Disadvantages usually outweigh advantages but may be used with caution (WHO category 3)

Advantages broadly outweigh disadvantages (WHO category 2)

⚠ Ask women to report ↑ in headache frequency or onset of focal symptoms when taking the COC pill.
If new focal symptoms, discontinue immediately and if not typical of migraine aura and last >1h., admit.

Figure 4.1 is reproduced with permission from the *British Journal of Family Planning* (1998); **24**: pp.54–60

170

Figure 4.2 Combined contraceptives currently available in the UK

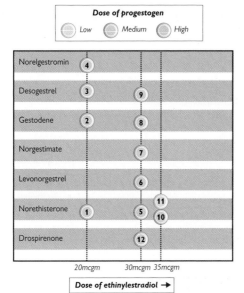

Dose of progestogen

◉ Low ◉ Medium ◉ High

	Dose of ethinylestradiol →
Norelgestromin	
Desogestrel	
Gestodene	
Norgestimate	
Levonorgestrel	
Norethisterone	
Drospirenone	

20mcgm   30mcgm 35mcgm

Dose of ethinylestradiol →

Progestogen*	Ethinylestradiol*		
	20mcg	30mcg	35mcg
Norethisterone 500mcgm			Brevinor[11®] Ovysmen[11®]
Norethisterone 1mg	Loestrin 20[1®]		Norimin[10®]
Norethisterone 1.5mg		Loestrin 30[5®]	
Levonorgestrel 150mcg		Microgynon[6®] Microgynon ED[6®] Ovranette[6®]	
Norgestimate 250mcg			Cilest[7]®
Gestodene 75mcg	Femodette[2®]	Femodene[8®] Femodene ED[8®] Minulet[8®]	
Desogestrel 150mcg	Mercilon[3®]	Marvelon[9®]	
Drospirenone 3mg		Yasmin[12®]	
Norelgestromin 150mcg/24h.	Evra[4®]		

* **Phased preparations** 📖 p.175

Choosing a COC: *BNF 7.3.1.* COCs differ by oestrogen content, type of progestogen and method of administration (pill or patch).

COC pills: Most COC pills come in packets of 21 pills. The woman takes the entire packet starting on the first day of her cycle and then has a 7-day 'pill-free' break before starting the next packet. Pills vary by:

Oestrogen content: Ranges from 20–35mcg – choose a pill with the lowest oestrogen and progestogen content which gives good cycle control with minimal side-effects:

- *Low-strength preparations* – contain ethinylestradiol 20mcg. Appropriate for women with risk factors for circulatory disease where the COC is not contraindicated or if oestrogen-related side-effects.
- *Standard strength preparations* – contain ethinylestradiol 30, 35, or 30–40mcg in phased preparations. Use for most women.
- *Phased preparations* – where dose of oestrogen/progestogen varies through the cycle (Table 4.5, 📖 p.175). Suitable for women who:
  - do not have withdrawal bleeding or
  - have breakthrough bleeding with monophasic products.
- *Every day (ED) preparations* – have 21 active pills and 7 'inactive' pills to cover the 'pill-free' week. They are taken continuously and can be helpful for women who find remembering to start a new packet difficult.

Progestogen type: COC pills containing:
- *Levonorgestrel and norethisterone* – suitable for most women. Choose for 1st time COC pill users.
- *Desogestrel* (Marvelon®), norgestimate (Cilest®) and gestodene (Femodene®) – consider if women have side-effects with other progestogens, e.g. acne, headache, depression, weight ↑, breast symptoms, breakthrough bleeding. ❶ Desogestrel and gestodene have both been associated with ↑ risk of venous thromboembolism.
- *Drospirenone* (Yasmin®) – has anti-androgenic and anti-mineralo-corticoid activity. ❶ May ↑ serum K⁺ in women at risk.
- *Cyproterone acetate* (Dianette®) – licensed for treatment of acne but not for contraception, though does provide effective contraception. Use for 3–4mo. after resolution of symptoms. Associated with 4x ↑ risk of venous thromboembolism compared to COC containing levonorgestrel.

Contraceptive patch (Evra®): 20mcg ethinylestradiol and norelgestromin in a transdermal patch. Alternative if compliance with daily pill-taking is problematic.

Starting routines for the COC pill: Table 4.4

Starting routines for the contraceptive patch

Changing from the COC pill: Apply patch the day after taking the last active pill in the packet. If started at any other time in the cycle, use additional precautions (barrier methods) concurrently for the first 7d.

Table 4.4 Starting routines for the COC pill

Circumstances	When to start the COC pill	Additional contraception required?
Women having normal menstrual cycles	Start COC up to and including day 3 of the menstrual cycle*	None
	Any other time if it is reasonably certain the woman is not pregnant	For 7d.
Amenorrhoeic woman	Start the COC at any time if it is reasonably certain the woman is not pregnant	For 7d.
After miscarriage/TOP	Start <7d. after miscarriage/TOP (ideally the same day)	None
	>7d. after miscarriage/TOP	For 7d.
After childbirth	Start 3wk. after birth if not breast feeding (↑ risk of thrombosis if started earlier)	None
	If started >3wk. after birth	For 7d.
Breast feeding – <6mo. post-partum COC is not recommended	If >6mo. post-partum and no periods – start as for other amenorrhoeic women	
	If >6mo. post-partum and normal menstruation – start as for women with normal cycle	
Switching from other methods of contraception		
From another brand of COC	Continue the current pack until the last tablet then start the first tablet of the new brand the following day. If changing from an 'ED' preparation, omit the 'inactive pills' and start the first 'active' tablet of the new brand the day following the last 'active' tablet of the old brand	None
	If a 7d. break is taken before starting the new brand	For 7d.
From the POP	Start on day 1 of menstruation or any day if amenorrhoea is present and pregnancy has been excluded	None
From injectable progestogen/ implant	Start when the next injection is due or the day an implant is removed	For 7d.
From non-hormonal methods (excluding IUCD)	Start COC up to and including day 5 of the menstrual cycle	None
	Any other time if it is reasonably certain the woman is not pregnant	For 7d.
From IUCD or IUS	Start on day 1–3 of cycle. Remove IUCD/IUS when COC started	None
	Any other time in cycle – leave IUS/IUD in situ until next bleed or use additional barrier method for 7d.	

* WHO guidelines suggest no additional contraception up to and including day 5 of the cycle.

Changing to the COC patch from progestogen-only method
- *From an implant* – apply first patch on the day implant removed
- *From an injection* – apply first patch when next injection due
- *From oral progestogen* – apply first patch the day after stopping pill

⚠ For all these methods additional precautions (barrier methods) should be used concurrently for the first 7d.

After childbirth (not breast feeding): Start 4wk. after birth; if started >4wk. after birth additional precautions (barrier methods) should be used for the first 7d.

After TOP or miscarriage
- *<20wk. gestation* – start immediately. No additional contraception required if started <7d. after TOP/miscarriage.
- *>20wk. gestation* – start on day 21 after TOP/miscarriage or on the first day of first spontaneous menstruation. Use additional precautions (barrier methods) for first 7d. after applying the patch.

Instructions for use

COC pill: Take each tablet at approximately the same time each day. If delayed by >24h. treat as a missed pill (📖 p.177).
- *21d. combined (monophasic) preparations* – take 1 tablet daily for 21d. Subsequent courses are repeated after a 7d. interval. Withdrawal bleeding occurs in the 7d. interval.
- *Every day (ED) combined (monophasic) preparations* – start active tablets on day 1 of cycle then 1 tablet daily. Withdrawal bleeding occurs when the 'inactive' tablets are being taken. Subsequent courses are repeated without interval.

174

⚠ If the woman vomits <2h. after taking a COC pill or has very severe diarrhoea, assume the COC pill has not been absorbed and treat as a missed pill (📖 p.177).

Contraceptive patch: Apply patch on day 1 of cycle; change patch on days 8 and 15; remove 3rd patch on day 22 and then apply a new patch after a 7d. 'patch-free' interval to start the subsequent cycle.

Short-term side-effects: Usually resolve within 2–3 cycles.

Relative oestrogen excess: Breast tenderness (3.6% women); nausea (1.5% women); dizziness; cyclical weight ↑; bloating; vaginal discharge without infection. Use a more progestogen-dominated pill (Figure 4.2, 📖 p.171).

Relative progestogen excess: Depression (3.9% women); PMT; dry vagina; sustained weight ↑; ↓ libido; lassitude; acne. Use a more oestrogen-dominant pill (Figure 4.2, 📖 p.171).

Headache: Affects 2.9% of women taking the COC pill. Ask women to report ↑ in headache frequency or onset of focal symptoms when taking the COC pill. If new focal symptoms, discontinue immediately and, if not typical of migraine aura and lasts >1h., admit. If headaches continue, consider switching brand/alternative method of contraception.

⚠ **Reasons to stop the COC immediately** (pending investigation if needed)
- Sudden severe chest pain (even if not radiating to left arm)
- Sudden breathlessness (or cough with bloodstained sputum)
- Unexplained severe pain in calf of one leg
- Acute abdominal pain
- Serious neurological effects including:
  - unusual severe, prolonged headache, especially if first time or getting progressively worse or
  - sudden dysphasia, partial or complete loss of vision, disturbance of hearing, or other perceptual disorders
  - bad fainting attack or unexplained collapse
  - first unexplained epileptic seizure
  - weakness, motor disturbances, or numbness affecting one side or one part of body
- Hepatitis, jaundice, liver enlargement
- BP >160/100mmHg
- Prolonged immobility after surgery or leg injury
- Detection of a risk factor/contraindication (📖 p.168)

Table 4.5 Phased COC pill preparations available in the UK

Preparation	Content
Logynon®, Logynon ED® and Trinordiol®	6x ethinylestradiol 30mcg; levonorgestrel 50mcg 5x ethinylestradiol 40mcg; levonorgestrel 75mcg 10x ethinylestradiol 30mcg; levonorgestrel 125mcg [7x inactive tablets] ED preparation only
Binovum®	7x ethinylestradiol 35mcg; norethisterone 500mcg 14x ethinylestradiol 35mcg; norethisterone 1mg
Synphase®	7x ethinylestradiol 35mcg; norethisterone 500mcg 9x ethinylestradiol 35mcg; norethisterone 1mg 5x ethinylestradiol 35mcg; norethisterone 500mcg
Trinovum®	7x ethinylestradiol 35mcg; norethisterone 500mcg 7x ethinylestradiol 35mcg; norethisterone 750mcg 7x ethinylestradiol 35mcg; norethisterone 1mg
Triadene® and Triminulet®	6x ethinylestradiol 30mcg; gestodene 50mcg 5x ethinylestradiol 40mcg; gestodene 70mcg 10x ethinylestradiol 30mcg; gestodene 100mcg

175

GP Notes: Long journeys and DVT

Women taking COCs are at ↑ risk of DVT during travel involving long periods of immobility (>5h.). Advise women:
- to drink plenty of non-alcoholic fluids
- to keep their legs moving whilst sitting, or walk up and down the aisle.

Graduated compression hosiery is available for purchase OTC and does ↓ risk of DVT.

Breakthrough bleeding: Most common in the first few months of COC use – after 6 cycles affects 1.1% women (spotting affects 3.3% women). If no vomiting/diarrhoea and no missed pills, breakthrough bleeding does not indicate ↓ efficacy. If breakthrough bleeding persists:

Check for gynaecological causes

- Exclude sexually transmitted diseases – chlamydial cervicitis is the most common cause of breakthrough bleeding in young sexually active women.
- Examine the cervix – check smear is up to date and take smear if overdue.
- Check the woman is not pregnant.

Check compliance

- Have there been any missed pills? Breakthrough bleeding may start 2–3d. after a missed pill.
- Has there been any diarrhoea/vomiting?
- Does the woman drink heavily? Women who drink a lot of alcohol are more likely to miss COC pills and less likely to remember they have missed one.

Management: ↑ oestrogen content of COC pill if on low-dose preparation. If problem persists, change progestogen. If still persists, ↑ progestogen and/or try phased preparation.

Missed pills: Figure 4.3

Missed patches

- ***If patch is partly detached for <24h.:*** Reapply to the same site or replace with a new patch immediately – no additional contraception is needed and the next patch should be applied on the usual change day.
- ***If patch is detached for >24h. or unaware when detached:*** Stop the current contraceptive cycle and start a new cycle by applying a new patch, giving a new 'day 1'. Use additional non-hormonal contraception for the first 7d. of the new cycle.
- ***If first patch of a new cycle is delayed:*** Contraceptive protection is lost. Apply a new patch as soon as remembered, giving a new 'day 1'. Advise additional non-hormonal contraception for the first 7d. of the new cycle. If intercourse has occurred during the patch-free interval, consider emergency contraception.
- ***If patch in the middle of the cycle is delayed*** (i.e. the patch is not changed on day 8 or day 15) for:
  - ≤48h. – apply a new patch immediately; next patch change day remains the same and no additional contraception is required.
  - >48h. – protection may have been lost. Stop the current cycle and start a new 4-week cycle immediately by applying a new patch, giving a new 'day 1'. Use additional non-hormonal contraception for the first 7d.
- ***If patch is not removed at the end of the cycle*** (day 22): Remove as soon as possible and start the next cycle on the usual 'change day' (i.e. after day 28) – no additional contraception is needed.

Figure 4.3 Advice for women missing COC pills

If ONE or TWO 30–35mcg eithinylestradiol pills have been missed at any time OR ONE 20mcg ethinylestradiol pill is missed	If THREE or MORE 30–35mcg ethinylestradiol pills have been missed at any time OR TWO or MORE 20mcg ethinylestradiol pill are missed
The women should take the most recent missed pill as soon as she remembers	The women should take the most recent missed pill as soon as she remembers
She should continue taking the remaining pills at her usual time*	She should continue taking the remaining pills at her usual time*
She does not require additional contraceptive protection	Advise her to use condoms or abstain from sex until she has taken pills for 7d. in a row
She does not require emergency contraception	IN ADDITION Because extending the pill-free interval is risky

If pills are missed in week 1 (days 1–7)	If pills are missed in week 3 (days 15–21)
Because the pill-free interval has been extended, emergency contraception should be considered if the woman had unprotected sex in the pill-free interval or week 1	To avoid extending the pill-free interval, advise the woman to finish the pills in her current pack and start a new pack the next day, thus omitting the pill-free interval

* Depending on when she remembers her missed pill she may take 2 pills on the same day (one at the moment of remembering and the other at the regular time) or even at the same time.

GP Notes: Surgery

COCs should be discontinued, and alternative contraceptive arrangements made (e.g. depo-injection, barrier methods), 4wk. before major elective surgery and all surgery to the legs/surgery which involves prolonged immobilization of a lower limb. Restart the COC on the first day of the next period occurring ≥2wk. after full mobilization.

Drug interactions: Many drugs affect efficacy of the COC pill and contraceptive patch. These broadly fall into 2 categories:
- Hepatic enzyme-inducing drugs:
  - Antibacterials: rifamycins (rifampicin, rifabutin)
  - Antidepressants: St John's wort
  - Anticonvulsants: phenytoin, carbamazepine, oxcarbazepine, phenobarbital, primidone, topiramate
  - Antifungals: griseofulvin
  - Antivirals: nelfinavir, nevirapine, ritonavir
  - Modafinil
- Broad-spectrum antibiotics: interfere with absorption by affecting gut flora, e.g. amoxicillin, tetracyclines.

Management: Table 4.6

Follow-up
- 3mo. after starting or changing COC or contraceptive patch – earlier if complications.
- Once established, review every 6–12mo.

At follow-up:
- Assess risk factors and side-effects.
- Give health education, e.g. smoking cessation advice, information about STDs.
- Check BP.

Further information
Family Planning Association (FPA) ☎ 0845 310 1334
🖥 www.fpa.org.uk
Faculty of Family Planning & Reproductive Health Care
🖥 www.ffprhc.org.uk
World Health Organization (WHO) 🖥 www.who.int

> **GP Notes: Long-term antibiotics**
>
> - If long-term antibiotics are prescribed, additional barrier precautions are needed for the first 3wk. with omission of the pill-free week.
> - Additional precautions are unnecessary if a woman starting a COC has been on a course of antibiotics for ≥3wk.
> - If the antibiotic type is changed or the dose is increased, an additional barrier method is required for 3wk. with omission of the pill-free week.
>
> **Antibiotics which do *not* affect pill efficacy:** Erythromycin, cotrimoxazole, sulphonamides
>
> **Anticonvulsants which do *not* affect pill efficacy:** Sodium valproate, lamotrigine – but seizure frequency may ↑ when the COC and lamotrigine are used together and side-effects of lamotrigine may be ↑ when the COC is stopped.

Table 4.6 Management of drug interactions with the COC pill and contraceptive patch

Circumstances	Advice
COC pill	
<3wk. course of a non-enzyme-inducing broad-spectrum antibiotic e.g. amoxicillin	Use additional contraception during the course and for 7d. afterwards. Omit the pill-free interval if the 7d. runs beyond the end of the packet. Omit the inactive tablets if using an 'ED' preparation.
Short course (<7d.) of enzyme-inducing drug	Advise additional barrier contraception whilst taking the enzyme-inducing drug and for 4wk. after stopping it. Omit pill-free week or inactive tablets if using an 'ED' preparation. If breakthrough bleeding occurs, ↑ the dose of ethinylestradiol to provide ≥50mcg ethinylestradiol/d. (unlicensed).
Longer courses of enzyme-inducing drugs, excluding rifamycins e.g. anticonvulsants, St John's wort	Encourage use of alternative methods of contraception. If the woman still choses the COC, advise of ↑ failure rate and adjust the dose of COC to provide ≥50mcg ethinylestradiol/d. (unlicensed). Tricycling the packs, with no withdrawal bleed for 3–4 packs and then a ↓ pill-free interval of 4d. is also recommended (unlicensed). If breakthrough bleeding occurs, ↑ the dose of ethinylestradiol further. Continue additional contraceptive measures for 4–8wk. after stopping the drug.
Longer course of rifamycin	Use alternative non-hormonal method, e.g. IUCD.
Contraceptive patch	
Enzyme-inducing drugs	Advise additional barrier method whilst taking the enzyme-inducing drug and for 4wk. after stopping. If treatment with enzyme-inducing drug is for >3wk., start a new treatment cycle immediately without a patch-free break. If prolonged course of an enzyme-inducing drug, consider another form of contraception, e.g., IUCD.

Advice for patients: Further information for patients

Family Planning Association ☎ 0845 310 1334 🖥 www.fpa.org.uk

Progestogen-only contraceptives

Progestogen-only contraceptives thicken cervical mucus, ↓ endometrial receptivity and inhibit ovulation. They ↓ risk of pelvic infection and can be used when oestrogen is contraindicated.

Progestogen-releasing intrauterine device (intrauterine system, Mirena®): 📖 p.186

Progestogen-only pill (POP or 'mini-pill'): *BNF 7.3.2.1.* Oral POPs are a suitable alternative for women for whom oestrogen-containing pills are contraindicated:
- Older women
- Heavy smokers
- Women with past history/predisposition to venous thromboembolism
- Patients with hypertension, valvular heart disease, DM or migraine
- Breast-feeding women <6mo. post-partum. ❶ Delay until ≥ 3wk. post-partum to avoid risk of heavy bleeding.

Choice of POP: 5 brands are currently available in the UK:
- etynodiol 500mcg – Femulen®
- norethisterone 350mcg – Micronor® or Noriday®
- levonorgestrel 30mcg – Norgeston®
- desogestrel 75mcg – Cerazette® – consider if compliance problems, history of ectopic pregnancy or ovarian cysts (Cerazette has a stronger ovarian suppressive effect than other POPs) and/or weight >70kg.

Side-effects and risks
- **Failure rate:** Higher failure rate than COC pills.
- **Menstrual irregularities:** Oligomenorrhoea, menorrhagia, amenorrhoea – examine to exclude a pathological cause ± do a pregnancy test. Menstrual irregularities tend to resolve with long-term use. If necessary, consider changing progestogen or ↑ to 2 pills/d. (unlicensed).
- **Ectopic pregnancy:** ↑ risk. If a patient presents with abdominal pain, treat as an ectopic pregnancy (📖 p.236) until proven otherwise.
- **Others:** Nausea and vomiting; headache; dizziness; breast discomfort; depression; skin disorders; disturbance of appetite; weight changes; changes in libido.
- **Long term:** Small ↑ risk breast cancer – risk reverts to normal <10y. after stopping the POP.

Starting the POP
- *No previous hormonal contraception* – Start on day 1 of cycle – no additional contraception needed.
- *Changing from a COC* – Start the day following completion of the course of COC without a break (omitting the 'inactive' pills if ED preparation) – no additional contraception needed.
- *After childbirth* – Start any time >3wk. post-partum (↑ risk of breakthrough bleeding if started earlier). Does not affect lactation. No additional contraception needed.

❶ If weight >70kg consider Cerazette® or prescribing 2 tablets/d. of one of the other POPs (unlicensed).

Contraindications to all progestogen-only methods
(WHO 3/4)

- Undiagnosed abnormal PV bleeding
- Hormone-dependent tumour (women with a past history of breast cancer may use the POP after 5y. if no evidence of current disease)
- Porphyria
- Liver adenoma/severe liver disease
- Current or high-risk of arterial disease
- Pregnancy
- ↑ HCG due to trophoblastic disease.

Advice for patients: Further information

Family Planning Association ☎ 0845 310 1334 🖳 www.fpa.org.uk

Directions for taking the POP
- Take 1 tablet every day with no pill-free breaks.
- Take each tablet at the same time each day (>4h. before usual time for intercourse to give maximum protection). If delayed >3h. (>12h. for Cerazette®), treat as missed pill (see below).

Missed pills: If a pill is missed or delayed >3h. (>12h. for Cerazette®), continue taking the POP at the usual time and use additional barrier methods for 2d.

⚠ Give emergency contraception if ≥1 POPs have been missed or taken >3h. late (>12h. late for Cerazette®) and unprotected intercourse has occurred in the 2d. following this.

Diarrhoea/vomiting: Continue taking the POP but use an additional barrier method during the episode and for 2d. afterwards.

Interactions with other drugs
- Efficacy of POPs is not affected by antibacterials that do not induce liver enzymes.
- Efficacy is ↓ by enzyme-inducing drugs (📖 p.178) – advise women to use an additional barrier or alternative contraceptive method during treatment and for >4wk. afterwards.

Follow-up
- Review patients 3mo. after starting the POP or changing from COC pill – earlier if complications.
- Once established, review every 6–12mo. – assess risk factors and side-effects; give health education, e.g. smoking cessation advice, information about STDs; check BP.

Injectable progestogens: *BNF* 7.3.2.2. Useful if oestrogen-containing preparations are contraindicated or compliance is a problem. Failure rate is <4/1000 women over 2y.

Contraindications: 📖 p.181

Advantages
- Can be used to age 50y. if no other risk factors for osteoporosis.
- ↓ ectopic pregnancy, functional ovarian cysts, and sickle cell crises.
- ↓ risk of endometrial cancer. Provides endometrial protection as part of HRT regime (unlicensed).
- May alleviate premenstrual syndrome and ↓ menorrhagia.

Disadvantages
- May ↓ bone density in first 2–3y. of use – see CSM warning for Depo-Provera® (opposite). Consider DEXA scan in older women if result would influence choice.
- Can mask natural menopause.
- May be a delay in return of fertility of up to 1y. on stopping.
- Can cause menstrual disturbance. If troublesome, give next injection early (8–11wk. after the previous injection for Depo) or add oestrogen if no contraindications.
- Other side-effects, e.g. weight ↑ (up to 2–3kg), mood swings, acne.

CSM advice about Depo-Provera®

- In all women, weigh benefits of use for >2y. against risks.
- In women with risk factors for osteoporosis, consider a method of contraception other than Depo-Provera®.
- In adolescents, Depo-Provera® should only be used only when other methods of contraception are inappropriate.

GP Notes: Counselling for women before injectable contraception

All women should be counselled that:
- Periods may change and may be irregular, heavy or even stop. Irregular bleeding may continue for some months after stopping the injections.
- Women may put on weight and some women report headaches, abdominal pain or discomfort, dizziness, spotty skin, tender breasts, bloating, and/or changes in mood and/or sex drive.
- Injections work for 12 or 8 weeks, depending on which type is given, and cannot be removed from the body. If there are any side-effects, they will probably continue for this time and some time afterwards.
- Periods and fertility may take a few months to return after stopping injections. Sometimes it can take more than a year for periods and fertility to get back to normal.
- Contraceptive injections do not protect against sexually transmitted infections, so consider using condoms as well.

Advice for patients: Further information

Family Planning Association ☎ 0845 310 1334 🖳 www.fpa.org.uk

Preparations available

Depo-Provera® – medroxyprogesterone acetate 150mg/ml.

- Give 1x1ml by deep IM injection into the buttock/lateral thigh or deltoid up to day 5 of the cycle. Don't rub the injection site afterwards.
- If given after day 5, check the woman is not pregnant and provide and advise an additional method for 7d.
- Post-partum: delay until >6wk. after childbirth. If not breastfeeding, 1st dose can be given <5d. after childbirth but may cause heavy bleeding.
- Repeat every 12wk. If interval is >12wk. and 5d. – see Table 4.7.

Noristerat® – norethisterone enantate 200mg/ml.

- Warm first then give 1x1ml by deep IM injection into the gluteal muscle before day 6 of the cycle or immediately after childbirth (avoid breast feeding if baby has jaundice requiring treatment). Don't rub the injection site afterwards.
- May be repeated once only after 8wk. Unlicensed if repeated further.

Interactions

- Effectiveness is not ↓ by antibacterials that don't induce liver enzymes.
- Effectiveness of Noristerat® (but not Depo-Provera®) is ↓ by enzyme-inducing drugs (📖 p.178) – advise additional contraception whilst taking enzyme-inducing drugs and for 4wk. after stopping *or* alternative method.

Progestogen implant: *BNF 7.3.2.2.* One implant is currently available in the UK. Implanon® is a semi-rigid rod (40mm x 2mm) releasing 30–40mcg of etonogestrel/d. The rod is inserted subdermally into the lower surface of the upper arm before day 6 of the cycle. If inserted after day 5, check the woman is not pregnant and use an additional method for 7d.

Contraindications: 📖 p.181

Advantages

- Lasts 3y. and once inserted no compliance required.
- Can be used for women at risk of ectopic pregnancy.
- No effect on bone density.
- Once removed, fertility returns immediately to normal.

Disadvantages

- A minor operation is needed for insertion/removal. Special training is needed and complications of minor surgery can occur (e.g. infection, scarring).
- ↓ efficacy with liver enzyme-inducing drugs – advise additional method for duration of treatment and 4wk. afterwards or alternative contraception if enzyme-inducing drugs are being used long-term.
- Cannot be used as part of a HRT regime.
- May cause menstrual disturbances – exclude other causes. Treat with oestrogen (Marvelon® contains the same progestogen), additional progestogen or NSAID.
- Other side-effects include acne, mood swings, breast tenderness, change in libido – treat symptoms as needed.

Timing of Depo-Provera	Has un-protected sex occurred?	Can the injection be given?	Is emergency contra-ception needed?	Are condoms or abstinence advised?	Should a pregnancy test be done?
Table 4.7 Late Depo-Provera® guidelines					
Up to 12wk. and 5d. since date of previous injection	N/A	Yes	No	No	No
When an injection is overdue	No	Yes	No	Yes – for the next 14d.*	No
	Yes – but only in the last 3d.	Yes – or give Cerazette® for 21d.	Yes	Yes – for the next 14d.*	Yes – 21d. later
	Yes – but only in the last 3–5d.	Yes – or give Cerazette® for 21d.	Yes – offer copper IUD	No	Yes – 21d. later
	Yes – >5d. ago	No	No	Yes – for 21d. until a pregnancy test is confirmed negative and for a further 14d.* after giving Depo injection	Yes – at initial presenta-tion and 21d. later

☞ * WHO/FFPRHC recommendations state that injections of Depo-Provera® can be given up to 14wk. and Noristerat® can be given up to 10wk. after the previous injection without the need for additional barrier contraception. These guidelines also state that, when needed, additional contraception is only necessary for 7d.

Advice for patients: Further information

Family Planning Association ☎ 0845 310 1334 🖥 www.fpa.org.uk

Further information

NICE Long-acting reversible contraception (2005) 🖥 www.nice.org.uk

185

Intrauterine devices (IUDs)

Intrauterine contraceptive device (IUCD): *BNF 7.3.4.* Plastic carrier wound with copper wire/fitted with copper bands. Suitable for older parous women, as 2nd line contraception in young nulliparous women, or for emergency contraception. Acts by inhibiting fertilization, sperm penetration of the cervical mucus and implantation. Pregnancy rate with IUCDs containing $380mm^2$ copper is <20/1000 over 5y.

Emergency contraception: 📖 p.166

Intrauterine system (IUS): *BNF 7.3.2.3.* The progestogen-only intra-uterine system (Mirena®) releases levonorgestrel 20mcg/24h. directly into the uterine cavity. It acts by preventing endometrial proliferation, thickening cervical mucus and suppression of ovulation (some women and some cycles). Licensed uses include:
- contraception – particularly suitable for women with heavy periods
- primary menorrhagia – menstrual bleeding is ↓ significantly in 3–6mo.
- prevention of endometrial hyperplasia during oestrogen therapy.

Choice of devices: Table 4.8

Contraindications
Applying to IUCD only
- Allergy to copper
- Wilson's disease
- Heavy/painful periods

Applying to IUCD and IUS
- Pregnancy or <4wk. post-partum (WHO 3/4)
- Current or high risk of sexually transmitted infections or pelvic inflammatory disease (includes severe immunosuppression) – a woman should not have an IUCD/IUS fitted <3mo. after treatment of a pelvic infection (WHO 3/4). Following treatment of a sexually transmitted infection suitability depends on ongoing risk
- Undiagnosed uterine bleeding (WHO 4)
- Distorted uterine cavity (WHO 4)
- Current endometrial, ovarian or cervical cancer, or trophoblastic disease (WHO 3/4)
- Anticoagulation – caution – use another method if possible
- Risk of subacute bacterial endocarditis – see opposite.

Advantages
Applying to IUCD only
- No systemic side-effects
- Does not mask the menopause
- If fitted in a woman of >40y., can remain in the uterus until menopause.

Applying to IUS only
- ↓ menorrhagia/dysmenorrhoea
- ↓ risk of pelvic inflammatory disease – particularly younger age groups
- ↓ risk of ectopic pregnancy compared to the IUCD
- If 45y. and amenorrhoeic, can be left *in situ* for 7y. for contraception (unlicensed) – change after 4y. if using IUS for endometrial protection.

Table 4.8 Intrauterine devices currently available in the UK

Device	Licence	Uterine length	Comment
Flexi-T® 300	5y.	>5cm	Easy insertion
GyneFix®	5y.	Any	Frameless. Special training needed for insertion. ↓ expulsion if fitted correctly
Load® 375	5y.	>7cm	
Multiload® Cu375	5y.	6–9cm	
Nova-T® 380	5y.	6.5–9cm	Small insertion diameter
T-Safe® Cu380 A	8y.	6.5–8cm	Gold standard
TT 380 Slimline®	10y.	>7cm	Easy insertion
UT 380 Short or Standard®	5y.	Short – <7cm Standard – >7cm	
Mirena®	5y. (4y. if being used for prevention of endometrial hyperplasia)	>6.5cm	Intrauterine system releasing levonorgestrel 20mcg/24h. Does *not* contain copper

> ⓘ **Discontinued IUCDs**
- Gyne-T® 380 – some women may have the device in place until 2009.
- Multiload® Cu250 and Multiload® Cu250 Short – some women may have the devices in place until 2011.

GP Notes:

Subacute bacterial endocarditis (SBE): The IUCD/IUS can be fitted for women with risk factors for, or past history of, SBE. No antibiotic prophylaxis is required for insertion/removal *unless* high-risk of subacute bacterial endocarditis (SBE), i.e. complex cyanotic congenital heart disease, prosthetic heart valve or history of SBE.

⚠ If in doubt, or prophylaxis is required for high-risk patients, ask advice from the cardiologist in charge of the patient's care or a specialist in infectious diseases.

Further information
BNF 5.1
British Heart Foundation Factfiles Infective endocarditis (12/2003 & 1/2004) ▣ www.bhf.org.uk
European Heart Journal Horstkotte D. *et al.* Guidelines on prevention, diagnosis and treatment of infective endocarditis (2004) 25(3) 267–76

Applying to IUCD and IUS:
- Long-lasting – Table 4.8, 📖 p.187.
- Can be used up to the menopause.
- Once fitted, no compliance needed.
- Easily and immediately reversible by removal.
- Can be used for women who are breast feeding.
- Can be used for women who are obese.
- Can be used for women with concurrent illness – migraine, venous thromboembolism, DM, cardiovascular disease (or ↑ risk of cardiovascular disease), or women taking long-term hepatic enzyme-inducing drugs (e.g. anticonvulsants, antivirals).
- Can be used for HIV +ve women – but screen for STDs first and advise condom use.

Disadvantages and problems
Applying to IUCD only
- *Ectopic pregnancy* – risk (0.02/100 women years) is higher than if using a hormonal contraceptive method but not compared to women using no contraception at all (risk 0.3–0.5/100 women years). If pregnancy occurs, ↑ risk of ectopic pregnancy (1:20) – consider ectopic pregnancy in any woman with an IUCD presenting with abdominal pain.
- ↑ *dysmenorrhoea/menorrhagia* – up to 50% discontinue use of IUCDs in <5y. The most common reason cited is dysmenorrhoea or menorrhagia. Exclude infection and malposition of the IUCD. Exclude other gynaecological causes. Treat with NSAID or tranexamic acid or consider changing to the IUS.

Applying to IUS only: Progestogenic side-effects:
- Changes in pattern/duration of menstrual bleeding (spotting/prolonged bleeding) are common – warn women prior to insertion. Bleeding usually becomes light/absent within 3–6mo. of insertion.
- Mastalgia, mood changes, change in libido – usually resolve in <6mo.
- Functional ovarian cysts – usually resolve spontaneously – monitor with USS.
- Cannot be used for emergency contraception.

Applying to IUCD and IUS
- *Fitting and removal:* Requires specialist training and can be uncomfortable for the woman.
- *Expulsion/malposition:* Risk of expulsion is ≈ 1:20. Usually occurs <3mo. after insertion – teach women to feel for IUD threads after each period. If threads can't be felt, advise other contraception until checked by health professional (Figure 4.4, 📖 p.191).
- *Perforation of the uterus:* Risk <1:1000.
- *Pelvic inflammatory disease:* Excess risk of infection occurs in the first 20d. after insertion and is related to existing carriage of sexually transmitted infections. Always consider pre-screening for sexually transmitted infection (especially Chlamydia) ± antibiotic prophylaxis, e.g. azithromycin 1g stat prior to insertion. Advise women to contact their doctor immediately if any sustained pain is experienced in the first 3wk. after insertion.

Advice for patients:

Frequently asked questions about intrauterine devices

What is an intrauterine device (IUD)? It is a small device made from plastic. The intrauterine system (Mirena®) also contains a progesterone-like hormone. Other devices do not contain hormones but are wound with copper wire or fitted with copper bands instead.

How does the IUD work? The intrauterine system (IUS) works differently from other IUDs. The progestogen it contains makes the cervical mucus thicker so sperm cannot get through and makes the lining of the womb thinner, stopping any eggs from implanting. Other IUDs work through the action of copper which prevents fertilization and may also inhibit implantation.

How effective is the IUD? Both the copper-containing IUDs and IUS are very effective with less than one in 100 women becoming pregnant each year of use – without contraception more than 80 women out of 100 would become pregnant within a year.

What are the advantages of the IUD? Once fitted you don't have to worry about contraception any more. IUDs do not interfere with sex and your fertility returns to normal as soon as the IUD is removed. Copper-containing IUDs do not have any effects on the rest of the body. With the IUS your periods usually get lighter and may even stop.

What are the disadvantages? Most women have no problems once the IUD is fitted. Possible problems include:
- *Periods* – some women find that their periods become heavier, longer, or more painful with an IUD. This often settles within a few months. If you have heavy periods, talk to your doctor about having an IUS fitted as that usually makes periods lighter.
- *Infection* – there is a small risk of pelvic infection, particularly in the first 3 weeks after the IUD is fitted. You may be checked for infection before an IUD is fitted to prevent this. See your doctor if you develop pain, heavy bleeding or a smelly vaginal discharge.
- *Ectopic pregnancy* – the chance of becoming pregnant is very small if you use an IUD, but if you do become pregnant there is a higher than normal chance that the pregnancy will be ectopic. See a doctor urgently if you miss a period and develop lower abdominal pain.
- *Expulsion* – rarely the IUD may come out without you noticing. Feel for its threads inside the vagina after each period to check it is in place. If you cannot feel the threads then use other contraceptive methods (such as condoms) until you have been checked by a doctor or nurse.
- *Damage* – rarely fitting of an IUD can cause damage to the uterus.

What if I want my IUD removed? IUDs can be removed at any time by a trained professional. If you want to have your IUD removed, but do not want to get pregnant, use other methods of contraception (such as condoms) for 7days before removal.

Further information

Family Planning Association ☎ 0845 310 1334 🖳 www.fpa.org.uk

189

- *Actinomyces-like organisms (ALOs) on cervical smear:* Assess to exclude pelvic infection. If no signs of pelvic infection offer choice of leaving IUD *in situ* or changing it. If symptomatic, discuss antibiotic treatment with microbiology and refer to GUM/gynaecology for further management.
- *Intrauterine pregnancy:* Confirm intrauterine pregnancy with USS. Remove IUD at <12wk. gestation whether or not the woman intends to continue the pregnancy (↓ miscarriage rate by 50% and ↓ risk of infection – but miscarriage rate associated with removal). If pregnancy is >12wk. or no threads are visible, refer to obstetrics/gynaecology.

Insertion: Special training is required. Check BP and pulse before and after fitting. Perform a pelvic examination to determine shape and orientation of the uterus. Provided it is reasonably certain the woman is not pregnant (📖 p.165), the IUS/IUD may be inserted:
- <7d. after onset of menstruation – though tail end of a period is the optimum time and the heaviest days of a period are best avoided.
- At any other time in the cycle – if replacement IUS/IUD. If first IUD, ensure not pregnant. If first IUS and not in the first 7d. of the cycle, ensure not pregnant and advise additional method for 7d.
- Immediately after TOP/miscarriage or any time thereafter.
- >4wk. post-partum (unlicensed <6wk. post-partum), irrespective of the mode of delivery[N].

🕐 Consider a NSAID (e.g. ibuprofen 400mg) 30min. before insertion or using of topical local anaesthetic gel during insertion to ↓ discomfort.

⚠ **Cervical shock:** Rare complication of IUD insertion. Presents with pallor, sweating, and bradycardia. Immediately tip the woman head down with legs raised. If symptoms/bradycardia persist, give 0.6mg atropine IV.

⚠ **Women with epilepsy:** ↑ risk of seizure at the time of cervical dilation – ensure emergency drugs are available.

Follow-up: Review after 1st period, then annually. Ask about periods, pelvic pain, vaginal discharge and discomfort to partner. Perform pelvic examination to check threads.

Removal
- If pregnancy desired – remove at any time.
- If pregnancy not desired – remove after establishing a hormonal method or use barrier methods/abstinence for ≥7d. prior to removal. If urgent removal is necessary, provide emergency contraception if midcycle and intercourse has occurred in the previous 7d. (📖 p.166).
- Menopause – remove after 1y. amenorrhoea if aged >50y. or after 2y. if aged <50y. If there is difficulty removing the IUD, try again after a 5d. course of oestrogen (e.g. Premarin® 1.25mg od po).

Further information
FFPRHC The copper intrauterine device as long-term contraception (2004) 🖥 www.ffprhc.org.uk
NICE Long-acting reversible contraception (2005) 🖥 www.nice.org.uk

GMS contract

Intrauterine devices (including Mirena®) may be fitted as a *national enhanced service*. A payment is available for fitting the intrauterine device and a further payment is made for annual review.

Figure 4.4 Missing IUD threads

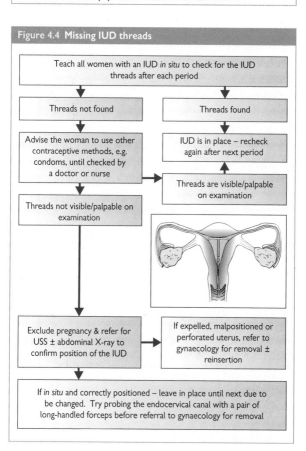

Teach all women with an IUD *in situ* to check for the IUD threads after each period

↓ Threads not found | ↓ Threads found

Threads not found → Advise the woman to use other contraceptive methods, e.g. condoms, until checked by a doctor or nurse

Threads found → IUD is in place – recheck again after next period

Threads are visible/palpable on examination

Threads not visible/palpable on examination

Exclude pregnancy & refer for USS ± abdominal X-ray to confirm position of the IUD

If expelled, malpositioned or perforated uterus, refer to gynaecology for removal ± reinsertion

If *in situ* and correctly positioned – leave in place until next due to be changed. Try probing the endocervical canal with a pair of long-handled forceps before referral to gynaecology for removal

GP Notes: Training in IUD insertion

The Faculty of Family Planning and Reproductive Health Care run a training scheme leading to the Letter of Competence in Intrauterine Contraception Techniques. The Letter of Competence must be updated every 5y. ☎ 020 7724 5669 🖳 www.ffprhc.org.uk

Other methods of contraception

Condoms: Give protection against STDs. Male and female versions. Condoms lubricated with spermicide do not ↓ pregnancy rates and the irritant effect of the spermicide may ↑ rates of transmission of STDs. Advise about emergency contraception in the event of an accident. Certain lubricants (e.g. petroleum jelly (Vaseline®), baby oil and oil-based vaginal/rectal preparations) can ↓ effectiveness. Water-based lubricants are safe (e.g. K-Y jelly).

Vaginal diaphragms or caps: *BNF 7.3.4.* Flat metal spring, coiled metal rim or arcing spring diaphragms are available. Motivation is crucial.
- Fitting must be performed by a doctor or nurse trained to fit diaphragms. Arcing diaphragms are useful when the cervix is posterior or there is mild prolapse.
- After fitting, a woman should practise inserting, wearing, checking the diaphragm is over the cervix, and removing the diaphragm for >1wk. using another form of contraception.
- Spermicides must always be used in combination with diaphragms and the diaphragm must be left *in situ* for at least 6h. after intercourse.
- Some vegetable/mineral oil-based lubricants (e.g. petroleum jelly (Vaseline®), baby oil) can damage caps. Water-based lubricants are safe (e.g. K-Y jelly®).

Follow-up: Check fit and comfort after ~1wk. and discuss again the routine for its use, especially the importance of spermicide. See after 3mo. and then annually, but more frequently if there are difficulties, if there is a weight change of >4kg, if the woman has a baby, or after pelvic surgery. Prescribe a new diaphragm yearly.

Cervical/vault caps: *BNF 7.3.4.* Attach by suction. Otherwise used in the same way as a diaphragm. Useful for women with poor muscle tone, absent retropubic ledge or recurrent cystitis when using a diaphragm.

Spermicides to use in combination with caps: *BNF 7.3.3.* Ortho-Creme, Orthoforms (pessaries).

Avoidance of intercourse during times of fertility: 3 methods of estimating time of ovulation are used:
- Urine testing – a commercial kit (Persona®) is available to buy.
- Temperature – taken orally in the morning before drinking/getting up (thermometer available on FP10). ↑ 0.2–0.4°C indicates progesterone release from the corpus luteum. Unprotected intercourse can take place only from the 3rd day of the ↑ until the next period.
- Mucus texture (Billing's method) – texture of vaginal secretions is felt between finger and thumb daily. Prior to ovulation the mucus becomes profuse and slippery, then abruptly changes to being thicker and more tacky. No unprotected intercourse from the day the mucus becomes more profuse until 3d. after it becomes tacky. Patients with cycles >or <28d. must vary timings.

Coitus interruptus: Penis is withdrawn prior to ejaculation.

Sterilization: There are no contraindications to sterilization of men or women provided they:

- make the request themselves
- are of sound mind *and*
- are not acting under external duress.

Take additional care if:

- <25y
- no children
- pregnant woman
- reacting to loss of a relationship
- at risk of coercion by partner or others.

ⓘ Prior sanction by a high court judge must be sought in all cases where there is doubt over mental capacity to consent.

Method

- Women – laparoscopic tubal occlusion with clips or rings. Usually done under general anaesthetic as a day case.
- Men – vasectomy. Usually done under local anaesthetic as a day case.

Pre-referral counselling

- Alternative long-term contraceptive methods (include sterilization of partner as an alternative)
- Reversibility – sterilization is intended to be permanent, reversal is only 50–60% successful
- Post-procedure pregnancy rate ('failure rate' – 1:200 for women; 1:2000 for men)
- ↑ risk of ectopic pregnancy post-tubal occlusion
- Risk of operative complications
- Effect on long-term health – no proven long-term risks
- Need for contraception before and after operation:
  - *Women:* other contraception until 1st post-procedure period
  - *Men:* other contraception until 2 consecutive semen analyses, 2–4wk. apart and ≥8wk. after the procedure shows azoospermia.

ⓘ All counselling should be supported by accurate, impartial information.

Further information

RCOG Male and female sterilization (2004) ⌨ www. rcog.org.uk.
Faculty of Family Planning and Reproductive Health Care Male and female condoms (2007) ⌨ www.ffprhc.org.uk

---

GP Notes: Advice for women using a diaphragm

- Insert before intercourse and leave in place ≥6h. afterwards.
- Place a ribbon of spermicide ≈ 4cm long on each side of the diaphragm before insertion. If intercourse takes place ≥3h. later, more spermicide is needed either as cream or pessary.
- After use, wash the diaphragm in warm soapy water, dry and store in its container to maintain shape.

Advice for patients: Further information

Fertility UK ⌨ www.fertilityuk.org
Family Planning Association ☎ 0845 310 1334 ⌨ www.fpa.org.uk

Consultation with teenagers

Adolescents visit their GPs on average 2–3x/y. but their needs are often poorly addressed. Aspects of general practice important to them include:

Confidentiality and consent: Posters/leaflets in the surgery about confidentiality help ↑ confidence. Usual principles of confidentiality and consent apply. In particular, an adolescent judged competent:
- can withhold permission for their parents to have access to medical information about them
- can request to be seen alone without a parent.

🕛 Ensure confidentiality isn't breached when appointments are booked (e.g. for emergency contraception) and when telephoning about results, appointments or prescriptions.

Accessibility: Access to the primary care team can be a problem for teenagers, – especially about issues they don't want to tell their parents about. To make services more accessible consider:
- *Timing and availability of appointments:* Special teenage clinics after school hours can help.
- *Friendliness:* Ensure reception staff welcome teenagers when they come to the surgery without their parents. Listen to what teenagers say they want from the practice and try to be as accommodating as possible in providing those facilities/services.
- *Information:* Provide leaflets and posters using language and presented in ways which are attractive for teenagers.
- *Offer a choice of doctor:* Gender of the doctor is particularly important for sexual health matters. Often teenagers *don't* want to see the doctor they've always seen since being a small child or the doctor their mother always takes them to.
- *Non-judgemental attitudes:* Teenagers often push the boundaries. They won't consult for help if they know they will be judged when they go too far or make mistakes. Listen and offer support, help, advice and treatment without being judgemental wherever possible.

Specific problems to look out for in teenagers:
- *Behavioural problems*
- *Psychiatric disease* – may present for the first time.
- *Eating disorders* – 📖 p.326
- *Drugs, solvent and/or alcohol abuse* – 📖 p.18 & p.10
- *Sexual health problems* – >½ have had sexual intercourse aged <16y. and so fear and risk of pregnancy are part of adolescent life. Those who have intercourse early are at greater risk of early pregnancy and health problems such as sexually transmitted disease and cervical cancer. Worries about sexuality for some can add to the pressure. Sensitive support, clear guidance and accurate information about contraception, sexuality and sexually transmitted disease is helpful.
- *Teenage pregnancy* – The UK has the highest teenage pregnancy rate in Western Europe. Not all are unplanned. Pregnant teenagers need information and non-judgemental support to help them reach a decision whether or not to continue with the pregnancy.

Contraception and the under-16s: In England and Wales, a doctor is allowed to give advice to a girl aged <16y. without parental consent if:
- she has sufficient maturity to understand the moral, social and emotional implications of treatment
- she cannot be persuaded to inform (or allow the doctor to inform) her parents
- she is very likely to begin, or continue, sexual intercourse with or without contraception
- she is likely to suffer if no contraceptive advice or treatment is given
- it is in her best interest that contraceptive advice or treatment is given with or without parental consent.

Choice of contraceptive method

- Condoms are adolescents' most commonly used form of contraception but have a relatively high failure rate. Suggesting their use in addition to another form of contraception will help prevent STDs.
- The low-dose combined oral contraceptive (COC) pill is the most suitable method of contraception for the under 16s. Poor compliance can be a problem and leads to a high failure rate.
- Progestogen implants/injectables – alternative to COC pill but the CSM advises that, in adolescents, medroxyprogesterone acetate (Depo-Provera®) should only be used when other methods of contraception are inappropriate. May ↑ osteoporosis risk (use alternative if other risk factors and try not to use >2y.), menstrual irregularity and ↑ weight.
- The progestogen-containing intrauterine contraceptive device (IUCD) is less likely to cause pelvic inflammatory disease and ectopic pregnancy than other IUCDs but can be difficult to insert in a young woman.
- 'The morning after pill' (Levonelle) is not suitable as a regular method but valuable in preventing unwanted pregnancy. Information on availability and ability to make an urgent appointment are essential.

Do's and don'ts

- Don't insist on vaginal examination or taking a smear unless there is a problem that necessitates it.
- Do discuss the merits of delaying sexual intercourse until older.
- Do stress the need for protection against sexually transmitted diseases.
- If prescribing the COC pill for dysmenorrhoea or cycle control in young women, do explain its use for contraception too.

Advice for patients: Information and support for teenagers

Childline 24h. confidential counselling ☎ 0800 1111
🖥 www.childline.org
Brook Advisory Service Contraceptive advice and counselling for teenagers ☎ 0800 0185 023 🖥 www.brook.org.uk
Sexwise For under-19s ☎ 0800 28 29 30 🖥 ruthinking.co.uk
Teenage Health Freak 🖥 www.teenagehealthfreak.org

Further information

BMJ McPherson. Adolescents in primary care (2005) 330 465–7.
NICE Preventing sexually transmitted infections and reducing under 18 conceptions (2007). 🖥 www.nice.org.uk

Termination of pregnancy (TOP)

Legal constraints: The 1967 and 1990 Human Fertilization/Embryology Acts govern termination of pregnancy in the UK. Termination is allowed at <24wk. gestation if it:

- ↓ risk to the woman's life
- ↓ risk to the mother's physical/mental health (90% TOPs are carried out under this clause)
- ↓ risk to the physical/mental health of the mother's existing children
- the baby is at serious risk of being physically or mentally handicapped.

There is no upper time limit if there is:

- real risk to the mother's life
- risk of grave, permanent injury to the mother's physical or mental health *or*
- the baby would be born seriously physically or mentally handicapped.

TOPs >24wk. can only be carried out in NHS hospitals. 99% TOPs take place <20wk. Those taking place >20wk. are usually performed when foetal abnormality is found on USS (or amniocentesis) or if pregnancy is concealed in the very young.

Procedure

- *Medical:* Oral mifepristone followed by vaginal prostaglandin.
- *Surgical:* Suction termination <15wk.; dilation and evacuation >15wk.

Follow-up: In many areas post-procedure follow-up is undertaken by the GP. Worrying symptoms are:

- excessive blood loss
- pain *and/or*
- high temperature.

Assess, consider the possibility of infection and treat if reasonably well – admit if you are worried.

ⓘ Check anti-D has been given if needed (📖 p.241) and chosen method of contraception has been started.

Complications

- Infection
- Haemorrhage
- Uterine perforation
- Cervical trauma
- Failed procedure and ongoing pregnancy
- Psychological sequelae.

ⓘ There is no association between TOP and subsequent infertility or miscarriage/pre-term delivery.

Contraception post termination or miscarriage <24wk

- *Combined pill/patch, POP, progestogen injection/implant:* Start on the day of surgical or second part of medical abortion. No additional method required. If started >7d. after abortion an additional method is required for 7d. (combined pill/patch or progestogen injection/implant) or 2d. (POP).
- *IUCD or IUS:* Insert at time of surgical or second part of medical abortion. No additional method required. Otherwise delay insertion to 4wk. post-abortion – use another method in the interim.

GP Notes: The role of the GP

- The earlier in pregnancy an abortion is performed, the lower the risk of complications. General practice is often the 1st stage of the referral procedure – have arrangements which minimize delay.
- Termination of pregnancy, especially for 'social' reasons, is a difficult ethical area for many GPs. We do not sit in moral judgement. Whatever your views, be sympathetic and if not prepared to refer yourself, arrange for the patient to see someone who will as soon as possible.
- Confirm pregnancy if unsure. Assess dates by bimanual palpation or arrange dating USS.
- Counselling – unbiased counselling to allow a woman to reach a decision she feels is right for her – this is an important decision she will have to live with for the rest of her life. Why does she want a termination? Has she considered alternatives? Does her partner/do her parents know? What are their views?
- Ideally the woman should be given some time once she has all the information to make her decision (e.g. follow-up in a few days). Offer a let-out clause – she can always change her mind right up until the time of the procedure and you will support whatever decision she makes.
- Consider signing form HSA1.
- Discuss contraception after TOP (ideally do this before TOP so it can be started immediately after).
- Arrange follow-up after the procedure.

Advice for patients: Information and support for women about termination of pregnancy

Marie Stopes International ☎ 0845 300 8090
🖳 www.mariestopes.org.uk
British Pregnancy Advisory Service (BPAS) ☎ 0845 730 40 30
🖳 www.bpas.org
Brook Advisory Centres (patients <25y. only) ☎ 0800 0185 023
🖳 www.brook.org.uk
Antenatal Results and Choices (ARC) Supports parents faced with termination for fetal abnormality ☎ 0207 631 0285
🖳 www.arc-uk.org

Further information

RCOG The care of women requesting induced abortion (2001)
🖳 www. rcog.org.uk

Chapter 5

Pregnancy

Pre-pregnancy and antenatal care
Pre-conception & early pregnancy counselling *200*
Antenatal care *204*
Who should deliver where? *212*
Screening in pregnancy *214*

Symptoms
Symptoms arising in pregnancy *220*
Rashes in pregnancy *226*
Bleeding in pregnancy *232*

Problems in pregnancy
Haemolytic disease and rhesus isoimmunization *240*
A–Z of medical conditions in pregnancy *242*
Epilepsy and pregnancy *248*
Diabetes in pregnancy *250*
Hypertension in pregnancy *252*
Infection in pregnancy *256*
Intrauterine growth *260*
Breech babies and multiple pregnancy *262*

Labour 264

Obstetric emergencies 268

Postnatal care
Maternal postnatal care *274*
Common postnatal problems *276*
The neonatal check *282*
Neonatal bloodspot screening *288*
Feeding babies *292*
The 6-week checks *294*
Stillbirth and neonatal death *296*

Pre-conception and early pregnancy counselling

The aim of pre-pregnancy care is to give a woman enough information for her pregnancy to occur under the optimal possible circumstances. Areas to cover include the following.

Smoking: ↓ ovulation, ↓ sperm count, ↓ sperm motility.

Once the woman is pregnant, smoking:
- ↑ miscarriage rate (x2) and risk of ectopic pregnancy
- ↑ risk of placenta praevia and placental abruption
- ↑ risk of premature rupture of membranes and pre-term delivery
- ↑ risk of cleft deformities
- ↑ perinatal mortality and ↓ birth weight (by an average of ≈ 200g).

Once the baby has delivered, smoking is associated with:
- ↑ rate of cot death
- ↑ chest infections and otitis media in children.

27% of pregnant women are smoking at the time of delivery. Explain risks and advise on ways to stop – 📖 p.14.

Alcohol: Fetal alcohol syndrome is rare and tends to occur in babies of heavy drinkers, especially those who binge drink. Effects of smaller quantities of alcohol are less clear but even 1 drink/d. is associated with a small ↓ in growth and intellect. Miscarriage rates are ↑ in moderate drinkers. Current advice is to avoid alcohol in pregnancy.

Illicit drugs: Cannabis (used by 5% mothers) is possibly associated with poorer motor skills in children and strongly linked with cigarette smoking – discourage. If taking other illicit drugs, refer for specialist care.

Diet: See opposite.

Folate supplementation: ↓ risk of neural tube defect (open spina bifida, anencephaly, encephalocoele) by 72%.
- *If no previous neural tube defects:* 0.4mg od when pregnancy is being planned and for 12wk. after conception.
- *If 1 parent/sibling affected, mother is affected herself, on anti-epileptic medication, diabetic, or previous child affected:* Advise 5mg od from the time the pregnancy is being planned until 13wk. after conception.

Only ~1:3 women take folic acid prior to conception. Effect of starting in early pregnancy is unevaluated. Supplements can be prescribed or are available OTC from chemists/supermarkets. Introduction of folic acid-fortified flour has recently been approved.

Other supplements
- *Vitamin D:* The DoH recommend 10mcg (400iu)/d. but limited evidence for general use. Consider for women from the Indian subcontinent (deficient due to poor sun exposure and diet), coeliacs and those on heparin.
- *Iron:* Don't routinely offer – for most, side-effects outweigh benefits.

Advice for patients:

Healthy eating tips: Eat a variety of foods including:
- plenty of fruit and vegetables – at least 5 portions per day
- plenty of starchy foods, e.g. bread, pasta, rice or potatoes
- protein-rich foods, e.g. lean meat, chicken, fish, eggs, beans, lentils
- fibre, e.g. wholegrain bread, pasta or rice, fruit & vegetables
- dairy foods containing calcium, e.g. milk, cheese & yoghurt

Folic acid (folate): Reduces risk of conditions such as spina bifida. Take folic acid supplements (400mcg) every day from stopping contraception until you are 12 weeks' pregnant. Eat foods containing folate, e.g. green vegetables, brown rice, fortified bread & cereals.

Iron: Eat iron-rich foods, e.g. red meat, beans, lentils, green vegetables, & fortified cereals. Fruit, fruit juice & vegetables help with iron absorption.

Avoid

Pâté & some unpasteurized dairy products: All pâtés (including vegetable), Camembert, Brie, other ripened soft cheeses, & blue cheese may contain *Listeria* which causes miscarriage, stillbirth & infections in newborn babies.

Raw or undercooked meat, eggs & ready meals: Risk of food poisoning.
- Wash your hands after handling raw meat.
- Keep raw meat separate from foods ready to eat .
- Only eat well-cooked meat – hot right through with no pink bits left.
- Only eat eggs cooked until white and yolk are solid. Shop mayonnaise and mousses are safe but avoid home-made dishes containing raw egg.
- Ensure ready meals are piping hot all the way through.

Liver products and vitamin A supplements: Too much vitamin A can harm a baby's development. Avoid eating liver (and liver products, e.g. pâté) and supplements containing vitamin A or fish liver oils.

Some types of fish: Eat 2 or more portions of fish per week (including 1 of oily fish – mackerel, sardines, fresh – not canned – tuna or trout) but:
- Avoid shark, swordfish or marlin and limit tuna to 2 steaks or 4 cans weekly. Mercury in these fish can harm a baby's nervous system.
- Only eat 1 or 2 portions of oily fish per week.
- Avoid raw shellfish as it can cause food poisoning.

Peanuts: If any close family members have allergies, asthma, eczema and/or hayfever, your baby may be at risk of nut allergy – avoid peanuts when pregnant and breast feeding.

Alcohol and caffeine: Avoid alcohol. High caffeine levels can cause miscarriage or low birth weight. There is caffeine in coffee, tea, chocolate, cola and some 'high energy' drinks. You can drink 4 cups of coffee, 6 cups of tea, or 8 cans of cola daily.

Gardening and changing cat litter: Toxoplasmosis can harm an unborn baby's nervous system and/or cause blindness. The parasite which causes it is found in meat, cat faeces & soil. Wear gloves when gardening or changing cat litter and wash your hands afterwards.

Contraception: Women contemplating pregnancy are usually still using contraception. Discussion about how to stop/what to expect may be helpful (e.g. injectables, IUCD).

Sexual intercourse: Not known to be harmful during pregnancy.

Chronic disease: Review of pre-existing medical conditions with referral for expert advice where necessary.

- Diabetes mellitus – refer for specialist diabetic review. Consider changing women taking sulphonylureas or metformin to insulin (📖 p.250).
- Epilepsy – refer for specialist review of medication (📖 p.248).
- Heart disease – refer for specialist advice if situation is not clear.
- Genito-urinary disease (e.g. HIV, genital warts, bacterial vaginosis) – refer for treatment/advice on mode of delivery if necessary (📖 p.256).

Review of medication: Drug handling by the body is altered during pregnancy and drugs can cause damage to the developing fetus.

- Discontinue known teratogens prior to conception
- Advise patients to avoid OTC medication unless they have checked safety with their doctor or midwife.
- Avoid prescribed medication as much as possible – few medicines have proven safety in pregnancy. If prescribing use only well-known and tested drugs at the smallest possible doses, and only when benefit to the mother outweighs risk.

Problems in previous pregnancies

- Recurrent miscarriage (📖 p.234)
- Cervical incompetence (📖 p.104)
- Congenital abnormalities/inherited disorders – pre-pregnancy counselling and detailed advice on genetic screening for high-risk pregnancies is available via regional genetics services.

Rubella status: If rubella status is unknown suggest it is checked. Rubella infection in early pregnancy carries a high chance (40–70%) of deafness, blindness, cardiac abnormalities or multiple fetal abnormalities (📖 p.226). If the woman is not rubella immune, suggest immunization with avoidance of pregnancy for 3mo. afterwards (live vaccine). Recheck rubella status 3mo. after immunization.

Work/benefits: Discussion of benefits available during pregnancy (Table 5.1) and employment law (📖 p.210) is necessary so that women may avoid possible hazards at work, attend for antenatal care and plan their maternity leave from early in pregnancy.

Discussion of antenatal care and screening available

- Brief discussion of antenatal screening and antenatal care procedures allows women to investigate their choices in pregnancy at their leisure.
- Brief discussion about miscarriage and possibility of infertility allows women to be more confident about asking for help if problems with conception/early pregnancy occur.

Advice for patients: Further information on maternity rights and benefits

Citizens' Advice Bureau 🖳 www.adviceguide.org.uk

Table 5.1 Benefits available to pregnant women

Benefit	Eligibility	How to apply	Benefits gained
Statutory Maternity Pay (SMP)*	• Worked for the same employer for 26wk. into the 15th wk. before the baby is due • Pregnant at (or have had the baby by) the 11th wk. before the baby is due • Earning ≥ NI lower earnings limit in the relevant period	• Inform employer at least 28d. before starting leave • Mat B1 form	Paid for up to 26wk. (Maternity Pay Period – MPP) – can start any time from 11th wk. before the baby is due until the week of birth • 1st 6wk. – 90% average earnings • 6–26wk. – 90% of usual earnings or £112.75/wk. – whichever is lower
Maternity Allowance (MA)*	• Employed/self-employed for ≥26wk. in the 66wk. preceding the baby's due date (test period) • Average weekly earnings of ≥£30/wk. for at least 13wk. of the test period • Do not qualify for SMP (e.g. changed jobs, became unemployed, self-employed)	Apply >26/40 and within 3mo. of date MA due to start. Need: • Form MA1 (available from social security offices, employer or DWP 🖥 www.dwp.gov.uk • MATB1; and, if employed, • Form SMP1 from employer	Paid for 26wk. (Maternity Allowance Period – MAP) – can start any time from 11th week before the baby is due until the day after birth. 90% of usual earnings or £112.75/wk. – whichever is lower
Sure Start Maternity Grant	• From 11wk. before baby is due to <3mo. after birth/adoption • Claiming Income Support or Income-based Job-Seekers Allowance; Child Tax Credit at a higher rate than the maximum family element or Working Tax Credit with a disability or severe disability element	Form SF100 from social security offices	£500 payment

Other benefits:
- *Free prescriptions/dentistry*: available to all mothers while pregnant and for 1y. after the expected date of delivery. Claim using form FW8.
- Women claiming Income Support, income-based Job-Seekers Allowance or Child Tax Credit may be able to claim *free milk and vitamin supplements* if >10wk. pregnant – details of how to claim are included in DoH booklet 'Free milk and vitamins: a guide for families', available from 🖥 www.dh.gov.uk
- *Incapacity Benefit and Income Support* may be available for women unable to claim SMP or MA.

GMS contract		
CON 2	The team has a policy for providing pre-conceptual advice	1 point

Antenatal care

Objectives of good obstetric care
- To provide a safe outcome for the mother and baby with the minimum of avoidable complications.
- To make the birth experience as satisfying as possible for the mother and her family.
- To make optimal use of available resources.

Pregnancy is a risky business for both mother and baby. Every year women die as a result of pregnancy, – the commonest causes being eclampsia, haemorrhage, pulmonary embolism and infection.

Definitions
- *Gravity* – number of pregnancies a woman has had (at any stage).
- *Parity* – number of pregnancies resulting in delivery >24wk. gestation (or live births <24wk.).
- *Primipara/multipara* – woman who has been delivered of a child for the 1st time (primipara) or 2nd or subsequent time (multipara).

Pregnancy tests: Detect urinary β-HCG. +ve from 1st day of missed period until ≈ 20wk. gestation. Remain positive for ≈ 5d. after miscarriage/termination or fetal death.

Antenatal care: Figure 5.1, 📖 p.208. Increased emphasis on antenatal screening means the 1st antenatal appointment should now be offered as early into pregnancy as possible. National guidelines suggest further appointments for healthy women should be offered at 16wk., 28wk., 34wk., 36wk., 28wk., and, if not already delivered, at 41wk. Additionally, healthy nulliparous women should be offered appointments at 25wk., 31wk., and 40wk. Provide additional appointments as needed for women with problems (Box 5.1).

First antenatal visit: The primary function of this visit is to identify those women needing additional care (Box 5.1). As there is so much information to be collected/discussed, consider 2 appointments.

History
- This pregnancy – LMP, usual cycle, fertility problems, contraception, desirability of pregnancy, any problems so far
- Estimated date of delivery (EDD) – Figure 5.2, 📖 p.209
- Past pregnancies – outcome and complications of previous pregnancies
- Past/current medical history – illness (including psychiatric illness), drugs, allergies, varicose veins, abdominal/pelvic surgery
- Family history – ↑ BP, DM, congenital/genetic abnormality, twins
- Social history – smoking, alcohol consumption, illicit drugs, support at home, work, housing, financial problems

Examination
- Check weight and calculate BMI – low BMI ↑ risk of pre-eclampsia, IUGR & pre-term delivery; high BMI is associated with pre-eclampsia.
- Listen to heart and lungs, check BP and examine abdomen.
- Fetal heart with a sonic aid per abdomen from 12–14wk. gestation.
- Fundus can be felt per abdomen from 12wk.

Box 5.1 Women who may need additional care

Women with

- Conditions such as ↑ BP, cardiac, renal, endocrine, autoimmune, psychiatric or haematological disorders, epilepsy, DM, cancer or HIV
- Factors that make the woman vulnerable, e.g. lack of social support
- Age ≥40y. or ≤18y.
- BMI ≥35kg/m^2 or <18kg/m^2
- Previous Caesarean section
- Severe pre-eclampsia, HELLP or eclampsia
- Previous pre-eclampsia or eclampsia
- ≥ 3 miscarriages
- Previous pre-term birth or mid-trimester loss
- Previous psychiatric illness or puerperal psychosis
- Previous neonatal death or stillbirth
- Previous baby with congenital abnormality
- Previous small-for-gestational-age or large-for-gestational-age baby
- Family history of genetic disorder

GP Notes: Provision and organization of care

- *Offer midwife- and GP-led care for uncomplicated pregnancies* – routine involvement of an obstetrician does not improve outcome.
- *Continuity of care* – extend into the post-partum/postnatal period if possible. Provide a small team of carers with whom the woman feels comfortable. Results in ↑ satisfaction, ↓ intervention rates and improved psychosocial outcome.
- *Ensure care is readily and easily accessible* – base care primarily in the community. Aim to create a safe environment in which women can discuss sensitive issues, e.g. domestic violence, sexual abuse, mental illness, drug abuse. ⓘ Women with physical/cognitive/sensory impairment, non-English speakers/readers, or special groups, e.g. teenage mothers, may need special consideration.
- *Use structured maternity notes* – preferably using a standardized, national maternity record. Women should carry their own notes.

ⓘ Beware of overloading the pregnant woman with information.

Advice for patients: Information and support for pregnant women

NHS Direct 🖳 www.nhsdirect.nhs.uk
National Childbirth Trust (NCT) ☎ 0870 444 8707 🖳 www.nctpregnancyandbabycare.com
Family Planning Association ☎ 0845 310 1334 🖳 www.fpa.org.uk
Birth Choice UK 🖳 www.birthchoiceuk.com
Mothers 35 plus 🖳 www.mothers35plus.co.uk
Emma's Diary 🖳 www.emmasdiary.co.uk
NHS Scotland 🖳 www.hebs.nhs.scot.uk/readysteadybaby
Baby World 🖳 www.babyworld.co.uk

Box 5.1 is reproduced with permission from NICE, 🖳 www.nice.org.uk

205

Investigations
- Offer early USS for dating purposes (<16wk. – ideally 10–13wk.).
- Arrange routine anomaly scan at 18–20wk. gestation – if the placenta extends across the internal cervical os, arrange another USS at 36wk.
- Check blood for:
  - Hb, blood group, Rhesus status and red cell antibodies.
  - Syphilis and rubella serology, HBsAg and HIV with pre-test counselling (📖 p.218).
  - Sickle test and/or Hb electrophoresis (if in high-risk group or area).
- MSU for protein and bacteriuria.
- Discuss and offer antenatal screening (📖 p.214) for all women.

Health promotion: 📖 p.200 and 📖 pp.210–11

Education
- Social security benefits (📖 p.203)
- Employment rights (📖 p.210)
- Free prescriptions and dental care (📖 p.203)
- Antenatal/parentcraft classes
- Local services (e.g. aquanatal classes, yoga for pregnancy)
- Choice of place of delivery and options available (📖 p.212)
- Procedure for antenatal care – Figure 5.1 (📖 p.208)
- Travel and limitations (📖 p.211).

Certification: Supply form FW8 which allows application for free prescriptions and dental care at the first antenatal appointment. Provide Mat B1 form at 20wk.

Information
- Give 'The Pregnancy Book' to all first-time pregnant women (order on ☎ 0870 155 54 55 – code 266528).
- Offer 'Emma's Diary' to all pregnant women (order from RCGP on ☎ 01628 640892) – contains information about pregnancy and vouchers.

Discussion: Worries about pregnancy or social situation – ask specifically about domestic violence.

Follow-up visits: Ask about problems and untoward symptoms. Provide the neonatal bloodspot screening leaflet at ~28wk.

Routine checks: Figure 5.1 (📖 p.208)
- BP
- Oedema
- Urine for protein
- Fundal height (from 24/25wk.)
- Fetal heart sounds
- Fetal lie and presentation (from 36wk.)

❗ Primiparous women are aware of movements from ≈ 20wk. but multiparous women often feel movements earlier.

Routine laboratory checks: Hb & antibodies at 28wk. (though see 📖 p.240).

Further information

NICE 🖥 www.nice.org.uk
- Antenatal care: routine care for healthy pregnant women (and patient information – 2003 – update due in 2007)
- Maternal and fetal nutrition – due for publication in 2007

GMS contract

Maternity services: Provided by practices as an additional service, i.e. most practices are expected to provide this service and payment is included in the global sum. If a practice 'opts out' global sum is ↓ by 2.1%.

Requirements: Practices should provide maternity services to pregnant women with exception of intrapartum care. This should include:
- routine antenatal care *and*
- postnatal care to mothers and babies (excluding the neonatal check) from birth or discharge from 2° care until the 14th day after delivery.

Intrapartum care: Intrapartum care and neonatal checks can be provided to women by GPs at home or in GP maternity units as a *national enhanced service*. One payment is payable for each woman who receives intrapartum care and a further payment for each neonatal check.

Quality and outcomes framework points

MAT 1	Antenatal care and screening are offered according to current local guidelines	6 points
Information 6	Information is available to patients on roles of the GP, community midwife, health visitor and hospital clinics in the provision of antenatal and postnatal care	½ point

Box 5.2 Interventions that are *not* part of routine antenatal care

- Repeated maternal weighing – only weigh if clinical management is likely to be influenced, e.g. concern about nutrition
- Breast examination
- Pelvic examination
- Screening for postnatal depression using the Edinburgh Postnatal Depression Score
- Iron supplementation
- Vitamin D supplementation
- Screening for the following infections:
  - *Chlamydia trachomatis*
  - Cytomegalovirus
  - Hepatitis C virus
  - Group B streptococcus
  - Toxoplasmosis
  - Bacterial vaginosis
- Screening for gestational diabetes mellitus – including dipstick testing for glycosuria
- Screening for pre-term birth by assessment of cervical length (either by USS or vaginal examination) or using fetal fibronectin
- Formal fetal movement counting
- Antenatal electronic cardiotocography
- USS >24wk.
- Umbilical artery Doppler USS
- Uterine artery Doppler USS to predict pre-eclampsia

Box 5.2 is reproduced with permission from NICE, 🖥 www.nice.org.uk

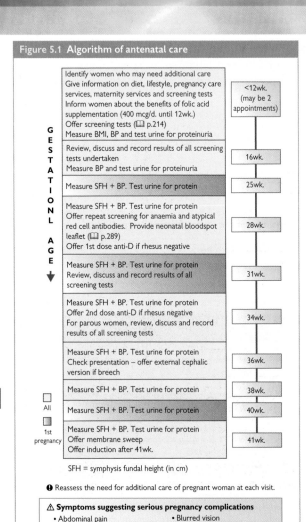

Figure 5.1 Algorithm of antenatal care

GESTATIONAL AGE →		
Identify women who may need additional care Give information on diet, lifestyle, pregnancy care services, maternity services and screening tests Inform women about the benefits of folic acid supplementation (400 mcg/d. until 12wk.) Offer screening tests (📖 p.214) Measure BMI, BP and test urine for proteinuria	<12wk. (may be 2 appointments)	
Review, discuss and record results of all screening tests undertaken Measure BP and test urine for proteinuria	16wk.	
Measure SFH + BP. Test urine for protein	25wk.	
Measure SFH + BP. Test urine for protein Offer repeat screening for anaemia and atypical red cell antibodies. Provide neonatal bloodspot leaflet (📖 p.289) Offer 1st dose anti-D if rhesus negative	28wk.	
Measure SFH + BP. Test urine for protein Review, discuss and record results of all screening tests	31wk.	
Measure SFH + BP. Test urine for protein Offer 2nd dose anti-D if rhesus negative For parous women, review, discuss and record results of all screening tests	34wk.	
Measure SFH + BP. Test urine for protein Check presentation – offer external cephalic version if breech	36wk.	
Measure SFH + BP. Test urine for protein	38wk.	
Measure SFH + BP. Test urine for protein	40wk.	
Measure SFH + BP. Test urine for protein Offer membrane sweep Offer induction after 41wk.	41wk.	

☐ All
☐ 1st pregnancy

SFH = symphysis fundal height (in cm)

❶ Reassess the need for additional care of pregnant woman at each visit.

⚠ **Symptoms suggesting serious pregnancy complications**
- Abdominal pain
- Vaginal bleeding
- Clear vaginal loss
- Severe headache
- Blurred vision
- Persistent itching
- Changed/↓ fetal activity

Figure 5.1 is reproduced from Antenatal Care: *Routine Care for the Healthy Pregnant Woman.* Clinical Guidline 2003, with permission from the Royal College of Obstetricians and Gynaecologists.

Figure 5.2 Expected date of delivery calculator

ⓘ As a rough guide, EDD = date of LMP + 1 year + 7 days − 3 months

Date of first day of last menstrual period							*Month →*					
Day ↓	Jan	Feb	Mar	Apr	May	Jun	Jul	Aug	Sep	Oct	Nov	Dec
1	8/10	8/11	6/12	6/1	5/2	8/3	7/4	8/5	8/6	8/7	8/8	7/9
2	9/10	9/11	7/12	7/1	6/2	9/3	8/4	9/5	9/6	9/7	9/8	8/9
3	10/10	10/11	8/12	8/1	7/2	10/3	9/4	10/5	10/6	10/7	10/8	9/9
4	11/10	11/11	9/12	9/1	8/2	11/3	10/4	11/5	11/6	11/7	11/8	10/9
5	12/10	12/11	10/12	10/1	9/2	12/3	11/4	12/5	12/6	12/7	12/8	11/9
6	13/10	13/11	11/12	11/1	10/2	13/3	12/4	13/5	13/6	13/7	13/8	12/9
7	14/10	14/11	12/12	12/1	11/2	14/3	13/4	14/5	14/6	14/7	14/8	13/9
8	15/10	15/11	13/12	13/1	12/2	15/3	14/4	15/5	15/6	15/7	15/8	14/9
9	16/10	16/11	14/12	14/1	13/2	16/3	15/4	16/5	16/6	16/7	16/8	15/9
10	17/10	17/11	15/12	15/1	14/2	17/3	16/4	17/5	17/6	17/7	17/8	16/9
11	18/10	18/11	16/12	16/1	15/2	18/3	17/4	18/5	18/6	18/7	18/8	17/9
12	19/10	19/11	17/12	17/1	16/2	19/3	18/4	19/5	19/6	19/7	19/8	18/9
13	20/10	20/11	18/12	18/1	17/2	20/3	19/4	20/5	20/6	20/7	20/8	19/9
14	21/10	21/11	19/12	19/1	18/2	21/3	20/4	21/5	21/6	21/7	21/8	20/9
15	22/10	22/11	20/12	20/1	19/2	22/3	21/4	22/5	22/6	22/7	22/8	21/9
16	23/10	23/11	21/12	21/1	20/2	23/3	22/4	23/5	23/6	23/7	23/8	22/9
17	24/10	24/11	22/12	22/1	21/2	24/3	23/4	24/5	24/6	24/7	24/8	23/9
18	25/10	25/11	23/12	23/1	22/2	25/3	24/4	25/5	25/6	25/7	25/8	24/9
19	26/10	26/11	24/12	24/1	23/2	26/3	25/4	26/5	26/6	26/7	26/8	25/9
20	27/10	27/11	25/12	25/1	24/2	27/3	26/4	27/5	27/6	27/7	27/8	26/9
21	28/10	28/11	26/12	26/1	25/2	28/3	27/4	28/5	28/6	28/7	28/8	27/9
22	29/10	29/11	27/12	27/1	26/2	29/3	28/4	29/5	29/6	29/7	29/8	28/9
23	30/10	30/11	28/12	28/1	27/2	30/3	29/4	30/5	30/6	30/7	30/8	29/9
24	31/10	1/12	29/12	29/1	28/2	31/3	30/4	31/5	1/7	31/7	31/8	30/9
25	1/11	2/12	30/12	30/1	1/3	1/4	1/5	1/6	2/7	1/8	1/9	1/10
26	2/11	3/12	31/12	31/1	2/3	2/4	2/5	2/6	3/7	2/8	2/9	2/10
27	3/11	4/12	1/1	1/2	3/3	3/4	3/5	3/6	4/7	3/8	3/9	3/10
28	4/11	5/12	2/1	2/2	4/3	4/4	4/5	4/6	5/7	4/8	4/9	4/10
29	5/11		3/1	3/2	5/3	5/4	5/5	5/6	6/7	5/8	5/9	5/10
30	6/11		4/1	4/2	6/3	6/4	6/5	6/6	7/7	6/8	6/9	6/10
31	7/11		5/1		7/3		7/5	7/6		7/8		7/10

Dates are given in the format day/month

Work: For most women, work in pregnancy is safe. By law:

- Employers must assess risks to the health/safety of the pregnant woman and adjust for risks accordingly
- Women are entitled to time off work for antenatal care
- Women cannot work >33wk. into pregnancy unless the woman's GP informs her employer she may continue
- Employers may not require/allow return to work <2wk. after childbirth
- Women who work for an employer qualify for 26wk. ordinary maternity leave (52wk. if she has worked for her employer for 26wk. before the 15th week before her EDD) and can apply for flexible/part-time working hours on return to work.

Further information

- Health and Safety Executive 🖳 www.hse.gov.uk/mothers
- Citizens' Advice Bureau 🖳 www.adviceguide.org.uk

Exercise: Moderate exercise is safe and healthy. Avoid:

- Contact sports, high-impact sports, and vigorous racquet sports
- Scuba diving – possible link with fetal birth defects and may cause fetal decompression disease.

❶ Advise women to wear gloves when/wash hands after gardening or changing cat litter.

Diet: Normal weight gain in pregnancy is 7–8kg. Do not routinely weigh unless worries about nutrition and/or weight.

Foods to avoid in pregnancy – 📖 p.201

Alcohol: 📖 p.10. Avoid alcohol in pregnancy. *Fetal alcohol syndrome* – a triad of growth retardation, CNS involvement and facial deformity – is rare (0.4/1000 live births) and tends to affect babies of heavy/binge drinkers. More common are lesser ↓ in growth/intellect.

Smoking: 📖 p.14. Stress benefits of quitting at any stage. Halving the number of cigarettes smoked results in an average 92g ↑ in birth weight.

NHS pregnancy smoking line ☎ 0800 169 0 169

Drugs: Avoid unnecessary medicines (including OTC) and illicit drugs.

Further information on drugs in pregnancy is available from the BNF (Appendix 4) and National Teratology Information Service ☎ 0191 232 1525

Complementary therapies: Use as little as possible.

- *Avoid* – oil of evening primrose (possible ↑ in PROM)
- *No benefit* – raspberry leaf tea[R] (but probably no risk either)
- *Possibly beneficial* – ginger[R], P6 acupressure[R] and acupuncture[C] for nausea and vomiting; moxibustion[C] for breech presentation; acupuncture[C] for backache/pelvic pain; acupuncture[R] for insomnia
- *No/limited evidence* – St John's wort (studies in progress), hypnosis, aromatherapy.

Travel

- *Car:* Seatbelt should go above and below – *not* across – the bump.
- *Air:* Check specific requirements of carrier. Most airlines will not accept pregnant women >32wk. (rarely 36wk. with a doctor's letter).

⚠ Travel involving long periods of immobility (>5h.) is associated with ↑ risk of venous thromboembolism. Advise women to drink plenty of non-alcoholic fluids; keep their legs moving whilst sitting or walk up and down the aisle; and purchase graduated compression hosiery OTC.

Travel abroad: Best time to travel is in the 2nd trimester. Travel to high-risk areas is best postponed/cancelled. Avoid travel to places at altitudes >2500m (↑ risk of IUGR/ pre-eclampsia).

Vaccines: Assess risk/benefit ratio on an individual basis.
- *Avoid live vaccines* – BCG, cholera, measles, mumps, rubella, varicella, smallpox, Japanese encephalitis. ❶ Inadvertent administration has not been shown to cause harm.
- *Inactivated vaccines* – can be given if needed (best after 1st trimester) – hepatitis A & B, influenza (consult consultant physician), meningococcal infection (only if significant risk of infection), inactivated poliomyelitis (normally avoided), rabies, tetanus/diphtheria, yellow fever (avoid unless at high risk).

Malaria: Infection in pregnancy – 📖 p.258. Travel to malaria areas is best avoided. If unavoidable:
- Sleep in screened accommodation, spraying screens with insecticide each evening, and use a prethroid vaporizer. If screens are not available use permethrin-impregnated bed net (kits available).
- In the evenings wear long-sleeved shirts and trousers; protect limbs with diethyltoluamide/lemon-eucalyptus repellant.

Chemoprophylactic drugs – regimes vary with location and time of year. Consult travel advice centres (e.g. National travel health network 🖥 www.nathnac.org) for up-to-date information on risk. Chloroquine and proguanil can be used in usual doses. Give folic acid 5mg od with proguanil. Consider mefloquine for travel to chloroquine-resistant areas. Avoid *Malarone*® and doxycycline.

Contaminated food/water
- Risk of listeriosis, toxoplasmosis and hepatitis E (avoid travel to hepatitis E areas – ~20% death rate in 3rd trimester).
- Severe dehydration due to diarrhoea may be harmful to the fetus.

Insurance for travel: Ensure adequate cover. Most companies insure pregnant women to 28wk., some to 32wk. In Europe:
- *Form E111:* Provides free emergency medical care. Does not cover costs of transport or repatriation.
- *Form E112:* Is required if >36wk. or planning to deliver in the European Economic Area (EEA) but outside the UK .

The UK has reciprocal agreements with some other countries for urgently needed medical treatment at ↓ cost/free. Countries and services available are listed on the DoH travel advice website (🖥 www.dh.gov.uk). Proof of British nationality or UK residence is needed.

Who should deliver where?

Since the publication of *'Changing Childbirth'*, all those offering maternity care must give women choices about type of care, place of care and birth and the information to make those choices 'avoiding personal bias or preference'. Who delivers where ultimately depends on the choice the woman makes. *Options:*

- Consultant unit
- Midwife or GP/midwife unit integral with/attached to a consultant unit
- 'Isolated unit' – distant from a specialist unit and manned by midwifes or midwifes and GPs
- Home ($\approx$ 1% deliveries in UK).

Legal position of GPs: GPs are often fearful of litigation if they accept a woman for delivery outside a specialist unit. Even women with no risk factors can run into problems – rapid intervention to save life is needed in $\approx$ 5% deliveries. Due to the low numbers of deliveries most GPs attend, they perceive they lack expertise which compounds this worry. Changes in the organization of out-of-hours cover and the time commitment to the GP entailed in home deliveries (and inadequate remuneration for that time) mean GP-attended home deliveries are uncommon.

The legal position is that
- GPs are responsible only for their own acts or omissions.
- Midwives are accountable for their own actions and decisions.
- The GP only becomes responsible for a woman's care in labour when the midwife attending seeks his/her advice. The GP is then bound by terms and conditions of service to offer advice (either over the telephone or by attending), whether or not the woman has been accepted for maternity care.
- If an accident occurs, the GP would be judged against standards of a colleague of similar skills and training, not a specialist obstetrician.

Duties of the GP
- Provision of impartial advice about available services locally.
- Discussion of the available options in a way to enable the woman to make an informed choice.
- To make arrangements for provision of care.

Specialist unit vs. community-based care: Although the perinatal and maternal death rates have $\downarrow$ as the proportion of hospital births has $\uparrow$ in the UK, no evidence exists that hospital is the safest place for healthy women to have low-risk births. In other countries (e.g. the Netherlands) there is some evidence to the contrary. For women with pre-existing illness or high-risk births, either advise to deliver in a consultant unit or refer to obstetrics for discussion of place of delivery (Box 5.3).

> ⚠ If a woman decides to deliver away from a specialist unit, she should be informed of what facilities and levels of skill and expertise are and are not available. Record the discussion in her notes.

Table 5.2 Reasons why women choose home or hospital births

Home birth	Hospital birth
To avoid intervention (31%)	
More in control in familiar surroundings (25%)	
Previous home birth (11%)	Safety (84%)
More relaxed at home (10%)	Previous hospital birth (6%)
Fear of hospitals (10%)	
Continuity of care with midwife (4%)	

Box 5.3 Women with pre-existing illness or high-risk births

Advise to deliver in a consultant unit
At booking if
- Pre-existing medical disorders – epilepsy, DM, cardiac, renal, respiratory, hepatitis B, HIV, active genital herpes, IV drug abuse, history of major gynaecological surgery, or known uterine abnormality
- Familial disorder with a high-risk of transmission
- ↑ BP
- Height <150cm and primigravida
- Weight at 1st examination <50kg or >100kg
- Past obstetric history of:
    - perinatal death
    - rhesus isoimmunization
    - pre-eclampsia or eclampsia
    - antepartum haemorrhage
    - IUGR
    - Caesarean section
    - post-partum haemorrhage
    - retained placenta
    - inverted uterus
    - shoulder dystocia

If any of the following develop during pregnancy
- Polyhydramnios
- Malpresentation
- Ante-partum haemorrhage
- Prolonged pregnancy (>40wk.+10d.)
- Pre-term labour <37wk.
- Suspected IUGR
- Pregnancy-induced ↑ BP
- Multiple pregnancy
- Gestational DM

Refer to obstetrics to discuss place of delivery if
- Primigravida <18y. and >35y. or ≥ para 5
- Excessive maternal weight gain
- Failure of engagement of the head near term in a primigravida
- Past history of prolonged labour, large baby, subfertility or cone biopsy

⚠ Other rarer medical or obstetric conditions may require specialist advice – if in doubt, refer.

Further information
NICE 🖳 www.nice.org.uk
- Antenatal care: routine care for healthy pregnant women (2003 – due for revision in 2007)
- Intrapartum care – due for publication in 2007
RCOG Home birth 🖳 www.rcog.org.uk

213

Screening in pregnancy

Most women undergo some form of screening in pregnancy, aiming to identify, prevent and treat actual or potential problems. Women and their partners must be given unbiased information verbally and in writing regarding screening and diagnostic tests, the meaning and consequences of both, what to expect in terms of results, and further options for management. The right to accept or decline should be made clear – and the decision recorded in the antenatal notes.

GPs need to be aware of techniques of prenatal diagnosis to:
- identify all women who might benefit from genetic counselling and/or early assessment by the obstetrician
- counsel patients about the accuracy and risk of prenatal diagnosis *and*
- ensure opportunities for prenatal diagnosis are not overlooked.

Pre-pregnancy genetic screening: There are many inherited diseases. Refer couples before pregnancy if they request referral or have factors which put them at high risk of having a baby with a genetic disorder (Box 5.4). Warn couples that most tests give no absolute 'yes' or 'no' but are a risk assessment.

Tools of antenatal screening

Basic screening tests: Blood and urine tests – many women are not aware these tests have been done, let alone their purpose or results. Ensure women are given information about the reasons for, significance of, and results of routine tests and record in the notes that permission has been given to do them. Usual tests are:
- Hb estimation
- Blood group
- Antibody screening (📖 p.240)
- Haemoglobinopathy screening (📖 p.218)
- MSU (📖 p.259)
- Urine dipstick for proteinuria (📖 p.218)
- Rubella immune status (📖 p.202)
- HIV status (📖 p.218)
- Syphilis status (📖 p.258)
- Hepatitis B status (📖 p.257)

ⓘ Rubella immune status is not strictly a screening test for this pregnancy but does identify susceptible women (~2.5%) so that post-partum vaccination may protect *future* pregnancies.

α-fetoprotein (AFP): Glycoprotein synthesized by the fetal liver. Can be measured in maternal blood and amniotic fluid. AFP is a non-specific test requiring those with abnormal values (Table 5.3) to undergo further investigation. Routinely offered in most centres as part of the Down's syndrome screening programme.

Ultrasound scan (USS)
- *Early USS* – Offer to all pregnant women at 10–13wk. for accurate gestational age assessment.
- *High-resolution 'anomaly' scan* – Offer at 18–20wk. to detect fetal structural abnormalities. Abnormalities are found in 2% of anomaly scans and 45% of structural abnormalities are found antenatally on USS (rate varies according to abnormality, i.e. 100% of babies with anencephaly are detected, but only 17% of cardiac abnormalities).

Box 5.4 Risk factors that warrant pre-pregnancy genetic screening

Personal or family history of genetic abnormality: e.g.
- Cystic fibrosis
- Down's syndrome
- Sickle cell disease
- β-thalassaemia
- Haemophilia
- Fragile X syndrome
- Duchenne and other muscular dystrophies
- Huntington's chorea
- Polycystic kidneys

High-risk ethnic groups
- Afro-Caribbean origin – sickle cell anaemia
- Indian subcontinent, Far East, Southern Europe – thalassaemia
- Ashkenazi Jew – Tay-Sachs disease

Older women: ↑ risk of Down's syndrome (📖 p.216).

Consanguinous couples: 1st degree cousins who have a baby together have an ↑ risk of congenital malformations in their offspring.

Table 5.3 Results of AFP testing

↑ AFP levels are associated with:	↓ AFP levels are associated with:
• Twins • Fetal malformation (10%) – neural tube defect, exomphalos, posterior urethral valves, nephrosis, GI obstruction, teratomas or Turner's syndrome • Adverse outcome (e.g. abruption, stillbirth) in those with ↑ levels but no detectable reason	• Diabetic mothers • Chromosomal abnormality, e.g. Down's syndrome (📖 p.216)

GP Notes:

Routine antenatal screening is NOT recommended for

Vaginal/genital infections
- Bacterial vaginosis
- Chlamydia
- Streptococcus B
- Genital herpes

Genetic conditions – refer for screening if a family member is affected
- Cystic fibrosis
- Familial dysautonomia
- Fragile X

Other infections
- Cytomegalovirus
- Hepatitis C
- HTLV-1
- Toxoplasmosis

Others
- Domestic violence
- Gestational diabetes
- Postnatal depression
- Pre-term labour
- Thrombocytopoenia
- Thrombophilia

Diagnostic tests

Chorionic villus sampling (CVS): At 10–12wk. gestation the developing placenta is sampled per abdomen or transcervically with ultrasound guidance. Used to detect genetic or metabolic abnormality in high-risk pregnancies.

- *Advantages:* undertaken earlier than amniocentesis to allow termination of affected pregnancies at an earlier stage.
- *Risks:* 2% miscarry; limb defects (rare).

Amniocentesis: Sampling of amniotic fluid via transabominal needle under ultrasound guidance. When undertaken for screening purposes takes place from 15wk. gestation. May be routinely offered to women at high-risk of fetal abnormality (e.g. women >35y. of age to exclude Down's syndrome) or to clarify abnormalities found with other screening tests (e.g. abnormal AFP or abnormality found on USS associated with genetic syndrome). 1% miscarriage risk.

Spina bifida: USS at 17–19wk. gestation detects 90–95% spina bifida and 100% anencephaly. AFP detects 80% of open defects and 90% of those with anencephaly. Confirmation with USS is required.

Down's syndrome:
The commonest single cause of mental handicap in children of school age. Incidence: 3/2000 births. Various screening measures may be used including:

- *Age:* Incidence ↑ with age – Table 5.4. Offer CVS or amniocentesis to all pregnant women >35y. (refer immediately if >40y.). Amniocentesis combined with routine anomaly scanning identifies ≈ 70% of all cases of Down's syndrome.
- *AFP alone:* Non-specific test. ↓ serum AFP may indicate chromosomal abnormality. Necessitates further evaluation in all cases.
- *Double/triple/quadruple test:* Blood test which measures AFP and human chorionic gonadotropin (hCG) ± oestriol (uE₃) ± inhibin A. Blood is taken at 16wk. gestation and a risk value calculated for the individual woman, taking into account age, exact gestation and weight. The result is expressed as a risk assessment (e.g. 1:300) or as a +ve or –ve result. A +ve result usually means the risk of having a Down's syndrome baby is >1:250 and amniocentesis is offered. Using a cut-off of 1:250 for amniocentesis, ~5% women require amniocentesis which turns out to be normal.
- *Nuchal translucency (NT) test:* USS measurement of the translucency of the nuchal fold in the neck of the fetus at 10–14wk. gestation (Figure 5.3). Detection rate ≈ 80%, false +ve rate ≈ 8%.
- *Integrated test:* Combines blood tests and USS to produce a single estimate of the woman's risk of having a child with Down's syndrome. Uses: woman's age; measurement at 10–13wk. gestation of nuchal translucency and maternal serum level of pregnancy-associated plasma protein A (PAPP-A); measurement 2–4wk. Later of maternal serum AFP, unconjugated oestriol, hCG and inhibin A. Detection rate: 85%. Only 1% of women require unnecessary amniocentesis.

⚠ The UK National Screening Committee has recommended all pregnant women, irrespective of age, should be offered screening for Down's syndrome. Recommended tests:

Gestation	11–14wk.	14–20wk.
Tests	• Nuchal translucency • Combined test (NT, hCG, PAPP-A)	• Triple test (AFP, hCG and uE_3) • Quadruple test (AFP, hCG, uE_3 and inhibin A)
	• Integrated test (NT, PAPP-A, AFP, hCG, uE3 and inhibin A) • Serum integrated test (PAPP-A, AFP, hCG, uE_3 and inhibin A) – used if NT measurement is not available	

ⓘ Test results are adjusted for age and gestation. If risk >1:250, refer for further investigation.

Table 5.4 Levels of risk of having a Down's syndrome pregnancy in relation to a woman's age

Woman's age (y.)	Risk as a ratio	% risk
20	1:1500	0.066
30	1:800	0.125
35	1:270	0.37
40	1:100	1.0
≥45	≥1:50	2.0

Reproduced with permission from Cuckle HS et al. Estimating a woman's risk of having a pregnancy associated with Down's syndrome using her age and serum alpha-fetoprotein level. *Br J Obstet Gynaecol.* (1987) 94(5) 387–402.

Figure 5.3 USS image of a fetus showing nuchal translucency

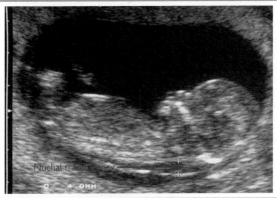

Nuchal translucency

217

Permission sought to reproduce figure 5.3.

Antenatal HIV testing: HIV testing is now offered as a routine part of antenatal screening in the UK.

Benefits of screening: Without intervention, ~20% babies born to mothers infected with HIV will become infected with HIV themselves. Administration of zidovudine to HIV-infected women from 28–32wk. into pregnancy until and including labour, and to the baby for the first 4–6wk. of life, together with delivery by Caesarean section and avoiding breast feeding, ↓ risk of transmission to ~2%.

ⓘ All pregnant women who are HIV +ve should be screened for genital infection – chlamydia, gonorrhoea and bacterial vaginosis, done as early as possible in pregnancy and at around 28wk. – as co-infection is common in certain subgroups of these women and can ↑ rate of mother-to-child transmission, as well as adversely affecting the pregnancy itself. Also check hepatitis B & C serology unless already done.

Haemoglobinopathies: Antenatal screening, performed as early in pregnancy as possible, is now offered to all women in the UK. Women identified as having a trait, or the disorder, should be referred for specialist counselling and their partners offered screening. Follow local guidelines for management in pregnancy and the puerperium.

Placenta praevia: Because most low-lying placenta detected at the routine 18–20wk. anomaly scan will resolve by the time the baby is born, only women with placenta praevia extending over the internal cervical os should be offered another transabdominal scan at 36wk. If this is unclear, a transvaginal scan should be offered.

Pre-eclampsia: At first contact, assess the pregnant woman's level of risk for pre-eclampsia. Risk factors for developing pre-eclampsia are:
- Nulliparity
- Age ≥40y.
- Family (e.g. mother, sister) or past history of pre-eclampsia
- BMI ≥35 or <18kg/m^2 at first contact
- Multiple pregnancy
- Pre-existing vascular disease, e.g. hypertension, DM

Consider ↑ frequency of BP monitoring in pregnancy for these women, though optimum frequency of BP checks is unclear. Whenever BP is measured, check a urine sample at the same time for proteinuria.

Psychiatric illness: Ask about family history of perinatal mental illness and if the woman has a current or past history of psychiatric illness. At first contact and booking, screen all women for depression (📖 p.244). Women with a current or past history of serious psychiatric disorder should be referred for a psychiatric assessment during the antenatal period.

Tay-Sachs disease: Genetic condition carried by 1:25 Ashkenazi Jews. Offer genetic screening *whether or not* there is a family history. Offer screening for other diseases commonly carried in this population (e.g. Gaucher's disease, familial dysautonomia, cystic fibrosis, Canavan's disease) *only* if there is a family history.

Table 5.5 High-risk groups for haemoglobinopathy	
Haemoglobinopathy	High-risk groups
Sickle cell disease	Blacks of African or Caribbean origin; Saudi Arabians; Indian and Mediterranean populations
Thalassaemia	Mediterranean, Middle Eastern, Indian and South East Asian populations

⚠ Warn pregnant women of the symptoms of advanced pre-eclampsia:
- headache
- problems with vision, e.g. blurring or flashing before the eyes
- bad pain just below the ribs
- vomiting
- sudden swelling of face, hands or feet.

If a pregnant woman experiences any of these symptoms in pregnancy, she should seek advice from a doctor or midwife as soon as possible.

Advice for patients:

Information and support for patients
Antenatal Results and Choices (ARC) ☎0207 631 0285
🖳 www.arc-uk.org
Perinatal Institute 🖳 www.preg.info
DIPEx patient experience database – women's experiences of antenatal screening 🖳 www.dipex.org
Department of Health Testing for Down's syndrome in pregnancy booklet. Available from 🖳 www.dh.gov.uk
Genetics Interests Group ☎020 7704 3141 🖳 www.gig.org.uk
Down's Syndrome Association ☎ 0845 230 0372
🖳 www.downs-syndrome.org.uk
Association for Spina Bifida and Hydrocephalus (ASBAH) ☎ 01733 555988 🖳 www.asbah.org
Sickle Cell Society ☎ 020 8961 7795 🖳 www.sicklecellsociety.org
UK Thalassaemia Society ☎ 0800 731 1109 🖳 www.ukts.org
Tay-Sachs and Allied Disease Association ☎ 01473 404 156

Further information
NICE 🖳 www.nice.org.uk
- Antenatal care: routine care for the healthy pregnant woman (2003 due for update 2007)
- Antenatal and postnatal mental health: Clinical management and service guidance (2007)

RCOG Amniocentesis and chorionic villus sampling (2005)
🖳 www.rcog.org.uk
National Screening Committee Antenatal and newborn screening programme 🖳 www.screening.nhs.uk/an

Symptoms arising in pregnancy

Abdominal pain: A relatively common symptom in pregnancy. Non-obstetric causes of abdominal pain may be forgotten or signs may be less well localized than in the non-pregnant patient – Figure 5.4.

Backache: Affects 60% of pregnant women – usually from the 2nd trimester onwards and worse in the evenings – may interfere with sleep/activities. Due to ↑ joint laxity in lumbar spine and sacro-iliac joints, exaggerated lumbar lordosis and poor posture.

Management: Encourage light exercise (unless contraindicated, e.g. pre-eclampsia) – special land and water-based classes are run for pregnant women. Treat with simple analgesia, physiotherapy ± massage.

Bleeding: 📖 p.232

Breast soreness: Commonest early in pregnancy. Good support bras are essential (can be purchased from specialist clothing stores). Nipples enlarge and darken at ≈ 12wk.

Carpal tunnel syndrome: Affects ~28% pregnant women. Due to compression of the median nerve as it passes under the flexor retinaculum. Symptoms are typically bilateral and arise in the 3rd trimester. They include pain in the radial 3½ digits of the hand ± numbness, pins and needles ± thenar wasting. Worse at night. Symptoms are improved by shaking the wrist.

Diagnosis: Hyperflexion of wrist for 1min. triggers symptoms (Phalen's test). Tapping over the carpal tunnel causes paraesthesiae (Tinel's test).

Management: Reassure usually resolves after pregnancy. Night splints may help. If severe consider steroid injection. Diuretics do not help. If does not resolve after pregnancy, refer for orthopaedic assessment.

Constipation: Affects up to 40% of pregnant women. ↑ fluid and fibre intake. If necessary use a bulk-forming laxative, e.g. ispaghula husk. Avoid bowel stimulants as they ↑ uterine activity.

Cramp: Leg cramp affects 1:3 in late pregnancy. Worse at night. Raising the foot of the bed by 20cm (e.g. 1–2 bricks under the bed) can help.

Fatigue

Early pregnancy: Almost universal symptom. Reaches peak at 12–15wk. Advise rest and adjustment of lifestyle. Reassure.

Late pregnancy: Due to ↑ physical effort needed to do everyday tasks and sleep deprivation. Check not anaemic, else reassure.

Haemorrhoids: Affect 8% of women in the 3rd trimester. May be associated with itching, pain and bleeding. Advise ↑ fibre intake. Treat prolapse with ice packs and replacement. Topical haemorrhoid applications are commonly used but lack of evidence of safety or efficacy.

Headache: Usually tension headache – check BP and urine for protein to exclude pre-eclampsia (📖 p.252). Treat with rest and analgesia. Migraine may ↑ or ↓ in pregnancy.

Figure 5.4 Abdominal pain in pregnancy

In all cases consider:

UTI: (📖 p.259)

Constipation: See opposite page

Gastritis/heartburn: 📖 p.222

Appendicitis: 1/1000 pregnancies. Mortality is higher in pregnancy and perforation commoner (15–20%). Fetal mortality is 5–10% for simple appendicitis but rises to 30% when there is perforation. Due to the pregnancy, the appendix is displaced and pain is often felt in the paraumbilical region or subcostally. Admit immediately if suspected.

Cholecyctitis: 1–6/10,000 pregnancies. Pregnancy encourages gall stone formation. Symptoms include right upper quadrant pain, nausea and vomiting. Diagnosis can be confirmed on USS. Treatment is the same as outside pregnancy, aiming for interval cholecystectomy after birth.

Fibroids: Torsion or red degeneration. Fibroids ↑ in size in pregnancy. They may twist if pedunculated. Red degeneration occurs usually >20wk. gestation and may occur until the puerperium. It presents as abdominal pain ± localized tenderness ± vomiting and low-grade fever. Treatment is with rest and analgesia. Pain resolves within 1wk.

Ovarian tumours/torsion: 1/1000 pregnancies. Torsion or rupture of a cyst may both cause abdominal pain, as may bleeding into a cyst. USS can confirm the presence of a cyst. Management depends on the nature of the cyst and the severity of the pain. Admit for assessment.

In addition consider:

If <20wk. gestation →

> **Miscarriage:** (📖 p.234)
> **Ectopic pregnancy:** (📖 p.236)

If ≥20wk. gestation

> **Labour:** (📖 p.264)
> **Pubic symphysis dysfunction:** (📖 p.224)
> **Pre-eclampsia:** May present with epigastric pain – check BP and dipstick urine for proteinuria (📖 p.252)
> **Haematoma of the rectus abdominis:** Rarely bleeding into the rectus sheath and haematoma formation occurs spontaneously or after coughing in late pregnancy. May cause swelling and abdominal tenderness. USS can be helpful. If unsure of diagnosis, admit to exclude acute surgical or obstetric cause of pain.
> **Uterine rupture:** (📖 p.271)
> **Abruptio placentae:** (📖 p.271)

Heartburn: Affects 70% of women in the 3rd trimester. Reassure not harmful. Advise low-fat, bland food, small portions and frequent meals. Avoid eating late at night if worse at night and consider raising the head of the bed (1–2 bricks under the bed). Avoid gastric irritants, e.g. caffeine. Antacid preparations, e.g. magnesium trisilicate are helpful if lifestyle modifications are ineffective but may worsen constipation.

⚠ Pre-eclampsia can present with epigastric pain – check BP and urine for protein. If epigastric/right upper quadrant pain not relieved by antacids refer for same-day assessment even if BP is normal and no/trace proteinuria (📖 p.252).

Hypotension: Common symptom of early pregnancy due to normal physiological fall in BP caused by ↑ peripheral circulation and venous pooling in lower limbs. Check no bleeding. Advise to avoid standing suddenly and to avoid hot baths.

Insomnia: Avoid drug treatment. Reassure. Relaxation techniques and mild physical exercise prior to sleep can help.

Itching: Common symptom. Diagnosis/management – Figure 5.5.

Nausea and vomiting: >80% from 4–6wk. – ≈ ½ vomit. Occurs at any time of day ('morning' sickness in <20%) and made worse by odours associated with preparation/sight of food. If severe exclude multiple pregnancy, trophoblastic disease and UTI. Symptoms usually improve by 14–16wk. though persist in some.

Management: Reassure – normal part of pregnancy. Adjust lifestyle, e.g. ask partner to do the shopping. Advise frequent small meals – avoid greasy/spicy foods, eat foods you can face (varies). Self-help measures include ginger^{CE} and P6 acupressure^{CE}. If severe/disabling consider anti-emetics^{CE}, e.g. cyclizine 50mg tds. Suppositories are an effective method of administration if po route is not tolerated. If dehydrated or >2–5kg weight loss (*hyperemesis gravidarum* – 1% pregnancies), admit for rehydration.

Peripheral paraesthesia: Abnormalities of sensation (e.g. tingling, pins and needles) of hands/feet are common. Reassure. Symptoms usually resolve after delivery. Carpal tunnel syndrome – 📖 p.220.

Skin changes: Pregnancy is associated with:
- Pigmentation – particularly the linea nigra – Figure 5.7 (a), 📖 p.225
- Spider naevi – Figure 5.7 (b), 📖 p.225
- Abdominal striae – Figure 5.7 (c), 📖 p.225
- Chloasma/merasma – Figure 5.7 (d), 📖 p.225
- Palmar erythema
- Pruritus – see itching (Figure 5.5)
- PUPPP – Figure 5.5 and Figure 5.6, 📖 p.224
- Pemphigoid gestationis (rare) – Figure 5.5
- Impetigo herpetiformis – rare – 3rd trimester. Mild itch. Systemically unwell. Refer. Remits after delivery but may recur in later pregnancies.

Other rashes: 📖 p.226

Sweating and feeling hot: Common. Check apyrexial. If apyrexial, reassure normal in pregnancy. If pyrexial, look for a source of infection.

Figure 5.5 Investigation and management of itching in pregnancy

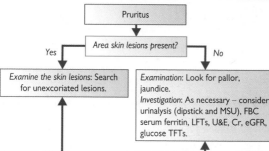

Pruritus

Area skin lesions present?

Yes → *Examine the skin lesions*: Search for unexcoriated lesions.

No → *Examination*: Look for pallor, jaundice.
Investigation: As necessary – consider urinalysis (dipstick and MSU), FBC serum ferritin, LFTs, U&E, Cr, eGFR, glucose TFTs.

Consider:
Non-pregnancy-related causes
• Urticaria
• Contact dermatitis and allergies to food or drugs
• Prickly heat
• Skin infestations, e.g. scabies, pediculosis, insect bites
• Infections – viral, e.g. chicken-pox, fungal
• Dermatitis herpetiformis
• Lichen planus
❶ Don't forget psychological causes in which excessive excoriation causes lichenification of the skin.
Pregnancy – related causes
• Abdominal striae may itch
• Pruritic papules and plaques of pregnancy (PUPP – 1.240 pregnancies) – urticarial wheals may develop into vesicles (Figure 5.6. 📖 p.224)
• Pemphigoid gestationis – rare – starts in mid-pregnancy and appears as a generalized, intensely itchy rash with bullous lesions (tense vesicles/blisters). Refer for specialist management. May recur in subsequent pregnancies and with the COC pill
• Impetigo herpetiformis – (📖 p.222)

Large differential diagnosis. Consider:
Hepatic causes – pruritus gravidarum or recurrent cholestasis of pregnancy – Affects 2–20:100 pregnancies and sometimes runs in families. Usually begins in the 3rd trimester, reaching a peak in the last 1mo.
• Frank jaundice – rare – refer urgently to an obstetrician
• No jaundice – check LFTs and bile acids. Refer to obstetrics if abnormal. Otherwise treat with moisturizers (e.g. aqueous cream) ± oily calamine. Antihistamines do not help
Disappears after delivery but recurs in subsequent pregnancies (40–50%) and with the COC pill
Endocrine causes – DM thyrotoxicosis, hypothyroidism
Renal causes – Chronic renal failure
Haematological causes – Iron deficiency
Drug allergies
Psychological causes – Obsessive states, schizophrenia

❶ If still undiagnosed – refer.

Swelling: Fluid retention affects 80% – ankles, hands/fingers, face. If severe or sudden ↑ in oedema, exclude pre-eclampsia (check BP, dipstick urine for protein).

Symphysis pubis dysfunction: 3%. Symphysis separates causing discomfort/pain in lower abdomen/pelvic area radiating to lower back, upper thighs and perineum. Pain is constant and worse on movement, resolves on rest. Treat with simple analgesia. Consider referral to physiotherapy for pelvic support belt or elbow crutches. Advise rest in a semi-recumbent position when in pain. Generally resolves after delivery but if persists, refer to orthopaedics.

Urinary frequency: Check MSU – UTI is common in pregnancy and associated with premature delivery – 📖 p.259.

Varicose veins: Cause aching legs, fatigue, itch and ankle/foot swelling. If ankles are swollen, exclude pre-eclampsia (check BP, dipstick urine for proteinuria). Elevate legs when sitting, provide support stockings, and encourage walking/discourage standing still. Complications include *thrombophlebitis* – treat with ice packs, elevation, support stockings and analgesia – and DVT (📖 p.246). If veins do not settle <2–3mo. after delivery, consider referral for surgery.

Vaginal discharge: Usually ↑ in pregnancy, Investigate if smelly, itchy, sore or associated with dysuria.

Vomiting: See nausea and vomiting.

Figure 5.6 Pruritic urticarial papules and plaques of pregnancy (PUPPP)	
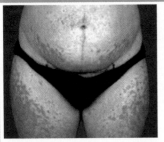 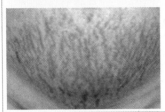	Associated with first and/or multiple pregnancies and/or excessive weight gain in pregnancy. Develops >35wk. and appears as a rash usually confined to the lower abdomen/buttocks. Treat with calamine and/or topical steroids (limit use to a few days and do not prescribe unless sure of diagnosis). Usually clears spontaneously <6wk., and often just a few days, after delivery. Does not recur in subsequent pregnancies.

Figure 5.6 is reproduced with permission from DermNet NZ, 🖳 http://dermnetnz.org

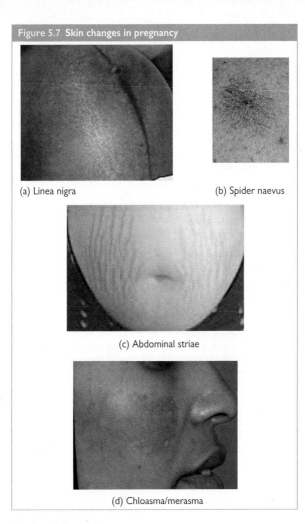

Figure 5.7 Skin changes in pregnancy

(a) Linea nigra

(b) Spider naevus

(c) Abdominal striae

(d) Chloasma/merasma

Further information

NICE Antenatal care: routine care for healthy pregnant women (and patient information – 2003 – due update in 2007) 🖥 www.nice.org.uk

Advice for patients: Advice and support for pregnant women

National Childbirth Trust (NCT) ☎0870 770 3236. Info line 0870 444 8707 🖥 www.nctpregnancyandbabycare.com

Rashes in pregnancy

At booking:
- Enquire if the woman has had chickenpox and/or shingles in the past. If not, advise her to make urgent contact if she develops a chickenpox-type rash or has contact with chickenpox or shingles.
- Advise the woman to inform the midwife/GP urgently if she develops any rash during pregnancy or has contact with anyone who has a rash.

Presentation with a rash: If a woman presents with a rash, consider:
- Rubella
- Parvovirus B19
- Chickenpox/shingles
- Measles
- Enterovirus infection
- Infectious mononucleosis (EBV or rarely CMV)
- Syphilis (📖 p.258)
- Streptococcus infection
- Meningococcus
- Common skin diseases, e.g. eczema, contact dermatitis and urticaria
- Skin changes specific to pregnancy (📖 p.222).

Investigation of pregnant women with rash illness: Figure 5.8

Rubella

- Presents with fever, LNs (including suboccipital nodes), and a pink maculopapular rash which lasts 3d.
- 50% of mothers infected with rubella are asymptomatic.
- Incubation is 14–21d. and once infected, patients are infectious from 7d. before the rash appears until 7d. after.
- Asymptomatic reinfection of women who have received vaccination can also occur, so serology is essential in all pregnant rubella contacts.

Affects on the fetus: Abnormalities that can occur include: cataract, deafness, cerebral palsy, mental retardation, microcephaly, microphthalmia. If the mother is infected with rubella at >20wk. gestation, infection does not affect the baby.

Transmission rates to the fetus: Depends on gestation:
- <11wk. – 90% of fetuses affected have adverse outcome
- 11–16wk. – 55% – 20% have adverse outcome
- >16wk. – 45% – minimal risk of deafness only.

Transmission risk is much lower with reinfection (<5%). There is no treatment to prevent transmission.

Management
- Contact with a non-vesicular rash or rubella – Figure 5.9.
- Non-specific, non-vesicular rash/suspected rubella infection – send blood for serology for rubella and parvovirus B19. Refer if proven infection. After further investigation and discussion of risks, women infected at <20wk. may be offered termination of pregnancy.

Parvovirus B19 infection: Febrile illness often accompanied by tenderness of the joints/arthritis affecting hands, wrists and knees – usually lasts 1–2wk. but 1:10 continue to have symptoms for several months. There may be a fine rash over the trunk and extremeties. Infectious from 10d. before rash appears. Incubation period 13–18d.

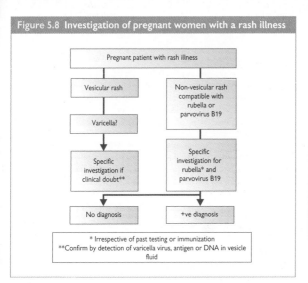

Figure 5.8 Investigation of pregnant women with a rash illness

Pregnant patient with rash illness

Vesicular rash

Varicella?

Non-vesicular rash compatible with rubella or parvovirus B19

Specific investigation if clinical doubt**

Specific investigation for rubella* and parvovirus B19

No diagnosis

+ve diagnosis

* Irrespective of past testing or immunization
**Confirm by detection of varicella virus, antigen or DNA in vesicle fluid

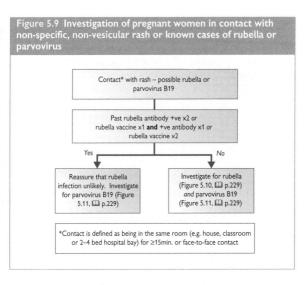

Figure 5.9 Investigation of pregnant women in contact with non-specific, non-vesicular rash or known cases of rubella or parvovirus

Contact* with rash – possible rubella or parvovirus B19

Past rubella antibody +ve x2 or rubella vaccine x1 **and** +ve antibody x1 or rubella vaccine x2

Yes

No

Reassure that rubella infection unlikely. Investigate for parvovirus B19 (Figure 5.11, p.229)

Investigate for rubella (Figure 5.10, p.229) *and* parvovirus B19 (Figure 5.11, p.229)

*Contact is defined as being in the same room (e.g. house, classroom or 2–4 bed hospital bay) for ≥15min. or face-to-face contact

227

Figures 5.8 and 5.9 are reproduced in modified format with permission from the Health Protection Agency (HPA), www.hpa.org.uk

Parvovirus B19 in pregnancy

- ~50% of young women in the UK are not immune.
- Risk of infection in pregnancy ≈ 1:400.
- Risk of a non-immune mother contracting the infection from a child who has Fifth disease (slapped cheek) ≈ 50%.

Affects on the fetus: After infection <20wk. gestation, there is a 9% ↑ miscarriage rate and 3% (14–56 babies/y. in the UK) develop hydrops fetalis 3–5wk. or more after infection, due to anaemia of the fetus – ½ of those babies die.

Tranmission rates to the fetus: Depend on gestation at the time of infection. There is no treatment to prevent transmission:
- <4wk. – 0%
- 5–16wk. – 15%
- >16wk. – 25–70%, increasing with gestation.

Management

- Contact with a non-vesicular, non-specific rash or known contact with parvovirus – Figure 5.9, 📖 p.227.
- Non-specific, non-vesicular rash/suspected parvovirus B19 infection – send blood for serology for rubella and parvovirus B19. Refer if proven infection. USS is started 4wk. post-onset of illness/date of seroconversion and then every 1–2wk. until 30wk. If there are any signs of hydrops fetalis on USS, the patient is referred to a regional centre for consideration of intrauterine transfusion. Early transfusion ↑ chances of the baby's survival. There are no long-term effects from an infection which does not cause miscarriage or hydrops.

Chickenpox[G]: Contact with chickenpox in pregnancy is common.

- People with chickenpox infection are infectious from 2d. before the rash appears until the rash has finished cropping and crusted over.
- Incubation period for chickenpox is 14–21d.
- If the mother has definitely had chickenpox there is no risk to herself or the baby.
- If she doesn't recall having chickenpox, check her immunity with a blood test – 80% have antibodies from silent infection.

Risk to the mother

- Chickenpox infection complicates 2–3:1000 pregnancies.
- Chickenpox pneumonia is more common (10%) and can be severe (1:1000 mortality).

Risks to the baby: Rates of transmission are higher later in pregnancy (~50% >36wk.; 5–10% <28wk.). Infection:
- <20wk.: miscarriage, fetal varicella syndrome (1–2% – segmental skin defects/scarring, limb hypoplasia ± paresis, low birth weight, microcephaly, neurological abnormalities, e.g. hypotonia, eye defects – may occur up to 28wk. gestation)
- 20–37wk.: intrauterine infection or death, shingles in childhood
- 1wk. before – 1wk. after delivery: onset 4d. before delivery – 2d. after delivery carries a 20% risk of overwhelming neonatal infection. The baby may need VZ-Ig treatment ± aciclovir. Seek specialist advice.

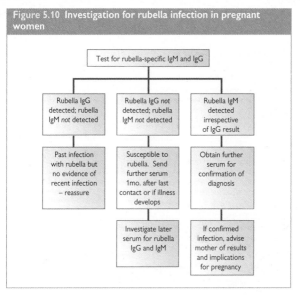

Figure 5.10 **Investigation for rubella infection in pregnant women**

Test for rubella-specific IgM and IgG

Rubella IgG detected; rubella IgM *not* detected → Past infection with rubella but no evidence of recent infection – reassure

Rubella IgG *not* detected; rubella IgM *not* detected → Susceptible to rubella. Send further serum 1mo. after last contact or if illness develops → Investigate later serum for rubella IgG and IgM

Rubella IgM detected irrespective of IgG result → Obtain further serum for confirmation of diagnosis → If confirmed infection, advise mother of results and implications for pregnancy

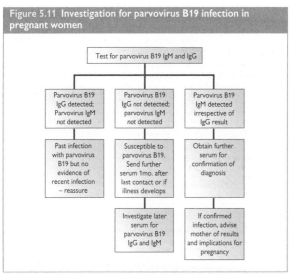

Figure 5.11 **Investigation for parvovirus B19 infection in pregnant women**

Test for parvovirus B19 IgM and IgG

Parvovirus B19 IgG detected; Parvovirus IgM *not* detected → Past infection with parvovirus B19 but no evidence of recent infection – reassure

Parvovirus B19 IgG *not* detected; parvovirus IgM *not* detected → Susceptible to parvovirus B19. Send further serum 1mo. after last contact or if illness develops → Investigate later serum for parvovirus B19 IgG and IgM

Parvovirus B19 IgM detected irrespective of IgG result → Obtain further serum for confirmation of diagnosis → If confirmed infection, advise mother of results and implications for pregnancy

229

Figures 5.10 and 5.11 are reproduced in modified format with permission from the Health Protection Agency (HPA), ⌨ www.hpa.org.uk

Management: Figure 5.12

In cases of 'at-risk' exposure: Arrange for VZ-Ig to be given to mother and/or baby. This can be life-saving and significantly ↓ disease severity if given ≤10d. after exposure. Babies are at risk if:

- The mother develops chickenpox from 7d. before to 7d. after delivery
- If the mother is not immune and the baby is exposed to chickenpox <7d. after birth
- The baby has been exposed to chickenpox and has potentially inadequate transfer of maternal antibodies, i.e. babies born at <28wk. gestation, babies born weighing <1000g and/or babies who have had repeated blood sampling with replacement by packed red cell infusion; or babies requiring intensive or prolonged special care nursing. VZ-Ig can be given without antibody testing to these babies but, where possible, test.

⊘ Duration of protection from VZ-Ig is limited. Give a 2nd dose if still at risk and further exposure occurs and ≥3wk. since 1st dose. Check antibody status again before giving 2nd dose.

☚ Some advocate use of prophylactic aciclovir for women with significant additional risk factors, e.g. immunosupression, smokers, did not receive early VZ-Ig, or in 2nd half of pregnancy.

If mother develops chickenpox: treat with aciclovir 800mg 5x/d. po for 1wk. or valaciclovir 1g tds po for 1wk. if presents <24h. after the rash appears and the mother is >20wk. gestation. Monitor daily. Admission criteria – Box 5.5. If <28wk. gestation, refer for detailed USS 5wk. after infection to exclude fetal varicella syndrome.

⊘ Warn pregnant women with chickenpox to avoid contact with anyone potentially at risk of developing severe chickenpox, especially other pregnant women or neonates.

Cytomegalovirus (CMV): More frequent cause of birth defect than rubella in the UK – 5:1000 live births – 10% develop handicap. The fetus is most vulnerable when infection occurs in early pregnancy. Maternal disease may be asymptomatic or a mild flu-like illness. Occasionally there is a rash. No effective prevention strategy.

Measles: Rare in the UK since introduction of routine MMR vaccination of children. Presents with coryza, lymphadenopathy, conjunctivitis and disseminated maculopaular rash which becomes confluent. Complications include pneumonia, otitis media and encephalitis. Infection in pregnancy can lead to intrauterine death and pre-term delivery. There are no associations with congenital infection or abnormalities.

Rash infections which cause no harm to the fetus

- Epstein-Barr virus (EBV)
- Enteroviruses – Coxsackievirus A, B; echovirus; enterovirus 68–71 – cause disease such as hand, foot and mouth. Some enteroviruses can cause severe neonatal infection and prophylactic immunoglobulin may be necessary – seek specialist advice.

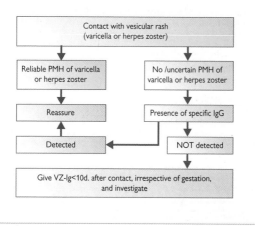

Figure 5.12 Investigation of pregnant women in contact with chickenpox

Contact with vesicular rash
(varicella or herpes zoster)

Reliable PMH of varicella or herpes zoster → Reassure

No /uncertain PMH of varicella or herpes zoster → Presence of specific IgG

Detected → Reassure

NOT detected

Give VZ-Ig<10d. after contact, irrespective of gestation, and investigate

Box 5.5 Criteria for admission of pregnant women with chickenpox

Admit if
- Chest symptoms
- Neurological symptoms other than headache
- Haemorrhagic rash or bleeding
- Severe disease – dense rash/numerous mucosal lesions
- Significant immunosuppression, e.g. HIV +ve

Consider admission if
- Pregnancy approaching term
- Bad obstetric history
- Smoker
- Chronic lung disease
- Poor social circumstances
- Unable to monitor the woman closely, e.g. homeless, traveller

Refer for urgent hospital assessment: if no deterioration but
- Fever persists *or*
- Cropping of the rash continues >6d.

231

Further information

Health Protection Agency (HPA) Guidance on the management of rash illness and exposure to rash illness in pregnancy 🖥 www.hpa.org.uk
RCOG Chickenpox in pregnancy (2001) 🖥 www.rcog.org.uk
DTB Volume 43.
- Chickenpox, pregnancy and the newborn (September 2005)
- Chickenpox, pregnancy and the newborn – a follow-up (December 2005)

Bleeding in pregnancy

Bleeding up to 14wk. into pregnancy: Bleeding in early pregnancy occurs in 1:4 pregnancies. *Causes:*

- Bleeding in normal pregnancy – largest group
- Miscarriage
- Ectopic pregnancy
- Trophoblastic disease
- Non-obstetric conditions, e.g. friable cervix, polyp, cervical neoplasia.

> ⚠ Any sexually active woman presenting with abdominal pain and vaginal bleeding after an interval of amenorrhoea has an ectopic pregnancy until proven otherwise.

Assessment

- Take a history of pain and bleeding – pain preceding bleeding suggests ectopic pregnancy is more likely. Have any products of conception been passed? 🛈 Clots/products can be difficult to distinguish.
- Check LMP and pregnancy test result (do a test if a pregnancy test has not been done).
- Check pulse (>100 bpm suggests shocked), BP and temperature (? toxic).
- Abdominal examination – guarding, peritonism and/or unilateral tenderness suggest ectopic pregnancy.
- Pelvic examination – with the advent of Early Pregnancy Assessment Units, the necessity of pelvic examination is debatable. If performed, assess uterine size, cervix – is the cervix open? (A closed cervix admits only 1 fingertip in a multiparous woman.) Is there any other cause for the bleeding?

Initial management

- If severe bleeding and/or pain, shocked or toxic, admit to gynaecology as an emergency. If shocked, give 1ml Syntometrine® IM and try to gain IV access.
- Otherwise, refer to the Early Pregnancy Assessment Unit (EPAU), if available, to check site and viability of pregnancy. USS is the definitive test of viability of pregnancy – at 5wk. gestation sac ± yolk sac is seen on scan; at 6wk. a fetal pole and fetal heartbeat is usually seen (occasionally not seen until 7wk.). Blood group and rhesus status is also checked at the EPAU (📖 p.240).

🛈 Advise women there is a strong possibility of a transvaginal ultrasound scan (~40%) – in practice, usually well tolerated.

Bleeding in early normal pregnancy: Often termed *threatened miscarriage.* If fetal heart is seen on USS then there is ~97% chance of the pregnancy continuing to progress. There is no evidence that rest or abstinence from sex improves outcome.

Complications of bleeding: Significant sub-chorionic haematoma is associated with ↑ risk of premature rupture of membranes and IUGR – refer early for specialist antenatal care.

⚠ Rhesus –ve women

Bleeding <12wk. gestation: Anti-D is not required for:
- threatened miscarriage unless heavy or repeated bleeding and/or abdominal pain *or*
- complete miscarriage where there is no medical or surgical uterine evacuation.

🛈 If there is any clinical doubt, give anti-D.

Bleeding >12wk. gestation, ectopic pregnancy and/or medical/surgical evacuation of the uterus at any gestation: Give anti-D immunoglobulin (250iu IM if gestation <20wk.) within 72h. of bleeding – *whether or not* the pregnancy is lost – 🕮 p.240.

GP Notes: Dealing with psychological effects of early loss of pregnancy

- Broach the subject with all women who have suffered a miscarriage or other early loss of pregnancy – one way of doing this is to telephone the patient after discharge and offer support.
- Include the woman's partner if possible.
- Not all women are grieved – adjust your approach accordingly.
- Legitimize any grief and acknowledge it.
- Provide information about the condition which caused the loss and reassure where appropriate about the future (if <3 miscarriages, risk of further miscarriage is not significantly ↑, risk of further ectopic pregnancy is ~1:10).
- Discuss worries and concerns of the woman and her partner.
- Warn of the anniversary phenomenon (sadness felt at the baby's due date or anniversary of the pregnancy loss) or sadness/jealousy they may feel on the birth of another's baby.
- Inform about self-help organizations, e.g. Miscarriage Association, Ectopic Pregnancy Trust.
- Provide ongoing support as needed. An easy access policy is useful as different women will want to discuss their feelings at different times after loss. If the woman already has young children, inform the health visitor.

Miscarriage: Also termed spontaneous abortion. Occurs in 1:5 pregnancies – 80% at <12wk. gestation. *Risk factors:*

- Maternal age
- BMI >29kg/m^2 – if >32kg/m^2, risk is ↑ by 30%
- Smoking
- Excess alcohol

Causes

- Fetal abnormality (50%)
- Multiple pregnancy
- Uterine abnormality – fibroids, polyps, congenital abnormality, cervical incompetence (☐ p.108 – late 2nd trimester miscarriages)
- Systemic disease – renal, autoimmune or connective tissue disease, particularly SLE, PCOS, DM, systemic infection
- Drugs – cytotoxics, stilboestrol
- Placental vascular abnormalities.

Management

- *Complete miscarriage* – psychological support.
- *Incomplete miscarriage* – products of conception remain in the uterus but there is no fetal heart – usually admitted for evacuation of retained products of conception (ERPC). Some women prefer a 'watch and wait' approach – at 3d. 86% will be complete.
- *Missed (or delayed) miscarriage* – usually discovered when no heartbeat is seen on routine antenatal scan. Treatment is with ERPC. A 'watch and wait' approach is possible but at 4wk. only 66% are complete, and associated with longer bleeding.

ⓘ Medical management with prostaglandin analogues ± antiprogesterone priming is an alternative to ERPC and offered in some units.

Rhesus negative women: ☐ p.233.

Complications

- *Early* – perforation of the uterus, retained products of conception, infection. Treat with antibiotics if infection is suspected (e.g. doxycycline 100mg od). Re-refer/readmit if shock, pain, heavy bleeding or bleeding is not settling.
- *Later* – uterine synechiae (Asherman's syndrome), cervical incompetence (☐ p.108), psychological sequelae.

Recurrent miscarriage: ≥3 miscarriages (1–2% couples). Check:

- Age – incidence of recurrent miscarriage ↑ with age
- How many miscarriages – confirmed pregnancies (not just late, heavy periods)? All with the same partner? What gestation? The more miscarriages, the lower the chance of successful pregnancy (Table 5.6)
- Infertility treatment? 25–30% of women who miscarry
- Past medical history – gynaecological problems (cervical instrumentation, PCOS), systemic disease
- Family history – recurrent miscarriage, thrombosis/thrombophilia.

Management: Refer for further investigation. No cause is found in ½ those referred. They have a 70% chance of successful pregnancy. Other causes include:

- Antiphospholipid antibodies (15%) – treatment with low-dose aspirin and low-molecular-weight heparin from 6wk.–34wk. improves outcome
- Chromosomal abnormality in 1 parent (3–5%).

Table 5.6 Probability of successful pregnancy after miscarriage				
Age (y.)	Number of previous miscarriages			
	2	3	4	5
20	92	90	88	85
25	89	86	82	79
30	84	80	76	71
35	77	73	68	62
40	69	64	58	52
45	60	54	48	42

GP Notes:

There is no evidence abstinence from pregnancy for time after miscarriage is helpful – fertility may actually ↑ immediately after miscarriage.

Advice for patients:

Experience of miscarriage

'I was in complete shock to find out I was pregnant. ... 8 weeks into the pregnancy I noticed light bleeding ... as I lay on the bed for my ultrasound, I knew that this was the moment of truth. As my heart cried silently, my hopes remained strong. I prayed that my baby had received strength from somewhere to cling onto its life. ... Unfortunately, this was not the case and I was informed I had had a complete miscarriage. For the second time in a few short weeks my life had performed a complete u-turn. ... I blamed myself and vigorously tried to work out what I had done wrong.'

'Over the next few weeks my emotions were mainly of confusion. ... you have an emotional period to go through into accepting the pregnancy, only to have that taken away again. ... I have not got over my loss, but I have learnt to live with it.'

'People think I should be over it by now, but I just feel so empty and I can't stop crying.'

Further information/support

The Miscarriage Association ☎ 01924 200799
🖥 www.miscarriageassociation.org.uk

Experiences are reproduced with permission from The Miscarriage Association.

Further information

RCOG 🖥 www.rcog.org.uk
- Management of early pregnancy loss (2000)
- Investigation and treatment of couples with recurrent miscarriage (2003)

Table 5.6 is reproduced with permission from Bricker, L and Farquharson, R. Recurring Miscarriage, The Obstetrician and Gynaecologist, October (2000); 2: 20.

Ectopic pregnancy[G]: A fertilized egg implants outside the uterine cavity — 95% in a Fallopian tube. Incidence ≈ 1:100 pregnancies and increasing due to ↑ *Chlamydia* infections and PID. Risk factors — Box 5.6.

History
- *Abdominal pain* (97%): Unilateral or bilateral, often starts before bleeding, may radiate to shoulder tip, ↑ on passing urine/opening bowels.
- *Amenorrhoea* (absent in 25%): Peak incidence after 7wk. amenorrhoea.
- *Irregular vaginal bleeding* (79%): Described as 'prune juice' but may be fresh blood, usually not heavy. May pass decidual cast.

Examination
- Shock in 15–20%
- Abdominal tenderness ± rebound or guarding (71%)
- Pelvis — enlarged uterus, adnexal mass, and/or cervical excitation.

Management: Admit immediately for further investigation. Resuscitate before admission as needed. Hospital management may be expectant (watch and pregnancy resolves spontaneously), medical (methotrexate) or surgical (laparotomy or laparoscopic surgery). Offer early USS in future pregnancies to confirm pregnancy is intrauterine.

Complications: Death if undetected, infertility (pregnancy rate post-ectopic pregnancy is 66% with 10% having a further ectopic pregnancy).

Psychological effects of early loss of pregnancy: 📖 p.233.

Trophoblastic disease[G]

Hydatidiform mole: Benign tumour of trophoblast containing 46 chromosomes all of paternal origin and no fetal material. Moles may become invasive and penetrate the uterus and/or metastasize to the lungs. 1:30 go on to develop choriocarcinoma.

Presentation
- Bleeding in early pregnancy ± exaggerated symptoms of pregnancy
- Rarely symptoms of metastatic spread — haemoptysis, pleurisy
- Uterus is usually large for dates and no fetal heart can be heard
- USS has a typical appearance
- Blood — ↑↑ serum β-HCG.

Management: Refer urgently to gynaecology. If mole is confirmed, women are followed up by specialist centres. Incidence in further pregnancies ≈ 1:120. Pregnancy is not advised for 1y. after mole — investigate with early USS and β-HCG estimation. COC pill is contraindicated.

Partial mole: Benign tumour of trophoblast containing 69 chromosomes, 1 maternal and 2 paternal sets, with some fetal tissue. Treat as for mole. No ↑ risk choriocarcinoma.

Choriocarcinoma: Malignant tumour of trophoblast which follows molar (rarely normal) pregnancy — often many years after. Presents with vaginal bleeding and/or metastases (shadows on CXR, dyspnoea, haemoptysis). Treated with chemotherapy — prognosis is excellent. Pregnancy is possible after 2y. free from disease.

Box 5.6 **Risk factors for ectopic pregnancy**

- PID (single episode ↑ risk x7)
- Infertility (15%)
- Copper-containing IUCD (14%)
- Previous ectopic pregnancy (11%)

- Tubal surgery
- POP
- Age
- Smoking

Advice for patients: Information and support

Ectopic Pregnancy Trust ☎ 01895 238025 ▭ www.ectopic.org
Hydatidiform Mole & Choriocarcinoma Support Service
▭ www.hmole-chorio.org.uk

Further information

RCOG ▭ www.rcog.org.uk
- The management of tubal pregnancy (2004)
- Management of gestational trophoblastic neoplasia (2004)

Antepartum haemorrhage (APH): Any bleeding in pregnancy >28wk. gestation (or the point of fetal viability). *Causes:*

Uterine
- Abruption (🕮 p.271)
- Placenta praevia (below)
- Vasa praevia
- Circumvallate placenta
- Placental sinuses

Lower genital tract
- Cervical
  - Polyp
  - Erosion
  - Carcinoma
  - Cervicitis
- Vaginitis
- Vulval varicosities

⚠ **Action**
- ALWAYS admit to a specialist obstetric unit. If bleeding is severe, admit via an emergency ambulance and whilst awaiting transport raise legs; give O_2 via face mask; if possible gain IV access, take blood for FBC and cross-matching and start IV infusion.
- NEVER do a vaginal examination – placenta praevia bleeds +++.

Placenta praevia[G]: Occurs when the placenta lies within the lower uterine segment. *Incidence:* 1:4 routine anomaly scans done at 19wk. gestation show a low-lying placenta – 5% stay low at 32wk.; <2% at term.

Associations
- ↑ with parity
- Age >35y
- Smoking
- Twins
- Endometrial damage (e.g. history of D&C, TOP)
- Pre-term delivery
- Previous Caesarean section
- Placental pathology (marginal/vellamentous cord insertions, succenturiate lobes, bipartite placenta)
- Previous placenta praevia (recurrence rate 4–8%).

Management: If discovered at routine USS at 17–19wk., follow-up USS at 36wk. reveals whether the placenta is moving out of the lower segment. When the placenta remains low, management depends on whether the placenta covers the internal os (major placenta praevia) or not (minor placenta praevia). Major placenta praevia always requires delivery by Caesarean section. Normal delivery in a specialist unit may be attempted with minor placenta praevia if the head lies below the lower edge of the placenta.

Complications
Maternal
- APH – typically painless bleeding with a peak incidence at 34wk
- Malpresentation – 35% breech presentation or transverse lie
- Placental problems – placenta accreta and percreta, especially with a history of previous Caesarean section; abruption
- PPH.

Fetal: IUGR (15%); premature delivery; death

Post-partum haemorrhage (PPH)

Primary PPH: Loss of >500ml blood within 24h. of delivery. Affects 1:100 deliveries. *Causes.*

- Uterine atony (90%)
- Clotting disorders (3%)
- Genital tract trauma (7%)

Risk factors

- Past history of PPH
- Retained placenta (📖 p.273)
- Large placental site
- Low placenta
- Overdistended uterus
- Abruption
- Uterine malformation
- Fibroids
- Prolonged labour
- >5 previous vaginal deliveries
- Trauma to uterus or cervix

⚠ Action

- Give high-flow O_2 via face mask as soon as possible.
- Call emergency ambulance for transfer to hospital.
- Gain IV access, take blood for FBC and cross-matching and start IV infusion if possible.
- Give in turn as necessary: oxytocin 5–10 units by slow IV injection, ergometrine 0.25–0.5mg IV, and then, if available and still bleeding, IV oxytocin infusion (5–30 units in 500mls) given at a rate that controls uterineatony.
- If the placenta has not been delivered, attempt to deliver it by controlled cord traction.
- Check for trauma and apply pressure to any visible bleeding point/repair any visible bleeding point. Bimanual pressure on the uterus may decrease immediate loss.
- Some community units keep misoprostol 400–800mcgm and carboprost 250mcgm in 1ml (e.g. Haemabate) for emergency use. Give misoprostol PR and/or carboprost by deep IM injection (can be repeated after >15min. to a maximum total dose of 2mg).

Secondary PPH: Excessive blood loss PV >24h. after delivery. *Peak incidence:* 5–12d. after delivery. *Causes:* Retained placental tissue or clot; post-partum infection.

⚠ Action

- Refer for assessment and possible USS.
- If bleeding is slight and USS normal, manage conservatively. If any suggestion of infection, take a swab and start oral antibiotics – amoxicillin 500mg tds and metronidazole 400mg tds until sensitivities known.
- If the uterus is tender and the os open, if loss is heavy or there is any suggestion of retained products on USS, admit to an obstetric unit for further investigation/evacuation of retained products of conception.

Further information

RCOG 🖥 www.rcog.org.uk

- Management of post-partum haemorrhage (1997 and update, 2002)
- Placenta praevia and placenta praevia accreta: diagnosis and management (2005).

239

Haemolytic disease and rhesus isoimmunization

15% of women are RhD −ve. Development of anti-D antibodies results from fetomaternal haemorrhage (FMH) in RhD −ve women carrying a RhD +ve fetus. In later pregnancies these antibodies cross the placenta, causing rhesus haemolytic disease of the fetus which gets successively worse with each pregnancy.

All RhD −ve mothers are tested for D-antibodies at booking, at 28wk. and 2 weekly thereafter. Testing is not performed once women are given anti-D prophylaxis — see below. Anti-D titres <4iv/ml (<1:16) are unlikely to cause serious disease. If ≥4u/ml refer for specialist advice.

Effects on fetus
- Hydrops fetalis (oedematous fetus)
- Intrauterine death.

Effects on neonate
- Jaundice
- Heart failure (oedema, ascites)
- Anaemia
- Yellow vernix
- Hepatosplenomegaly
- CNS signs

🚺 All neonates with haemolytic disease should be managed by specialist paediatricians. Treatment usually involves UV light for jaundice ± exchange transfusion.

Immunoprophylaxis: Immunoprophylaxis for RhD −ve mothers using anti-D immunoglobulin (anti-D Ig) is given IM into the deltoid muscle as soon as possible after the sensitizing event — preferably within 72h., though there is evidence of benefit up to 9d. Women already sensitized should not be given anti-D Ig.

Test for the size of feto-maternal haemorrhage: In the UK blood is taken from the mother (anticoagulated sample) as soon as possible (preferably <2h.) after the sensitizing event if >20wk. gestation. A Kleihauer acid elution test (which detects fetal haemoglobin (HbF)) identifies women with large feto-maternal haemorrhage who need additional anti-D Ig.

Other causes: Anti-D antibodies are the commonest cause of rhesus disease. Other causes include: Rh C, E, c, e, Kell, Kidd, and Duffy. Anti-Du antibodies are relatively common but usually harmless. Follow advice of local transfusion service about follow-up.

🚺 Anti-D Ig rarely causes allergic reactions. If the woman is worried about use of blood products, an alternative approach is to check rhesus status of the father — if he is Rh −ve, then the baby is Rh −ve as well, so anti-D prophylaxis is not required.

Further reading
RCOG/NICE Use of anti-D immunoglobulin for rhesus prophylaxis (2002) 🖥 www.rcog.org.uk

When should anti-D be administered?

Following spontaneous miscarriage
- ≥20wk. – 500iu + test the size of the feto-maternal haemorrhage
- 12–19wk. gestation – 250iu
- <12wk. – only give anti-D if there has been an intervention (e.g. D&C) to evacuate the uterus

Following termination of pregnancy/ectopic pregnancy: All non-sensitized RhD –ve women.

If threatened miscarriage
- All non-sensitized RhD –ve women >12wk. gestation.
- If bleeding continues intermittently after 12wk. give anti-D Ig 6-weekly.
- <12wk. gestation – only administer if bleeding is heavy, repeated or there is associated abdominal pain (particularly if close to 12wk.).

Following sensitizing events before delivery: All non-sensitized RhD –ve women after:
- Invasive prenatal diagnosis (amniocentesis, CVS, fetal blood sampling) or other intrauterine procedures
- Ante-partum haemorrhage
- External cephalic version of the fetus
- Closed abdominal injury (e.g. RTA)
- Intrauterine death.

<20wk. – 250iu; >20wk – 500iu + test size of feto-maternal haemorrhage

Routine antenatal prophylaxis
- 1–1.5% of RhD –ve women develop anti-D antibodies during pregnancy due to feto-maternal haemorrhage which is usually small and silent – most commonly in the 3rd trimester.
- Routine antenatal prophylaxis ↓ sensitization to <0.2% and should now be routine practice in the UK. Give irrespective of whether a woman has had prior anti-D prophylaxis earlier in the pregnancy.
- Administration of 500iu anti-D Ig at 28wk. (after blood has been taken for routine antibody screening) and 34wk. gestation ↓ incidence of immunization after birth.
- Women who have been given antenatal prophylaxis may still be sensitized by a large feto-maternal haemorrhage so, following any potentially sensitizing event, additional anti-D Ig should be given and a Kleihauer test performed.
- Screening for anti-D antibodies after prophylaxis is uninterpretable.

Postnatal prophylaxis
- 500–1500iu (500iu in the UK) is given to every non-sensitized RhD –ve woman <72h. after delivery of a RhD +ve infant.
- >99% women have a feto-maternal haemorrhage of <4ml at delivery – a test to detect feto-maternal haemorrhage >4ml must be done so additional anti-D Ig can be given as needed.
- Risk factors for high feto-maternal haemorrhage include: traumatic delivery, LSCS, manual removal of placenta, stillbirth and intrauterine death, abdominal trauma during the 3rd trimester, twin pregnancy (at delivery), unexplained hydrops fetalis.

A–Z of medical conditions in pregnancy

Anaemia: Defined as Hb <11g/dl., or <10.5g/dl after 28wk. Common in pregnancy (20%). Some ↓ in Hb is physiological due to an ↑ in plasma volume but iron requirements ↑ x2–3 and folate requirements ↑ x10–20 during pregnancy. Anaemia is usually due to iron deficiency. Complications include excessive fatigue and poorer fetal outcome.

Risk factors
- Starting pregnancy anaemic
- Multiple pregnancy
- Frequent pregnancies
- Poor diet
- Haemoglobinopathy.

Screening: Haemoglobinopathy and low Hb are routinely screened for at booking. Hb is screened again at 28wk.

Management
- Routine use of oral iron for all pregnant women is of no proven benefit and may cause harm. Women in high-risk groups (e.g. multiple pregnancy) may routinely be given prophylaxis – follow local policies.
- If Hb is <11g/dl at booking or <10.5g/dl at 28wk., start iron (e.g. ferrous sulphate 200mg tds) and folate (5mg od) if indicated. Repeat Hb in 2wk.

If there is no response to oral iron
- Exclude occult infection (e.g. UTI).
- Check haematinics.
- Consider referral for parenteral iron.

Antiphospholipid syndrome: Antiphospholipid antibodies (lupus anticoagulant and/or anticardiolipin antibodies) and a history of ≥1 of:
- Arterial thrombosis
- Venous thrombosis
- Recurrent pregnancy loss (typically 2nd trimester – 📖 p.234).

Can be 1° (occurs alone) or 2° to another connective tissue disease – usually SLE. Associated with ↑ risk of thrombosis and ↑ pregnancy loss (<20% pregnancies result in live birth). Treatment is with low-dose aspirin and low-molecular-weight heparin usually from 6–34wk. Specialist referral is essential.

Asthma Affects ≈ 5% of pregnant women.
- Generally improves with pregnancy, especially into the 3rd trimester.
- In most cases, treat asthma as usual – there is no evidence most of the drugs commonly used cause birth defects, problems in pregnancy or with breast feeding. ⓘ Leukotriene receptor antagonists have limited safety data in pregnancy – seek specialist advice.
- Women with very badly controlled asthma are more at risk of early labour and IUGR and patients on oral steroids may require IV steroids to cover labour.
- Avoid Syntometrine® for 3rd stage of labour as it contains ergometrine which can cause a severe attack.
- There is a tendency to worsening of asthma after delivery.

Can start or continue in pregnancy: If clinically necessary and benefits outweigh risks:

- Analgesics – paracetamol, codeine-based preparations
- Antacids and ranitidine
- Antibiotics – except tetracyclines; avoid trimethoprim in 1st trimester and at term
- Anti-emetics – cyclizine, prochlorperazine, metoclopramide, domperidone
- Antihistamines – chlorphenamine
- Antihypertensives – methyldopa, nifedipine, labetalol, doxazosin
- β-agonists – salbutamol, ipratropium, terbutaline
- Inhaled steroids
- Hormones – thyroxine, insulin
- Laxatives
- Low-dose aspirin (75mg).

Discontinue or change in pregnancy

- NSAIDs – except low-dose aspirin
- Warfarin – may need to continue if prosthetic heart valves – liaise with obstetrician as may need to change to low-molecular-weight heparin
- Antibiotics – tetracycline, doxycycline
- Antihypertensives – ACE inhibitors, angiotensin receptor blockers
- Retinoids, e.g. isotretinoin.

Permission to reproduce sought from *The Practitioner*, January 2006.

Cardiac disease: Risk of death is greatest in conditions where pulmonary blood flow cannot be ↑, e.g. Eisenmenger's syndrome (maternal mortality 30–50%); 1° pulmonary hypertension (mortality 40–50%).

Management: Specialist obstetric care is required for all patients with a pre-existing cardiac condition. Where possible refer pre-conception to a cardiologist for discussion of risks. Antibiotic prophylaxis is necessary for women with structural cardiac disease for delivery.

Murmurs in pregnancy: Check heart sounds when primigravidas first present to the GP. Murmurs are common. Consider any heart murmurs detected during pregnancy significant and refer for further evaluation – 90% will be physiological.

Depression: A significant cause of maternal death.

Pre-existing depression: Consider referral for pre-conceptual psychiatric advice. When antidepressants are being used, weigh up the pros and cons of discontinuing treatment during pregnancy.

Screening for depression: Screen for depression at first presentation, booking, and 4–6wk. and 3–4mo. postnatally, with the questions:
- During the past month, have you often been bothered by feeling down, depressed or hopeless?
- During the past month, have you often been bothered by having little interest or pleasure in doing things?

If the woman answers 'yes' to either of the initial questions, ask: 'Is this something you feel you need or want help with?'

Depression in pregnancy: For women with mild/moderate depression consider self-help strategies and talking therapies (e.g. counselling) first. Monitor regularly using depression questionnaires (e.g. Hospital Anxiety and Depression questionnaire). Weigh up risks of antidepressant medication against benefits. Involve specialist psychiatric service early.

Postnatal depression: 📖 p.277

Diabetes: 📖 p.250   **Epilepsy:** 📖 p.248
Eclampsia: 📖 p.271   **Hypertension:** 📖 p.252
DVT: 📖 p.246   **Infection:** 📖 p.256

Jaundice: Any cause of jaundice may occur in pregnancy. Investigate as usual and treat according to cause. Common causes are:
- Viral hepatitis
- Gallstones
- Gilbert's or Dubin-Johnson syndrome.

Jaundice peculiar to pregnancy
- *Recurrent cholestasis of pregnancy/pruritus gravidarum* – 📖 p.223.
- *Acute fatty degeneration of the liver:* Rare. Usually >30wk. gestation. The mother develops abdominal pain, jaundice, headache and vomiting. Admit for specialist care. *Prognosis:* ≈ 15–20% maternal mortality; ≈ 20% fetal mortality.

244

- *Pre-eclampsia:* Jaundice is associated with severe pre-eclampsia ± HELLP syndrome – 📖 p.252.
- *Hyperemesis:* Jaundice is a complication of severe hyperemesis gravidarum – 📖 p.222.

Pre-eclampsia: 📖 p.252.

Renal disease: Refer all women for specialist obstetric care. Pre-eclampsia is more common – monitor carefully and refer early. Outcome depends on severity of disease.

Mild renal failure: Cr <125μmol/l and no ↑ BP. 96% have successful pregnancies without adverse effect on underlying disease. Low perinatal mortality.

Moderate (Cr 125–275μmol/l) and severe (Cr >275μmol/l) renal failure: Maternal complications occur in up to 70% and pregnancy-related loss of renal function in ~½ (10% progress to end-stage renal failure). IUGR in ~40% and pre-term delivery in ~60%.

Women on dialysis: Conception is uncommon. High rate of miscarriage and intra-uterine death. ~40–50% live birth rate. Mothers are prone to volume overload, polyhydramnios and severe exacerbations of ↑ BP ± pre-eclampsia. Women need a 50% ↑ in duration and frequency of dialysis during pregnancy.

Renal transplant: Risk of 1st trimester miscarriage is ↑, but pregnancies that survive are >90% successful. Immunosuppressant drugs must be continued – they are not harmful to the fetus. Pregnancy does not affect long-term survival of the transplanted kidney. Pelvic position of the transplant does not compromise vaginal delivery.

Rheumatoid arthritis: Symptoms often improve during pregnancy and worsen in the puerperium. Do not use NSAIDs for joint pain >24wk. gestation as can result in closure of the fetal ductus arteriosus. Paracetamol or paracetamol +codeine combinations are safe.

2nd line drugs
- Sulfasalazine – folic acid supplementation is recommended.
- Azathioprine – associated with IUGR.
- Penicillamine – may weaken fetal collagen.
- Methotrexate is contraindicated.

Systemic lupus erythematosus (SLE): Exacerbations are common in pregnancy.
- *Effects on fetus:* IUGR; neonatal lupus (from passively acquired maternal antibodies – usually self-limiting skin rash).
- *Effects on mother:* Renal complications may worsen and be associated with ↑ BP ± pre-eclampsia; oligohydramnios; premature delivery.

Management: If planning pregnancy refer for review of drugs. Once pregnant refer for specialist obstetric care. Pain control – as for rheumatoid arthritis (above).

Immunosuppressive drugs
- Azathioprine – associated with IUGR.
- Hydroxychloroquine – risk of deposits in fetal eye/ear.
- Cyclophosphamide and methotrexate are contraindicated.

Thromboembolism^G: Commonest direct cause of maternal death in the UK. Pregnancy ↑ risk of thromboembolism x10, even in very early pregnancy. *Incidence:* ≈ 1:100 pregnancies (20–50% antenatal).

> ⚠ Suspect DVT and/or PE in any woman who is pregnant or in the puerperium who has:
> * leg pain and/or swelling
> * mild unexplained fever
> * chest pain and/or breathlessness.

Major risk factors
* Age >35y.
* Obesity – BMI >30kg/m^2.

Other risk factors
* Smoking
* Parity >4
* Family history of venous thromboembolism
* Previous thromboembolism
* Thrombophilia
* Gross varicose veins
* Sickle cell disease
* Myeloproliferative disorders
* Inflammatory disorders, e.g. inflammatory bowel disease
* Prolonged bed rest/immobility for any reason
* Other medical disorders, e.g. nephritic syndrome, certain cardiac conditions
* Dehydration – including hyperemesis and ovarian hyperstimulation
* Severe infection, e.g. pyelonephritis
* Pre-eclampsia
* Prolonged labour
* Caesarean section
* High instrumental delivery
* Any other surgical procedure in pregnancy or puerperium.

Management: Warfarin is teratogenic when used in the 1st trimester of pregnancy and can ↑ miscarriage, maternal and fetal haemorrhage, and stillbirth rates. Avoid during pregnancy. Warfarin is safe post-partum and during breast feeding. Low-molecular-weight heparin (LMWH) is a safe alternative. Refer for expert advice.

Prevention: Ideally screen all women with a past history of thromboembolism for thrombophilia prior to conception. Prophylaxis is required if a patient has a thrombophilia or past history of pregnancy or COC-associated thromboembolism. LMWH is used antenatally and for up to 6wk post-partum – refer for expert advice.

Thyroid disease Refer for specialist obstetric advice.

Hyperthyroidism: Usually Graves disease. Severity ↓ through pregnancy. May be associated with neonatal goitre, hyperthyoidism or hypothyroidism. Continue treatment with carbimazole or propylthiouracil, aiming to keep plasma T$_4$ at the top of the normal range. Propylthiouracil is preferred post-partum if breast feeding, as less concentrated in breast milk.

Hypothyroidism: Rare (associated with infertility). If untreated associated with ↑ rate of miscarriage, stillbirth and fetal abnormality. T$_4$ needs to be ↑ in pregnancy and normal maintenance dose is ↑ to accommodate this – the fetus is not affected by maternal thyroxine. Check TFTs in each trimester.

Further information

RCOG 🖳 www.rcog.org.uk
- Thromboprophylaxis during pregnancy, labour and after vaginal delivery (2004)
- Thromboembolic disease in pregnancy and the puerperium (2001)

NICE Antenatal and postnatal mental health: Clinical management and service guidance (2007). 🖳 www.nice.org.uk

Epilepsy and pregnancy

90% epileptic women have normal pregnancies and healthy babies.

> ⓘ Notify pregnancies of women with epilepsy to the UK Epilepsy and Pregnancy Register (🖳 www.epilepsyandpregnancy.co.uk or ☎ 0800 389 1248) with consent of the pregnant woman.

Effects on the fetus

Antenatal: ↑ 1st trimester miscarriage and ↑ fetal malformation.
- Neural tube defect – ↑ risk with sodium valproate or carbamazepine.
- Cleft lip/palate – associated with phenytoin and phenobarbitone.
- Non-specific facial abnormalities – 5–30% exposed to anticonvulsants.

Peri/postnatal
- 2x ↑ perinatal mortality.
- Haemorrhagic disease of the newborn – associated with carbamazepine, phenytoin or phenobarbitone. All mothers on these drugs should have 10mg vitamin K od from 36wk. and all babies should have IM vitamin K at birth.
- Withdrawal symptoms – phenobarbitone (jittery, irritable, fits).
- Child has ↑ risk of developing epilepsy.

Effects on the mother

During pregnancy: 10% have ↑ fit frequency. The fetus is at slightly ↑ risk of harm during a generalized tonic-clonic seizure but absolute risk of harm is low. There is no evidence simple partial, complex partial, absence or myoclonic seizures harm pregnancy in any way, unless the patient falls. Status epilepticus is associated with high infant and maternal mortality.

During labour/puerperium: 1–2% have fit during labour and a further 1–2% <48h. post-delivery.

Management

Pre-pregnancy: Discuss risks of anti-epileptic medication/epilepsy with all women of child-bearing age – whether or not contemplating pregnancy. NICE advises caution in the use of sodium valproate in any woman of child-bearing age due to the risk of harm to the fetus. Advise folate supplementation (prescribe folic acid 5mg od) from the time the pregnancy is being planned until 13wk. after conception. Suggest referral to a neurologist for optimization of the anti-epileptic drug regime.

During pregnancy: Refer for specialist obstetric care – epileptic women are usually managed jointly by an obstetrician and neurologist during pregnancy. Drug doses may need to ↑ during pregnancy if fit frequency rises. Delivery should occur in a specialist centre where any fits can be managed.

Postnatally
- Breast feeding is not contraindicated with older anticonvulsants (e.g. phenytoin, sodium valproate, carbamazepine) – *BNF Appendix 5*.
- If drug dose has been ↑ in pregnancy, it may need to ↓ after delivery.
- All babies should have IM vitamin K due to ↑ risk of haemorrhage.
- Risk of injury to the child from maternal seizure is low. Discuss child care and minimizing risks to the child from the mother's epilepsy.

Advice for patients:

Practical information for mothers with epilepsy: New mothers with epilepsy often have particular concerns with safety issues. Identifying and introducing safety precautions can help reduce risks, build confidence and allow mothers to care for their babies safely. A mother who has seizures involving loss of consciousness will need to take more care than a mother who rarely has seizures or one who has reliable and sufficient warning before a seizure.

Overprotection: Although there may be concerns about how your epilepsy may affect your ability to safely care for your baby, avoid 'overprotection' as it affects vital bonding of mother and child.

Safety tips
- Identify a safe, convenient area for your baby if you should feel unwell, e.g. playpen, cot or other safe place.
- Risk of dropping your baby when feeding can be reduced by sitting on the floor with your back to the wall for support. Well-positioned cushions placed on either side decrease the risk of your baby falling far or onto a hard floor should you have a seizure.
- If you always fall in the same direction when you have a seizure, holding your baby on the opposite side whilst bottle feeding will ensure you always fall away from the baby.
- Bathing your baby is the one task you should never do whilst alone. A safer alternative is sponging your baby down on a changing mat or towel at floor level.
- If you are at risk of seizures always change your baby at floor level.
- If you have seizures involving loss of consciousness or awareness, carry your baby as little as possible. Ask another family member to carry your baby on the stairs. If it is unavoidable, carry your baby secured in a carrycot – this may reduce risk of injury to the baby in the event of being dropped.
- A length of cord tied to your wrist will stop the pram from running away should you lose awareness or consciousness. The cord should be long enough to ensure the pram is not pulled over. Alternatively, a brake can be fitted which halts the pram when the handle is released.

Information and support
Epilepsy Action ☎ 0808 800 5050. 🖳 www.epilepsy.org.uk
Epilepsy Scotland ☎ 0808 800 2200 🖳 www.epilepsyscotland.org.uk
Joint Epilepsy Council of the UK and Ireland
🖳 www.jointepilepsycouncil.org.uk

Further information
NICE The epilepsies: the diagnosis and management of the epilepsies in adults and children in primary and secondary care (2004)
🖳 www.nice.org.uk
SIGN Diagnosis and management of epilepsy in adults (2003)
🖳 www.sign.ac.uk

Diabetes in pregnancy

Pre-existing DM: Affects 2–3/1000 pregnancies. 95% have IDDM.

Effects on fetus
- *In utero* – large for dates or IUGR; fetal hyper-insulinaemia; ↑ congenital abnormalities (cardiac, renal and neural tube defects); hypoxia and intrauterine death (especially >36wk.)
- *Postnatally* – hypoglycaemia in the 1st few hours; transient tachypnoea of the newborn or respiratory distress syndrome; neonatal jaundice

Effects on mother: Problems are more common if control is poor.
- *In pregnancy* – 1st trimester miscarriage; premature labour; pre-eclampsia; pyelonephritis; polyhydramnios
- *In labour* – fetal distress; obstruction (especially shoulder dystocia)

Management
Pre-pregnancy: Suggest pre-pregnancy counselling via diabetic specialist normally involved with care.
- Careful attention to diabetic control (aim BM 4–6mmol/l pre-meals)
- Folate supplementation – 5mg od until 13wk.
- Stop drugs contraindicated in pregnancy, e.g. ACE inhibitors, biguanides and sulphonylureas – switch to insulin pre-conception if possible.

During pregnancy: Refer to an obstetrician early.
- Most women continue to use their pre-pregnancy insulin regime but requirements ↑ 2–3x in pregnancy.
- USS is routinely used to monitor fetal growth and exclude structural abnormalities.
- Delivery should always take place in a specialist unit with neonatal care facilities.

Postnatally
- ↓ insulin to pre-pregnancy levels (if breast feeding may need less).
- Oral hypoglycaemics are contraindicated if breast feeding.

Gestational diabetes: DM with onset/first recognition in pregnancy. Affects 2% of pregnancies and usually develops in the 2nd trimester. Lower risk of congenital malformation than if pre-existing DM. Intensive management can achieve almost normal rates of macrosomia and neonatal hypoglycaemia, but there is debate whether that is necessary.

Risk factors
- Obesity
- Family history of type 2 DM
- Past history of baby >4.5kg
- Unexplained stillbirth/neonatal death.

Management: Initially diet and, if well controlled, then management of pregnancy is otherwise normal. Up to 30% will require insulin. Insulin is stopped immediately post-partum. Check a 6wk. post-partum glucose tolerance test. Gestational DM usually recurs in future pregnancies and >30% develop DM in <10y.

🛈 Normal GTT in the 1st trimester does not exclude development of gestational DM in the 2nd/3rd trimester.

Glycosuria in pregnancy: Routine screening for glycosuria in pregnancy is no longer recommended. Pregnant women have a ↓ renal threshold for glucose and a physiologically ↑ plasma glucose level, so dipstick testing gives a high false +ve rate. However, if glycosuria is detected repeat the urine test – if still +ve arrange for a modified GTT.

Further information
Diabetes UK Professional and patient information on the management of pregnant women with gestational diabetes ⌨ www.diabetes.org.uk
NICE ⌨ www.nice.org.uk
- Antenatal care: routine care for healthy pregnant women (and patient information – 2003 – due to be updated in 2007)
- Diabetes in pregnancy – due for publication in 2007

Advice for patients:

Patient experiences of diabetes in pregnancy

Testing for gestational diabetes: 'I got picked up with a slightly raised glucose level, and so I had to go and do the test for whether I had gestational diabetes, which involves fasting for 12 hours and then drinking this disgusting like-Lucozade-gone-mad kind of drink – a really, really sweet, sickly drink – and then you wait for two hours and they test your glucose levels again. And that was kind of, you know, one more thing you just thought you could do without. And I was okay.'

Pre-pregnancy counselling for diabetic women: 'Another very important thing which I've never actually done is, they always say that you should have pre-planning counselling … whereby you tell them you want, you are trying to have, a baby. They then make sure that your sugars are at the optimum range before you actually conceive. And unfortunately with me that has never happened. Although all of my pregnancies have been planned in some way, I've never actually sat down with anyone before getting pregnant and made sure that my blood sugars were at a good level…. It wasn't a choice. It was just something that I never really thought about. I didn't think. [sigh] I suppose you don't actually think of what the consequences could be by not doing it.'

Diabetes in pregnancy: 'The most important thing that you have to be aware of is that you keep your blood sugars within a normal range, and by doing that it supposedly stops the baby from being too big and obviously causing further complications.'

Pregnancy complications caused by diabetes: 'Everything that happens to me is in some way put down to the diabetes. Children with heart defects are more prone to mothers with diabetes. Miscarriages are more prone to mothers with diabetes. Stillbirths are more prone to mothers with diabetes. And morning sickness again is probably more prone to people who have got diabetes.'

Information sheets and booklets for patients
Diabetes UK ☎ 0845 120 2960 ⌨ www.diabetes.org.uk

251

Hypertension in pregnancy

Chronic hypertension or essential hypertension: Present before or <20wk. into pregnancy. More common in older mothers and there may be a FH. Chronic hypertension may worsen in later pregnancy. Consider changing medication to drugs known to be safe in pregnancy pre-conceptually or as soon as pregnancy is confirmed (Table 5.7). Aim to keep BP <140/90. Risk of pre-eclampsia is ↑ x5 (see below).

Pregnancy-induced hypertension (PIH): ↑ BP appearing >20wk. into pregnancy and resolving <3mo. after delivery. Affects 10% of pregnancies and risk of pre-eclampsia is ↑. Treatment is the same as for chronic hypertension. ↑ risk of developing hypertension later in life.

Pre-eclampsia^G *(Pregnancy-induced hypertension and proteinuria or pre-eclamptic toxaemia (PET))*: Affects 5–7% of primigravida and 2–3% of all pregnancies. Multisystem disease of unknown cause, developing ≥20wk. into pregnancy and only resolving once the baby is delivered (<10d. after birth). Risk factors – Box 5.7. Untreated, may progress to eclampsia – one of the most common causes of death from pregnancy.

Criteria for diagnosis
- BP >140/90 or >+30/+15 from booking. The earlier in pregnancy the BP rises, the more likely the pre-eclampsia will be severe.
- Proteinuria ≥0.3g/24h. – urine dipstick is a useful screening tool – if ≥1+ protein then probably significant, but ~25% false +ve rate.

⚠ Pre-eclampsia is asymptomatic until its terminal phase, and onset may be rapid, so frequent BP screening is essential. Whenever you check BP in pregnancy, always check urine for protein.

Interval for routine BP checks
- If no risk factors for pre-eclampsia (Box 5.7) – routine antenatal care.
- If 1 risk factor for pre-eclampsia but no factor which requires referral in early pregnancy – from 24–32wk. gestation, recheck BP at least every 3wk., and >32wk. gestation, re-check at least every 2wk.
- If >1 risk factor or factor which requires referral in early pregnancy – refer <20wk. and then monitor as directed by the specialist.

Thresholds for further action: Table 5.8, 📖 p.254

Prevention
- Low-dose aspirin may be of benefit for high-risk women (i.e. those who have a past history of pre-eclampsia) – refer for advice.
- Other possible interventions (ongoing trials): rest, calcium supplements if low dietary calcium, antioxidants (especially vitamins C and E).

Risk of recurrence
- Risk of recurrence in subsequent pregnancy with the same partner is 10–15% but usually less severe.
- Women who have pre-eclampsia are at greater risk of developing ↑ BP later in life.

Eclampsia: 📖 p.271

Table 5.7 Drugs for hypertension that are safe in pregnancy	
Drug	**Notes**
Methyldopa	First choice. Doses <1g/d. cause less drowsiness
β-blockers	e.g. labetolol. Use with caution, preferably only in the 3rd trimester
Nifedipine	Modified-release preparations (unlicensed). Manufacturer advises use with caution
α-blocker	e.g. doxazosin. Manufacturer advises use with caution

Box 5.7 Risk factors for pre-eclampsia – evaluate at booking[G]

Refer early (<20wk.) for specialist care if:

- Pre-eclampsia/eclampsia in previous pregnancy
- Multiple pregnancy
- Underlying medical conditions:
  - Pre-existing hypertension or booking diastolic BP ≥90mmHg
  - Pre-existing renal disease or booking proteinuria ≥1+ on >1 occasion or quantified as ≥0.3g/24h.
  - Pre-existing DM
  - Antiphospholipid antibodies
- ≥2 other risk factors:
  - First pregnancy (or first time by a new partner)
  - Age ≥40y.
  - BMI ≥35 or <18kg/m^2
  - Family history of eclampsia/pre-eclampsia (particularly mother/sister)
  - Booking diastolic BP ≥80 but <90mmHg

⚠ Significant symptoms/signs of pre-eclampsia

- New hypertension
- New and/or significant proteinuria
- Maternal symptoms of headache and/or visual disturbance
- Maternal epigastric pain and/or vomiting
- Reduced fetal movements or small for gestational age infant

253

HELLP syndrome: Occurs in pregnancy or <48h. after delivery. Associated with severe pre-eclampsia.

- **H**aemolysis
- **E**levated **L**iver enzymes
- **L**ow **P**latelets

Signs
- Hypertension (80%)
- Right upper quadrant pain (90%)
- Nausea and vomiting (50%)
- Oedema

Management: Admit as for pre-eclampsia (opposite).

Table 5.8 Thresholds for further action		
Findings (BP readings are in mmHg)		**Action**
New hypertension without proteinuria >20wk. gestation	Diastolic BP ≥90 and <100mmHg	Refer for specialist assessment* in <48h.
	Diastolic BP ≥90 and <100mmHg with significant symptoms (below)	Refer for same-day specialist assessment*
	Diastolic BP ≥100mmHg	
	Systolic BP ≥160mmHg	
New hypertension and proteinuria >20wk. gestation	Diastolic BP ≥90 and new proteinuria ≥1+ on dipstick	Refer for same-day specialist assessment*
	Diastolic BP ≥90 and new proteinuria ≥1+ on dipstick and significant symptoms (below)	Immediate admission
	Diastolic BP ≥110 and new proteinuria ≥1+ on dipstick	
	Systolic BP ≥170 and new proteinuria ≥1+ on dipstick	
New proteinuria without hypertension >20wk. gestation	1+ on dipstick	Repeat pre-eclampsia assessment in <1wk.
	2+ on dipstick	Refer for specialist assessment* in <48h.
	≥1+ on dipstick with significant symptoms (below)	Refer for same-day specialist assessment*
Maternal symptoms or fetal signs/ symptoms without new hypertension or proteinuria	Headache and/or visual disturbance with diastolic BP <90 and trace or no proteinuria	Investigate cause of headache. ↓ interval to next pre-eclampsia assessment
	Epigastric pain with diastolic BP <90 and trace or no proteinuria	If simple antacids are ineffective, refer for same day specialist assessment*
	↓ fetal movements or small-for-gestational-age infant with diastolic BP <90 and trace or no proteinuria	Refer for investigation of fetal compromise. ↓ interval to next pre-eclampsia assessment

⚠ Significant symptoms
- Epigastric pain
- Vomiting
- Headache
- Visual disturbance
- ↓ fetal movements
- Small-for-gestational-age infant

* Most obstetric departments have a day-case 'step-up' assessment unit.

Further information
APEC Pre-eclampsia community guideline (2004) ⊞ www.apec.org.uk
RCOG Pre-eclampsia – study group recommendations (2003)
⊞ www.rcog.org.uk

Table 5.8 is reproduced with permission from APEC, ⊞ www.apec.org.uk

Advice for patients:

Frequently asked questions about pre-eclampsia

What is eclampsia and pre-eclampsia? Pre-eclampsia usually only occurs after the 20th week of pregnancy. It causes high blood pressure and protein to leak into the urine. Eclampsia may follow on from pre-eclampsia (1 in 2000 women with pre-eclampsia). It is a type of fit (or seizure) which is a life-threatening complication of pregnancy.

Why have I got pre-eclampsia? Any pregnant woman can develop pre-eclampsia (1 in 14 pregnancies). You have increased risk if you:
• are pregnant for the first time (1 in 30 women get pre-eclampsia), or are pregnant for the first time by a new partner
• have had pre-eclampsia before
• have a family history of pre-eclampsia, particularly if it occurred in your mother or sister
• had high blood pressure before the pregnancy started
• are diabetic, or have systemic lupus erythematosus (SLE), or chronic kidney disease
• are aged below 20 or above 35
• have a pregnancy with twins, triplets, or more
• are obese.

What causes pre-eclampsia? No one really knows. It is probably due to a problem with the placenta (the afterbirth).

How do you know I have pre-eclampsia? Most women do not feel ill or have any symptoms at first. Pre-eclampsia is present if:
• your blood pressure becomes high, *and*
• you have an abnormal amount of protein in your urine.

Severity of pre-eclampsia is usually (but not always) related to the blood pressure level. Other symptoms which suggest severe pre-eclampsia are:
• headaches
• blurring of vision, or other visual problems
• abdominal (tummy) pain – usually just below the ribs
• vomiting
• just not feeling right.

Swelling or puffiness of your feet, face, or hands (oedema) is also a feature of pre-eclampsia but is also common in normal pregnancy.

255

How is pre-eclampsia treated? Regular checks may be all that you need if pre-eclampsia remains relatively mild. If pre-eclampsia becomes worse, you are likely to be admitted to hospital. Tests may be done to check on your well-being, and that of your baby. As the only way of stopping the pre-eclampsia is to deliver the baby, in some cases babies are delivered early to prevent harm to mother or baby.

Will pre-eclampsia develop in my next pregnancy? If you had pre-eclampsia in your first pregnancy, you have about a 1 in 10 chance of it recurring in future pregnancies.

Further information

Action on Pre-EClampsia (APEC) ☎ 020 8863 3271
🖥 www.apec.org.uk

Infection in pregnancy

Bacterial vaginosis: Present in ≈ 10% of pregnant women – asymptomatic in ½. Associated with ↑ pre-term birth (x2). There is no screening policy in the UK, but if detected:

- Except in the first trimester of pregnancy, treat with metronidazole po (400mg bd for 7d.) or PV (5g bd for 5d)
- In the 1st trimester of pregnancy, treat with clindamycin 2% cream 5g nocte PV for 1wk.

ⓘ Treatment may not lower the risk to the pregnancy. There is some evidence that PV live yoghourt is almost as effective as metronidazole.

Chickenpox: 📖 p.228

Chlamydia: 1:20 pregnant women have Chlamydia infection. During pregnancy Chlamydia infection is associated with IUGR, pre-term birth and low birth weight. It can also pass to the baby during delivery, causing eye and/or chest infections. Post-partum, Chlamydia can cause womb infection. Treatable if detected (📖 p.122) – follow-up with swabs to confirm eradication. Refer any affected neonates for expert advice.

Screening: As part of the National Opportunistic Screening Programme for Chlamydia, women <25y. will be screened for Chlamydia in antenatal clinics. Otherwise there is no evidence of cost-effectiveness of routine antenatal screening for sexually transmitted diseases.

Coughs, colds & flu: Little threat to the pregnancy itself. *Advise:* fluids, paracetamol, rest and TLC. Inhaled decongestants are safe, but avoid cough linctus and OTC composite preparations. Treat any 2° infections as needed.

Cytomegalovirus (CMV): 📖 p.230

Enteroviruses: 📖 p.230

Genital herpes^G: Affects ≈ 10% of the UK population (diagnosis made in 1:3). Risk is greatest if the 1° attack occurs at >28wk. gestation. 2° attacks are much less of a problem.

Risks include:
- Passing the infection to the baby at the time of delivery
- Early labour
- IUGR (1° infection only).

ⓘ Elective Caesarean section is advised at term if a 1° attack occurs during pregnancy at >28wk. Gestation. It is controversial if Caesarean section is preferable if there is an active 2° attack at the time of labour.

Gonorrhoea: <1/1000 pregnancies. Can pass to the baby during delivery, causing eye infections. Treat if detected – 📖 p.122. Follow-up with swabs to confirm eradication. Refer any affected infants for expert advice.

Group B streptococcus (GBS)^G: Bacterium carried in the vagina by >1:4 pregnant women (20% of non-pregnant women). Usually harmless but if transmitted to the baby during delivery can cause neonatal septicaemia, pneumonia or meningitis.

Prevention of neonatal infection: A screening programme to detect women carrying group B streptococcal infection during pregnancy (at 35–37wk.) is under consideration but, at present, treatment with IV antibiotics during labour is advised in 'high-risk' scenarios only:

- early labour <37wk.
- prolonged (>18h.) or early (<37wk.) rupture of the membranes
- Group B streptococcus detected in urine in pregnancy
- if the woman has a temperature >37.8°C during labour
- if a previous baby has been affected with the condition (10x ↑ risk).

ⓘ If found incidentally during pregnancy, there is no evidence that treatment is effective. Give antibiotics during labour.

Hepatitis B: Prevalence of HBsAg in pregnancy is up to 1% (depending on geographical area). Women are routinely offered screening for hepatitis B infection in pregnancy. Transmission to the baby occurs during labour (up to 30% of infants of women seropositive for HBsAg and 90% of infants of women seropositive for both HBsAg and HBeAg). Infants infected are at high risk (~90%) of becoming chronic carriers and of developing chronic liver disease ± premature death.

Postnatally: Refer infected women for hepatology assessment. Infected mothers should not donate their milk.

Immunization: Give hepatitis B vaccine as soon as possible after birth to babies born to carrier mothers, with the addition of immunoglobulin (HBIG) if the mother carries the hepatitis B e-antigen or had acute HBV infection during pregnancy. 85–95% effective in preventing neonatal hepatitis B infection. Further doses of vaccine are required at 1 and 2mo. of age, and a booster dose at 1y. at the same time as follow-up testing.

Hepatitis C: Prevalence in pregnant women 0.14–0.8%. Except when initial infection of the mother occurs during pregnancy (when transfer rate is much higher), transmission rate to the fetus is 5%. To date there is no evidence HCV can be transferred to the child by breast feeding. Infants at risk can be screened for HCV infection at 12mo. (RNA screen) or 18–24mo. (HCV antibody test). The majority of infants who acquire HCV infection via their mothers develop chronic hepatitis. Treatment is with interferon and achieves viral clearance rates of 40%.

Advice for patients: Information

Department of Health Hepatitis B: how to protect your baby
▣ www.dh.gov.uk
Group B Streptococcus Support ▣ www.gbss.org.uk

HIV: Prevalence of HIV amongst pregnant women in the UK varies from 0.04% to 0.4% depending on geographical area. Up to 50% of infants of HIV seropositive mothers are pre- or perinatally infected with HIV, accounting for 90% of HIV infections in childhood. Risk can be ↓ to <5% by giving zidovudine to the mother antenatally, during delivery, and to the neonate for 1st 6wk. together with elective LSCS and advice against breast feeding. A detailed fetal anomaly scan is important if there is first-trimester exposure to antiviral treatment (including folate antagonists) as possible ↑ risk of congenital abnormality.

🚑 There is a theoretical concern of mother-to-child transmission with invasive pre-natal diagnosis. For those with advanced HIV, defer until the end of the first trimester.

Antenatal HIV testing: 📖 p.218

Fetal abnormalities include: wide-set eyes, short nose, patulous lips, 'box' forehead and growth failure. However, diagnosis is usually made between 6mo. and 2y. of age when the child presents with lymphadenopathy, recurrent or opportunistic infections, failure to thrive or progressive encephalopathy. Expert advice is needed throughout pregnancy and for neonatal follow-up.

Listeriosis: Rare. May occur in epidemics. Infection of the mother is usually via infected food, e.g. pâté, soft cheese, milk. Detection is with blood cultures. Suspect if unexplained fever >48h. and refer for expert advice.

Maternal symptoms: Fever, shivering, myalgia, headache, sore throat, cough, vomiting, diarrhoea, vaginitis

Consequences: Miscarriage (may be recurrent), stillbirth, premature labour, transmission to the fetus (in 2nd/3rd trimester). Infection in the newborn infant manifests in pneumonia ± meningitis.

Prevention: See opposite.

Malaria: Serious complications are more common in pregnancy (cerebral malaria has 50% mortality). Suspect in any pregnant woman who has a fever and has recently visited an infected area. Seek immediate expert advice.

Measles: 📖 p.230

Parvovirus B19: 📖 p.226

Rubella: 📖 p.226

Syphilis: Prevalence 0.07%. ~70–100% of pregnant mothers with primary, untreated syphilis transmit the disease to the fetus (1:3 die *in utero*). In the early latent phase, risk of transmission is ~40% and ~10–15% in late latent phase. Neurological abnormalities as a result of congenital syphilis include encephalopathy and sensorineural deafness. Treatment ↓ risk of transmission by >98%. Refer for specialist assessment if +ve result on routine testing. 🚑 +ve result is NOT specific to syphilis.

Thrush: More common in pregnancy. Not harmful to the fetus. Requires treatment only if causes troublesome itching, soreness or discharge. *Treatment:* Imidazole pessaries, for 1wk. optimally.

Toxoplasmosis: Caused by a parasite found in raw meat and cat faeces. Up to 90% of women have not had toxoplasmosis before pregnancy and ~2/1000 will catch it during pregnancy. 30–40% pass it to their fetus. Infection may result in miscarriage, stillbirth, growth problems, blindness, hydrocephalus, brain damage, epilepsy, or deafness. Risk of transmission to the fetus is related to gestation at the time of infection – 3rd trimester ≈ 70%, 1st trimester ≈ 15%. If infection is suspected, refer for specialist advice.

Urinary tract infections: 1:25 women develop UTI in pregnancy. If suspected, send MSU to confirm diagnosis and start antibiotics (e.g. cefalexin 250mg tds) immediately. Recurrent UTIs in pregnancy should be investigated – consider IVU >12wk. after delivery.

Screening for UTI: Routine screening with MSU for UTI is offered at booking. 2–5% of pregnant women have asymptomatic bacteriuria, defined as pure growth of $>10^5$ organisms/ml – 1:3 will develop symptomatic infection (acute cystitis, pylonephritis) if left untreated. Both untreated bacteriuria and frank UTI are associated with pre-term delivery and IUGR. Treat for at least 1wk. with suitable antibiotic (avoid trimethoprim). Check MSU following treatment to ensure infection has cleared.

Advice for pregnant women on prevention of toxoplasmosis and listeriosis

- Only eat well-cooked meat.
- Wash hands, cooking utensils and food surfaces after preparing raw meat.
- Keep raw meat and cooked foods on separate plates.
- Wash all soil from fruit and vegetables before eating.
- If possible, get someone else to clean cat litter or use gloves and wash hands afterwards.
- Use gloves when gardening and wash hands afterwards.

259

Further information

NICE Antenatal care: routine care for the healthy pregnant woman (2003 – due for update in 2007) 🖥 www.nice.org.uk

RCOG 🖥 www.rcog.org.uk
- Management of genital herpes in pregnancy (2002)
- Prevention of early-onset neonatal group B Streptococcal disease (2001)

National Screening Committee Antenatal and newborn screening programme 🖥 www.screening.nhs.uk/an

British HIV Association Management of HIV infection in pregnant women and the prevention of mother-to-child transmission of HIV (2005) 🖥 www.bhiva.org

Intrauterine growth

Intrauterine growth restriction[G]: Babies may be small because they are premature, small for their gestation or a combination of the two. Babies small for their gestational age (IUGR – weighing <10th centile weight for their gestational age) have different problems to those of premature babies.

Predisposing factors: The major antenatal indicator for IUGR is low maternal weight at booking (<51kg). *Others include:*

- Multiple pregnancy
- Malformation
- Infection
- Maternal smoking
- Maternal DM
- Pre-eclampsia
- Severe maternal anaemia
- Maternal heart or renal disease
- Previous history of small baby
- Low weekly maternal weight ↑ (<0.2kg).

Antenatal detection: Difficult to detect – ~½ are not detected until after birth. Most GPs will encounter IUGR when they do a routine antenatal check and find the symphysis – fundal height (SFH) is less than would be expected for the gestation (Figure 5.13). Other suspicious signs are oligohydramnios and poor fetal movements. Confirm suspicions with USS then seek specialist obstetric advice. Where the head circumference is relatively spared, suspect placental insufficiency.

Consequences

- *Labour:* More susceptible to hypoxia in labour so require monitoring in a specialist unit where Caesarean section facilities are available and there is paediatric back-up.
- *Postnatal problems:* Susceptible to neonatal hypoglycaemia and jaundice. Babies <2kg may have problems with temperature regulation and require incubator facilities.
- *Long-term effects:* More prone in later life to cardiovascular disease and NIDDM.

Oligohydramnios: Liquor volume <500ml. Rare. Associated with:

- Prolonged pregnancy
- PROM (📖 p.264)
- Placental insufficiency
- Fetal abnormality (renal agenesis, urethral aplasia).

Confirm diagnosis with USS then refer for specialist obstetric assessment.

Large for dates: Consider:

- Multiple pregnancy
- Large baby (>90th centile) – may have past history of large babies
- Maternal DM
- Fetal abnormality
- Polyhydramnios
- Molar pregnancy.

Refer for USS to confirm diagnosis and exclude fetal abnormality or multiple pregnancy. Check maternal fasting blood glucose ± GTT.

Polyhydramnios Liquor volume >2l. 1:250 pregnancies. *Causes:*
- *Fetal abnormality (50%):* hydrops fetalis; anencephaly (no swallowing reflex); spina bifida; oesophageal or duodenal atresia; umbilical hernia; ectopia vesicae
- *Maternal (20%):* DM; multiple pregnancy
- *No cause found (30%)*

Risks: Premature labour; malpresentation; cord prolapse; placental abruption; PPH

Management: Refer for USS to confirm diagnosis and exclude fetal abnormality or multiple pregnancy. Check maternal fasting blood glucose ± GTT. Refer for specialist obstetric advice.

Further information

RCOG The investigation and management of the small-for-gestational-age fetus (2002) ▣ www.rcog.org.uk

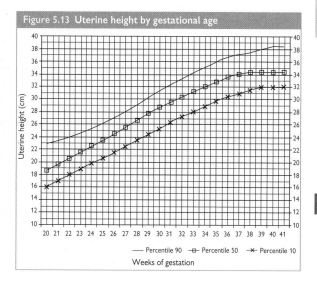

Figure 5.13 Uterine height by gestational age

Uterine height (cm) vs Weeks of gestation

—— Percentile 90 –□– Percentile 50 –✕– Percentile 10

Permission to reproduce Figure 3.12 sought from Belizan, J.M., Villar, J., Nardin, J.C. *et al.* (1978). Diagnosis of intrauterine growth retardation by a simple clinical method: measurement of uterine height. *The American Journal of Obstetrics and Gynaecology;* **131**(6):643–6, Elsevier.

Breech babies and multiple pregnancy

Breech babies[G]: 3–4% babies at term. Higher incidence <37wk. Associated with ↑ risk of cerebral palsy as breech presentation is more common in premature infants and those with congenital malformation.

Risk factors
- Bicornuate uterus
- Fibroids
- Placenta praevia
- Oligohydramnios.

Management
- Many turn spontaneously, especially if <36wk. gestation.
- If a baby is found to be breech at ≥36wk. gestation, confirm breech position and position of the placenta on USS and refer for specialist obstetric advice.

Specialist options
- Attempt to turn the baby (external cephalic version – ECV) – should only be attempted in specialist unit with facilities for fetal monitoring.
- Vaginal breech delivery – elective breech delivery should always take place in specialist units.
- Elective caesarean section.
- Moxibustion – some evidence for effectiveness[C]. Involves burning of herbs to stimulate acupuncture points beside the outer corner of the 5th toenail (acupoint BL67).

⚠ 10–15% of breech babies are discovered for the first time late in labour. If delivering at home or in a community unit, arrange transfer to a specialist unit immediately.

Follow-up: Congenital hip problems are more common in breech babies – refer all breech babies routinely for hip USS even if examination in the first 24h. is normal.

Multiple pregnancy: *Incidence:*
- twins – 1:105 ($1/3$ identical)
- triplets – 1:10,000

Predisposing factors
- Previous twins
- Family history of non-identical twins
- Race: most common amongst African blacks; least common in Japanese
- ↑ with maternal age
- Infertility treatment – induced ovulation (e.g. clomifene or gonadotrophin treatment); IVF and other assisted reproduction techniques

Diagnosis
- Hyperemesis (📖 p.222)
- USS
- Large for dates (📖 p.260)
- Polyhydramnios (📖 p.261)
- Palpation of 2 fetal heads ± multiple limbs
- 2 different fetal heart rates heard (>10bpm different).

Management: Refer for specialist obstetric care. Monochorionic twins are significantly higher risk than dichorionic twins.

Complications
- *In pregnancy:* Anaemia; polyhydramnios; pre-eclampsia (x3); APH; placenta praevia; placental abruption.
- *In labour:* Malpresentation; cord prolapse; fetal distress (↑ Caesarean section rate); PPH.
- *Fetus:* ↑ perinatal mortality (x5); prematurity; IUGR; malformations (x2–4); twin–twin transfusion may result in 1 twin being plethoric (and jaundiced later) and the other anaemic.

ⓘ Advise the mother to contact local nursery nurse training schemes. They may be able to allocate a student for learning experience who will be able to help her with the management of 2 babies.

Further information

RCOG The management of breech presentation (2001)
🖳 www.rcog.org.uk
Cochrane Coyle ME *et al.* Cephalic version by moxibustion for breech presentation (2005) Accessed via 🖳 www.library.nhs.uk

---

Advice for patients: Information and support for multiple pregnancy

Twins and Multiple Births Association (TAMBA) ☎ 0870 770 3305
🖳 www.tamba.org.uk

Labour

47% of deliveries are 'normal', i.e. occur without surgical intervention, use of instruments, induction, epidural or general anaesthetic.

Braxton-Hicks contractions: Irregular tightenings of the uterus. Start ≥30wk. gestation (common after 36wk.). May be uncomfortable but not painful.

Premature rupture of membranes (PROM): Rupture of membranes before labour starts. Usually presents with a gush of clear fluid (± an audible pop) followed by uncontrolled leakage. If chorioamnionitis is present the woman may have abdominal pain and feel unwell. Difficult to distinguish clinically from profuse vaginal discharge or incontinence of urine. Check temperature, pulse and BP and do a routine obstetric examination (including fetal heart).

ⓘ Do not perform a vaginal examination as repeated examinations can introduce infection.

Management
- *Evidence of infection* – admit for specialist obstetric care.
- *<37wk. gestation and suspected PROM* – admit to specialist obstetric unit for further assessment.
- *≥37wk. gestation* – if no signs of spontaneous labour admit for specialist obstetric assessment within 24h.

Premature labour: Any labour <37wk. gestation. *Prevalence:* 6% – 1:4 elective due to maternal/fetal problems. Largest contributor to neonatal morbidity/mortality in industrialized countries.

Causes of spontaneous premature labour: Unknown (40%).
- Cervical incompetence
- Multiple pregnancy
- Uterine abnormality
- DM
- Pyelonephritis or other sexually transmitted or urinary infection
- Polyhydramnios
- APH.

Presentation: Premature rupture of membranes or contractions. If suspected, admit immediately to obstetrics for further assessment.

Prolonged pregnancy/post-maturity: The due date is based on pregnancy lasting 40wk. or 280d. from the date of the LMP but at 40wk. only 58% of babies have delivered. It is normal to deliver between 37wk. and 42wk. At 40wk. gestation 65% will spontaneously go into labour in the next week but 15% of women have not gone into labour by 42wk. Perinatal mortality rate is ↑ x2 from 42–43wk. and x3 >43wk., so induction of labour is indicated if a pregnancy lasts >42wk.

Initial management
- Membrane sweep.
- If that is ineffective, refer for formal induction of labour (📖 p.266).
- If referral is declined, ↑ antenatal monitoring to 2x weekly CTG and USS (to measure maximum amniotic pool depth) as markers of fetal well-being.

Normal labour: Occurs ≥37wk. gestation and results in vaginal delivery of a baby in <24h. Often heralded by a 'show' consisting of mucus ± blood and/or spontaneous rupture of membranes ('waters going').

- *1st stage of labour:* Time from the onset of regular contractions until the cervix is fully dilated.
- *2nd stage of labour:* Time from complete cervical dilation until the baby is born. The mother has a desire to push.
- *3rd stage of labour:* Delivery of the placenta.

Pain relief for labour: Most women experience pain in labour. Strategies for pain relief include:
- Self-help – keep fit in pregnancy, relaxation techniques, breathing exercises, warm bath
- TENS – machines are available to hire from most obstetric units and some retail outlets
- Entonox – takes 30–45sec. to have effect – advise women to start inhaling it as soon as the contraction starts
- Injected opiates (e.g. pethidine)
- Epidural
- Pudendal block – used for instrumental delivery.

Advise women to discuss options with their midwife. Antenatal classes dealing with pain relief significantly ↑ a woman's confidence in managing her labour pains.

Epidural: Effective method of analgesia available in most hospital units. Initiated once in established labour (cervix >3cm dilated). Regular BP, pulse and fetal heart monitoring is required. *Particular indications:*
- Occipito-posterior position
- Breech
- Multiple pregnancy
- Pre-eclampsia
- Forceps delivery.
- Maternal medical conditions e.g. cardiac

Epidural complications during labour
- Postural hypotension
- Urinary retention
- ↑ need for instrumental delivery due to pelvic floor muscle paralysis

Epidural complications post-delivery: Urinary retention, headache (especially if dural puncture).

Meconium-stained liquor: Passage of fresh meconium (dark green, sticky and lumpy) during labour may be a sign of fetal distress. Transfer immediately to a consultant unit for further evaluation.

Management: Paediatrician should be present at delivery. Do not perform oropharyngeal suction if there is no evidence of foetal hypoxia.

Dystocia: Difficulty in labour. May be due to problems relating to the baby, birth passage or action of the uterus. Neonatal mortality and maternal morbidity both ↑ with duration of labour.

Possible causes
- Pelvic abnormality
- Shoulder dystocia (📖 p.272)
- Abnormal presentation
- Uterine dysfunction
- Cervical dystocia
- Cephalo-pelvic disproportion

Management: If a patient in labour at home or in a community unit fails to progress as expected, admit immediately to a specialist unit for consideration of intervention to speed the labour or Caesarean section. Shoulder dystocia is an obstetric emergency – 📖 p.272.

Induction of labour[G]: Performed when it is felt the baby is better off out than in (≈ 20% of deliveries). Only undertaken in units with facilities for continuous fetal monitoring and emergency Caesarean section.

Procedure involves: assessment of the cervix (+ vaginal prostaglandins if unfavourable); 'sweeping' of the membranes; artificial rupture of the membranes and/or IV oxytocin to maintain contractions.

Reasons for induction of labour include
- Post-maturity (most common)
- Diseases of pregnancy (e.g. pre-eclampsia)
- Maternal diabetes
- Premature rupture of membranes
- IUGR

Assisted delivery[G]: Table 5.9. Forceps and ventouse are used in ≈ 11% of deliveries in the UK (range 4–25% between hospitals). Assisted delivery should only be performed with adequate analgesia (usually epidural or pudendal block) and by experienced practitioners.

Caesarean section[G] (CS): Table 5.10. Rate in England and Wales is 21.5% (range 10–65% between different hospitals). 10% are elective and usually performed at >39wk. to minimize risk of respiratory complications, the other 11–12% occur after labour has started. Regional anaesthesia for CS is safer for mother and child than a GA.

Reasons for emergency CS: Failure to progress (25%); presumed fetal compromise (28%); breech (14%).

Planned CS is indicated for:
- Breech (where external cephalic version has failed)
- Multiple pregnancies where the first twin is not cephalic
- Placenta praevia (grade 3–4)
- HIV positive women, hepatitis C positive women and those with 1° HSV in 3rd trimester to ↓ virus transmission

GP Notes:

Maternal request is not, on its own, an indication for CS[G] but GPs should discuss risks and benefits if a request is made and, if the patient still requests a CS, refer for a consultant opinion.

Further information
RCOG 🖥 www.rcog.org.uk
- Induction of labour (2001)
- Instrumental vaginal delivery (2000)
NICE 🖥 www.nice.org.uk
- Caesarian section guidelines (2004)
- Intrapartum care – due for publication in 2007

GMS contract

Intrapartum care can be provided by practices as a *national enhanced service* – 📖 p.207.

Table 5.9 Forceps and ventouse

	Forceps	Ventouse
Indication	Delayed 2nd stage of labour	Delayed 2nd stage of labour
Procedure	• 'Wrigleys' forceps – for 'lift-out' deliveries • 'Neville-Barnes' forceps – for high deliveries • 'Keilland's' forceps – if rotation is required	• The vacuum extraction cup is applied to the baby's head, suction is applied and traction aids delivery • Ventouse allows rotation if the baby is malpositioned
Early complications	• Maternal trauma (episiotomy always needed) • Fetal facial bruising • Facial nerve paralysis	• 'Chignon' develops on the baby's head – resolves in ≤2d. • Cephalohaematoma • Retinal haemorrhage • Neonatal jaundice (but no ↑ need for phototherapy)
Longer-term complications	↑ risk of maternal faecal incontinence	
Comparison	Ventouse has ↑ failure rate compared to forceps but no ↑ CS rate ↓ requirement for regional anaesthesia with ventouse deliveries compared to forceps deliveries Forceps result in more maternal trauma than ventouse deliveries	

Table 5.10 Comparison of Caesarean section and vaginal birth

	Complications
↑ with CS	*Mother – this pregnancy*: abdominal pain; bladder or ureteric injury; hysterectomy; maternal death; need for further surgery; need for admission to intensive care/high dependency unit; thrombo-embolism; length of hospital stay; need for readmission *Mother – future pregnancies*: not having more children; ante-partum stillbirth, placenta praevia, uterine rupture *Baby*: neonatal respiratory problems
No difference	*Mother*: haemorrhage; infection; genital tract injury; faecal incontinence; back pain; dyspareunia; postnatal depression Baby: death (except breech); intracranial haemorrhage; brachial plexus injuries; cerebral palsy
↓ with CS	*Mother*: perineal pain; urinary incontinence; uterovaginal prolapse

Advice for patients: Information for women

NCT Information on labour and pain relief (including epidurals)
🖥 www.nctpregnancyandbabycare.com
RCOG About induction of labour – information for pregnant women, their partners and their families (2001) 🖥 www.rcog.org.uk

Obstetric emergencies

Resuscitation of the newborn: Follow the algorithm in Figure 5.14.

> *Rapid assessment of the infant at birth:* Start the clock. Assess colour, tone, breathing, heart rate.
>
> *A healthy baby*
> - Born blue
> - Good tone
> - Cries seconds after delivery
> - Good heart rate (120–150bpm)
> - Rapidly becomes pink during the first 90sec.
>
> *A less healthy baby*
> - Blue at birth
> - Less good tone
> - ± slow heart rate (<100bpm)
> - ± inadequate breathing by 90–120sec
>
> *An ill baby*
> - Born pale
> - Floppy
> - Slow/very slow heart rate (<100bpm)
> - Not breathing

Heart rate: Best judged by listening with a stethoscope – in many cases it can also be felt by palpating the umbilical cord – feeling for peripheral pulses is not helpful.

Airway
- Open the airway by placing the head in a neutral position – where the neck is neither extended nor flexed.
- If the occiput is prominent and the neck tends to flex, place a support under the shoulders – but don't overextend the neck.
- If the baby is very floppy, apply jaw thrust or chin lift as needed.

Breathing: Inflation breaths are breaths with pressures of ~30cm of water for 2–3sec.

If heart rate ↑: You have successfully inflated the chest. If the baby doesn't then start breathing alone, continue to provide regular breaths at a rate of ~30–40 breaths/min. until the baby starts to breathe on its own.

If heart rate does not ↑: Either you have not inflated the chest or the baby needs more help. By far the most likely is that you have failed to inflate the chest (the chest does not move). *Consider:*
- Is the baby's head in the neutral position?
- Do you need jaw thrust?
- Do you need a longer inflation time?
- Do you need a second person's help with the airway?
- Is there an obstruction in the oropharynx, e.g. meconium (laryngoscope and suction)?
- What about an oropharyngeal (Guedel) airway?

Chest compressions: Only commence after inflation of the lungs.
- Grip the chest in both hands in such a way that the thumbs of both hands can press on the sternum at a point just below an imaginary line joining the nipples and with the fingers over the spine at the back.
- Compress the chest quickly – ↓ the AP diameter of the chest by ~$\frac{1}{3}$ with each compression. The ratio of compressions to inflations is 3:1.

Drug support: For a few babies inflation of the lungs and effective chest compression is not sufficient to produce effective circulation. IV or interosseous drugs may be helpful. *Doses:*

- Adrenaline – 10mcg/kg (0.1ml/kg of 1:10,000 solution), increasing to 30mcg/kg (0.3ml/kg of 1:10,000 solution) if ineffective
- Sodium bicarbonate –1–2mmol/kg (2–4ml 4.2% bicarbonate solution)
- Dextrose – 250mg/kg (2.5ml/kg of 10% dextrose)

For emergency volume replacement (e.g. history of a bleed) – use 10ml/kg 0.9% saline given over 10–20sec. Repeat if needed.

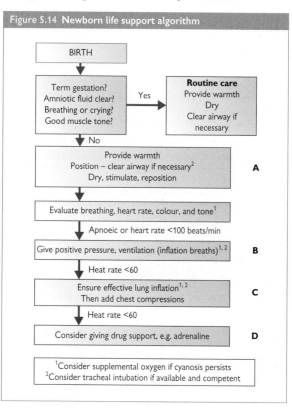

Figure 5.14 **Newborn life support algorithm**

269

Further information

Resuscitation Council (UK) Resuscitation guidelines (2005)
🖥 www.resus.org.uk

Figure 5.14 is reproduced with permission from the Resuscitation Council (UK) Resuscitation Guidelines (2005) 🖥 www.resus.org.uk

Obstetric shock: *Causes:*

- Haemorrhage – APH (📖 p.238); placental abruption (opposite – remember – bleeding may be internal and not seen per vaginum); PPH (📖 p.239)
- Ruptured uterus – see opposite page
- Inverted uterus – 📖 p.273
- Amniotic fluid embolism – 📖 p.272
- Broad ligament haematoma – 📖 p.273
- Pulmonary embolus
- Septicaemia
- Anaphylaxis (usually drugs).

> ⚠ **Action**
> - Call for help.
> - Arrange immediate admission to the nearest specialist obstetric unit (or A&E, if necessary).
> - Gain IV access and start IV fluids, give O_2 via face mask (if available).
> - Treat the cause if apparent.

Acute abdominal pain: Non-obstetric causes of abdominal pain may be forgotten or signs may be less well localized than in the non-pregnant patient. See 📖 p.221.

Appendicitis: 1/1000 pregnancies. Mortality is higher in pregnancy and perforation commoner (15–20%). Fetal mortality is 5–10% for simple appendicitis but rises to 30% when there is perforation. Due to the pregnancy, the appendix is displaced and pain often felt in the paraumbilical region or subcostally. Admit immediately if suspected.

Cholecystitis: 1–6/10,000 pregnancies. Pregnancy encourages gall stone formation. Symptoms include RUQ pain, nausea and vomiting. Diagnosis can be confirmed on USS. Treatment is the same as outside pregnancy, aiming for interval cholecystectomy after birth.

Fibroids: Torsion or red degeneration. Fibroids ↑ in size in pregnancy. They may twist if pedunculated. Red degeneration occurs usually after 20wk. and may occur until the puerperium. It presents as abdominal pain ± localized tenderness ± vomiting and low-grade fever. Treatment is with rest and analgesia. Pain resolves within 1wk.

Ovarian tumours/torsion: 1/1000 pregnancies. Torsion or rupture of a cyst may both cause abdominal pain as may bleeding into a cyst. USS can confirm the presence of a cyst. Management depends on the nature of the cyst and the severity of the pain. Admit for assessment.

If <20wk. gestation in addition consider:

- *Miscarriage:* 📖 p.234
- *Ectopic pregnancy:* 📖 p.236

If >20wk. in addition consider:

- *Labour:* 📖 p.264
- *Abruptio placentae:* see opposite page
- *Pubic symphysis dehiscence:* 📖 p.224
- *Uterine rupture:* see opposite page

- *Haematoma of the rectus abdominis:* Rarely bleeding into the rectus sheath and haematoma formation occurs spontaneously or after coughing in late pregnancy. May cause swelling and abdominal tenderness. USS can be helpful. If unsure of diagnosis, admit to exclude acute surgical or obstetric cause of pain.

Eclampsia: Occurs when the woman has a fit as a result of pre-eclampsia (2% women with pre-eclampsia). Incidence: 1:2000 pregnancies – 44% after delivery (usually <24h.). 35% of those who have a fit will have ≥1 major complication, e.g. stroke, and 1.8% die. Usually BP is very high – but may be normal or only mildly ↑, especially if the woman is non-Caucasian. If the baby is not yet born, it becomes distressed.

Symptoms and signs of impending eclampsia
- Restlessness/agitation
- ↓ urine output
- Hyperreflexia
- Retinopathy.

⚠ *Action*
- Call for help.
- Ensure the environment is safe, i.e. move any objects which could harm the woman.
- Turn onto side and place in the recovery position, if possible.
- Ensure airway is clear.
- If available, give magnesium sulphate 4g IV over 10–15min. then 1g/h. infusion. If not available, give one dose of diazepam 5–10mg IV or PR – repeated every 15 min. prn.
- Admit as 'blue light' emergency.

Abruptio placentae: 1:80–1:200 pregnancies. Part of the placenta becomes detached from the uterus. Consequences depend on the degree of separation and the amount of blood loss.

Presentation
- Typically constant pain – may be felt in the back if posterior placenta
- Woody hard, tender uterus
- Shock ± PV bleeding
- Fetal heart absent or signs of fetal distress (tachycardia or bradycardia).

⚠ *Action:* If suspected, admit as an acute emergency to the nearest specialist obstetric unit.

Uterine rupture: Rare in the UK (1:1500 deliveries). Associated with maternal mortality of 5% and fetal mortality of 30%. 70% are due to dehiscence of Caesarean section scars. Rupture occurs most commonly during labour but occasionally may occur in the 3rd trimester or after an otherwise normal delivery.

Presentation: Pain is variable but usually severe, bursting, constant lower abdominal pain ± heavy vaginal bleeding. Generally associated with profound shock in the mother and fetal distress. If in labour, the presenting part may disappear from the pelvis ± contractions stop.

⚠ *Action:* Admit as an acute emergency to a specialist obstetric unit.

Fetal distress: Signifies hypoxia. *Signs:*
- Passage of meconium during labour
- Fetal tachycardia (>160bpm at term)
- Fetal bradycardia (<100bpm–seek urgent obstetric assistance).

> ⚠ *Action:*
> - Give the mother oxygen via a face mask.
> - Turn the mother on her side.
> - Transfer immediately to a specialist obstetric unit for further assessment ± delivery.

Amniotic fluid embolism: Very rare. Mortality ~80%. Presents with profound shock, cyanosis, and dyspnoea. May occur at the height of a contraction.

> ⚠ *If suspected*
> - Call for help.
> - Resuscitate – Airway; Breathing; Circulation.
> - Transfer as a 'blue light' emergency to the nearest A&E or specialist obstetric unit.

Cord prolapse: 1:200–300 births. The cord passes through the os in front of the presenting part of the baby. If the presenting part squashes the cord, umbilical blood flow is restricted, causing fetal hypoxia and distress (fetal mortality 10–17%). *Risk factors:*

- Malpresentation – breech/transverse/oblique
- Cephalo-pelvic disproportion
- Multiple pregnancy
- Pre-term rupture of membranes
- Polyhydramnios
- Placenta praevia
- Pelvic tumours

> ⚠ *Action*
> - Minimize handling of the cord to prevent spasm.
> - Try to keep the cord within the vagina.
> - Call for help.
> - Aim to prevent presenting part from occluding the cord. Try:
> - Displacing the presenting part upwards with the examining hand
> - Get patient into knee/elbow position – head down
> - If possible, drop the head end of the bed
> - Fill the bladder with 500–750ml normal saline via a catheter and clamp the catheter.
>
> Admit as an emergency to the nearest specialist obstetric unit – usually treated with emergency Caesarean section.

Shoulder dystocia: Affects <1% deliveries but is a life-threatening emergency. Occurs when the anterior shoulder impacts upon the symphysis pubis after the head has delivered and prevents the rest of the baby following. Most cases of shoulder dystocia are unanticipated.

Clues
- Prolonged 1st or 2nd stage of labour.
- 'Head bobbing' – the head consistently descends then returns to its original position during a contraction or pushing in the 2nd stage.

If shoulder dystocia occurs in the community there is usually not time to transfer a woman to a specialist unit.

⚠ *Action:* Call for help. Consider episiotomy. Then try any of these procedures (no particular order):
- Roll the mother onto hands and knees and try delivering posterior shoulder first.
- Flex and abduct the mother's legs up to her abdomen (upside down squatting position) – try delivery again.
- Deliver the posterior arm – put a hand in the vagina in front of the baby – ensure the posterior elbow is flexed in front of the body and pull to deliver the forearm. The anterior shoulder usually follows.
- External pressure – ask an assistant to apply suprapubic pressure with the heel of the hand – a rocking movement can help.
- Adduction of the most accessible (preferably anterior) shoulder. Simultaneously put pressure on the posterior clavicle to turn the baby. If unsuccessful continue rotation through 180 degrees and try again.

Uterine inversion: Rare.

⚠ *Action:* Do not remove the placenta if attached until the uterus is replaced. If noted early, try to replace the uterus. Otherwise admit as an emergency. The mother may become profoundly shocked so set up an IV infusion before transfer if possible and give O_2 via a face mask.

Retained placenta: The 3rd stage of labour is complete in <10min. in 97% of labours. If the placenta has not been delivered in <30min. (to allow for cervical spasm), it will probably not deliver spontaneously.

⚠ **Action**
- Avoid excessive cord traction.
- Check the placenta is not in the vagina – remove if it is.
- Check the uterus.

If the uterus is well contracted: Cervical spasm is probably trapping an otherwise separated placenta – wait for cervix to relax to enable removal of the placenta.

If the uterus is bulky: The placenta may have failed to separate. Try:
- Rubbing up a contraction
- Putting the baby to the breast (stimulates uterine contraction)
- Giving a further dose of Syntometrine®
- If the placenta will still not deliver, admit as emergency for manual removal.

Broad ligament haematoma: Presents in a recently delivered woman as obstetric shock without excessive PV bleeding. Examination reveals pain and tenderness on the affected side. The uterus is deviated from that side.

⚠ *Action:* Admit as an acute emergency to the nearest specialist obstetric unit.

Maternal postnatal care

The puerperium is the 6wk. period after delivery. Most women in the UK spend ≥6h. after delivery in hospital. After discharge home, the midwife continues to visit for 2wk. after the birth and then the health visitor takes over. GPs usually see the mother and baby soon after discharge and again for the 6wk. postnatal check. Arrange additional reviews as needed.

The postnatal visit: Discuss problems during pregnancy/delivery and postnatal contraception (Table 5.11). Check:

- Rhesus status – if the mother is RhD -ve and the baby RhD +ve, ensure anti-D is given <72h. after delivery – 📖 p.241.
- Hb on day 5 after delivery (after the post-partum diuresis). If Hb is <10g/dl, continue iron supplements for 3mo.
- Rubella status – if non-immune, immunize as soon as possible and ensure effective contraception for 3mo afterwards. Reassure it is safe to breast feed after immunization.
- Temperature, pulse and BP. ↑ BP associated with pre-eclampsia usually resolves <48h. after delivery.
- Fundus – day 1 = 24wk. gestation size (up to umbilicus); day 5 = 16wk. gestation size; by day 10, uterus should not be palpable per abdomen. Persistent bulkiness suggests retained products of conception – refer for USS.
- Pain – breast, abdominal, perineal, legs.
- Vaginal loss – red, then brown, then yellowish over the first week, then serous for 3–6wk. Any fresh, red bleeding is abnormal.
- Moving about – women should try to get mobile as soon as possible after delivery to ↓ the risk of DVT.
- Feeding – 📖 p.292.
- Mental state – Screen for depression 4–6wk. and 3–4mo. postnatally (📖 p.277).

Further information

NICE Post-partum care – due for publication in 2007 🖥 www.nice.org.uk

---

GP Notes:

Postnatal visits from GPs: The first few days after having a baby can be very busy with visitors. If pregnancy and delivery were normal, the baby has had its neonatal check and the community midwife is visiting regularly and has no worries, a telephone call from the GP may be sufficient. Don't forget to mention contraception. Remind the mother to register the baby at the practice, and about the 6wk. checks.

Advice about driving and exercise (especially after CS): Resume driving when any pain is no longer distracting or restricting. Record 'fit to drive' in the notes, if required. Exercise is beneficial but 'sit-ups' are best avoided until at least 6wk. to ↓ risk of back strain.

Advice for patients: Information for women

Family Planning Association ☎ 020 7837 4044 🖥 www.fpa.org.uk
National Childbirth Trust 🖥 www.nctpregnancyandbabycare.com

Postnatal care, from hospital discharge until 14d. after delivery, excluding the neonatal check, is provided as an additional service (maternity services) and payment is included in the global sum. 'Opting out' → a 2.1% ↓ in global sum.

Table 5.11 Post-partum contraception

🛈 Contraception is *not* needed until 21d. post-partum

Method	If not breast feeding *	If breast feeding **
COC pill/ combined patch	Start ≥3wk. after delivery (patch states >28d.) as ↑ risk of thromboembolism. (🛈 Can be started immediately after miscarriage/termination). If starting on d.21 (or d.28 for patch) post-partum, immediate protection is provided. If starting after that time, use an additional method for 7d. If PET in pregnancy – start the COC pill *only* when BP and biochemical abnormalities have returned to normal.	Contraindicated <6wk. post-partum as it may inhibit lactation and enters breast milk in small quantities. >6wk. and <6mo. – use only if no other suitable method.
POP	Delay until ≥3wk. post-partum to avoid ↑risk of heavy bleeding. If started >3wk. after delivery, start on 1st day of period for immediate protection or, if cycle not established, use alternative protection for 1st 2d. For breast-feeding mothers, ↑ quantity of breast milk.	
Injectables/ implants	Preferably delay until ≥6wk. post-partum to avoid risk of heavy/irregular bleeding. If >3wk. (>4wk. for implant) post-partum, administer early in period or, if cycle not re-established, check pregnancy test before administration and use additional method for 7d. If breast feeding, delay giving injectable until ≥6wk. post-partum where possible.	
IUCD/IUS	Insert <48h. post-delivery (but ↑ risk of expulsion) or delay until >4wk. post-partum (Mirena® licence states 6wk.) – take care with insertion as the uterus may be soft and perforate easily. Use an additional method for 7d. if inserted >4wk. post-partum.	
Cap	Refit any time from 5–6wk. post-partum (even after CS). 🛈 May require a different size post-partum.	
Condoms	Useful until other methods are established and to prevent transfer of sexually transmitted diseases.	
Sterilization	↑ operative and failure rate at abortion or in post-partum period. Best delayed for a few months.	

* Ovulation can occur within 10d. of abortion and 28d. of delivery.
** Advise women <6mo. post-partum who are amenorrhoeic and fully breast feeding, there is only a low chance of pregnancy (≈ 2/1000 women) without contraception. If any supplementary bottle feeding, baby is weaned or any vaginal bleeding (except occasional spotting), then assume the woman is fertile.

Common postnatal problems

Abdominal pain: Cramping, 'period like' for the 1st 1–2wk. after delivery, especially when breast feeding. This is due to the uterus contracting down or involuting. Suspect infection if offensive lochia, fever, the uterus stops getting smaller day-by-day or is still palpable per abdomen 10d. after delivery.

Breast soreness: 3–5d. after birth the breasts become engorged ('the milk comes in') and may be quite painful. Support with a well-fitting maternity bra day and night. Express milk if still painful – a warm bath may help. *Other problems:*

Sore/cracked nipples: Try topical remedies, e.g. Kamillosan®, and/or nipple shields. Consider advice from a breast-feeding advisor – may be a 'positioning problem'.

Skin infection: Localized soreness, pain around the areola ± nipple or in the breast after a feed – usually due to candida infection. Treat mother and baby with miconazole oral gel.

🔾 Severe knife-like pain in breast during and for up to 1h. after feeding suggests deeper infection – treat mother additionally with fluconazole 150mg stat and then 50mg bd for 10d. (unlicensed use). Symptoms usually resolve in <3d.

Blocked duct: Hard, tender lump in the breast. Advise the mother to massage that area of the breast while feeding or expressing milk.

Mastitis: Tender, hot, reddened area of breast ± fever. Treat with flucloxacillin 250mg qds and NSAID, e.g. ibuprofen 400mg tds prn. Continue breast feeding or express the milk to prevent milk stagnation if too painful for feeding.

Breast abscess: Admit for incision and drainage.

Dyspareunia: Following perineal trauma. Almost always settles without need for surgery.

Haemorrhoids: Common and painful. *Try:*
- Local ice packs (frozen fingers of rubber gloves are the right shape)
- Topical preparations, e.g. proctosedyl
- Resting lying on 1 side
- Keeping stools soft using a stool softener
- Advising women to wash the haemorrhoids with cool water after opening bowels and gently push them through the anus (if possible).

Perineal bruising: Can be very painful. Advise regular analgesia, e.g. paracetamol 1g qds ± ibuprofen 400mg tds, ice packs. Ultrasound can help – consider referral to physiotherapy.

Hair loss: Hair becomes thicker in pregnancy and these hairs are all shed at about the same time ~5–6mo. post-partum. Reassure. Hair loss reverts to normal levels within 2–3mo. If severe, persistent or accompanied by tiredness, consider hypothyroidism – check TFTs.

Persistent lochia: Bleeding (lochia) >6wk. post-partum. *Causes:*
- Infection
- Resumption of normal cycle

- Retained products of conception
- Unhealed tears – cervical, vaginal or perineal
- Side-effects of contraception (e.g. POP, depot injection)
- Other cervical or uterine pathology.

Management

- Examine uterus per abdomen and do a bimanual vaginal examination to check involution. Perform a speculum examination and send a vaginal swab for M,C&S.
- If offensive loss or systemic symptoms/signs of infection, treat with antibitoics as for endometritis (🕮 p.278). Otherwise, arrange USS.
- If not settling and no cause is found, refer to gynaecology.

Poor abdominal and pelvic muscle tone: Classes for postnatal exercise to retone the body are available both on dry land and in the swimming pool at most leisure centres. Pelvic floor exercises can be started <1d. after delivery (🕮 p.145). Good leaflets explaining these are available from physiotherapists, local maternity units and the NCT.

Postnatal depression

Baby blues: Very common – women become tearful and low within the 1st 10d. of delivery. Be supportive. Usually resolves.

Depression: Common (10–15% mothers), reaching a peak ~12wk. after delivery – though symptoms are almost always present at 6wk. Often mothers do not report symptoms. NICE recommends screening all mothers for depression 4–6wk. and 3–4mo. postnatally by asking:

- During the past month, have you often been bothered by feeling down, depressed or hopeless?
- During the past-month, have you often been bothered by having little interest or pleasure in doing things?

If the woman answers 'yes' to either of the initial questions, ask: Is this something you feel you need or want help with?

Risk factors

- Depression during pregnancy
- A bad birth experience
- Social problems (e.g. poor social support, financial problems)
- Past medical history or family history of depression or postnatal depression
- Alcohol or drug abuse.

277

Management

- Talk through the problems. Refer to health visitor for support[CE].
- Give information, e.g. self-help groups, mother-and-baby groups.
- Consider checking TFTs, especially if presenting with tiredness.
- Consider counselling[CE] or referral for cognitive behaviour therapy.
- Consider antidepressant medication. If breast feeding, tricyclics are relatively safe but most manufacturers advise avoid (*BNF Appendix 5*). Of the SSRIs, sertraline 50mg od is the safest. In all cases, monitor the baby for unwanted side-effects (e.g. drowsiness, respiratory depression). If not breast feeding, fluoxetine 20mg od is the most effective antidepressant in trials[CE].
- Monitor progress using depression questionnaires e.g. Edinburgh postnatal depression scale – 🕮 p.280.
- Refer to the mental health team if these measures are not helping.
- Risk of recurrence in subsequent pregnancy is 30–50%. Women severely affected may benefit from an SSRI through their next pregnancy – seek expert advice.

> ⚠ Refer to the mental health team immediately if any risk of self-harm, suicide or harm to the baby.

Puerperal psychosis: Much rarer than postnatal depression (1:500 births). Suspect if:

- Severe depression
- High suicidal drive
- Mania
- Psychotic symptoms.

In all cases seek expert help from a psychiatrist. Consider admission – under a Section if necessary. Risk of recurrence is 20% – but 50% will never be mentally ill again.

Puerperal pyrexia: Temperature >38°C within 14d. of delivery or miscarriage. 90% infections are in the urinary or genital tracts. Ask about:

- Urinary symptoms
- Colour and smell of lochia
- Abdominal pain
- Breast symptoms
- Any other symptoms (e.g. cough, sore throat).

Examine fully, including bimanual VE, and send MSU and vaginal swabs for M,C&S. *Potential obstetric causes:*

Superficial perineal infection: Complicates tear or episiotomy – treat with flucloxacillin 250–500mg qds.

Endometritis: Presents with offensive lochia, lower abdominal pain and a tender uterus. Treat with amoxicillin 250–500mg tds and metronidazole 400mg tds or co-amoxiclav 375mg tds. If not settling in <48h. or very unwell admit for IV antibiotics.

Mastitis: See breast soreness – 🕮 p.276.

DVT or PE: Can present with pyrexia. Refer to exclude if any leg pain/chest pain/breathlessness.

Superficial thrombophlebitis: Affects 1% women. Presents with a tender (usually varicose) vein. Exclude DVT. Recovery usually occurs within a few days. Meanwhile advise the woman not to stand still and, when sitting, elevate the leg above waist height. Support the leg, e.g. with an elasticated stocking, and try applying an ice pack to the affected area. NSAIDs, e.g. ibuprofen 400mg tds prn, may help.

Tiredness: Very common in the 1st few months after delivery but it may be the presenting feature of postnatal depression, anaemia or hypothyroidism. Check FBC and TFTs.

Transient autoimmune thyroiditis: Up to 10% women 1–3mo. after delivery. Usually presents with fatigue and lethargy.

Hypothyroidism: Treat with thyroxine for 6mo. then stop for 6wk. and repeat TFTs. Follow up with annual TFTs – 1:5 go on to develop permanent hypothyroidism.

Hyperthyroidism: Refer to an endocrinologist – antithyroid treatment is not normally required but symptom control may be necessary.

Advice for patients:

Advice for carers of women with postnatal depression

- **Don't** expect the sufferer to have fears and worries that are reasonable. When you are depressed small things can upset you greatly.
- **Do** try to give her as much practical help as possible. Depression makes a sufferer feel very tired and small tasks feel like huge ones.
- **Don't** nag. Try to keep your patience even though it may be taxed.
- **Don't** point out shortcomings, unfinished jobs, unkempt appearance.
- **Don't** say 'Pull yourself together. You don't know how lucky you are. There are lots worse off than you.'
- **Don't** leave her alone with the baby if you feel there is the slightest possibility of her doing harm to the child or herself.
- **Do** try to let her express her own true feelings of anxiety and fear, even if she repeats herself.
- **Do** allow her to talk freely and express her innermost fears without showing shock or amazement.
- **Do** show consideration and sympathy for her predicament. Reassure her that she will recover, repeat this reassurance as often as you can.
- **Do** encourage her to have as much rest as possible.
- **Do** encourage and praise her when she makes an effort.
- **Do** encourage her to seek professional help.
- **Do** try to get out with friends, without the children if you can, but never force her to do anything she doesn't feel up to doing.
- **Don't** try to cope alone. You may find the present situation exhausting and stressful. Do talk about your own feelings as much as possible and accept any offers of help.

To partners – Remember she is still your wife/girlfriend, not just the mother of a child.

DON'T BE DISCOURAGED – Remember postnatal depression is an illness and mothers who suffer from it WILL recover.

General advice and support for postnatal women

National Childbirth Trust (NCT) ☎ 0870 770 3236 Info line 0870 444 8707 🖳 www.nctpregnancyandbabycare.com
NHS Direct 🖳 www.nhsdirect.nhs.uk
Baby World 🖳 www.babyworld.co.uk

Advice and support for women with postnatal depression

Royal College of Psychiatrists Information sheet on postnatal depression 🖳 www.rcpsych.ac.uk
Association for Postnatal Illness Support and befriending by women who have suffered postnatal depression/puerperal psychosis ☎ 020 7386 0868 🖳 www.apni.org
Meet-a-Mum Association Support and information for women with postnatal depression ☎ 0845 120 6162 🖳 www.mama.co.uk

Advice for carers is reproduced in modified format from the Association for Postnatal Illness website 🖳 www.apni.org.uk

Edinburgh Postnatal Depression Scale (EPDS)

Name of patient: _____

Date of test: _____

Age of baby: _____

As you have recently had a baby, we would like to know how you are feeling. Please UNDERLINE the answer which comes closest to how you have felt IN THE PAST 7 DAYS, not just how you feel today.

1. I have been able to laugh and see the funny side of things.
   - As much as I always could
   - Not quite so much now
   - Definitely not so much now
   - Not at all

2. I have looked forward with enjoyment to things.
   - As much as I ever did
   - Rather less than I used to
   - Definitely less than I used to
   - Hardly at all

3. I have blamed myself unnecessarily when things went wrong*.
   - Yes, most of the time
   - Yes, some of the time
   - Not very often
   - No, never

4. I have been anxious or worried for no good reason.
   - No, not at all
   - Hardly ever
   - Yes, sometimes
   - Yes, very often

5. I have felt scared or panicky for no very good reason*.
   - Yes, quite a lot
   - Yes, sometimes
   - No, not much
   - No, not at all

6. Things have been getting on top of me*.
   - Yes, most of the time I haven't been able to cope at all
   - Yes, sometimes I haven't been coping as well as usual
   - No, most of the time I have coped quite well
   - No, I have been coping as well as ever

7. I have been so unhappy that I have had difficulty sleeping*.
   - Yes, most of the time
   - Yes, sometimes
   - Not very often
   - No, not at all

8. I have felt sad or miserable*.
   - Yes, most of the time
   - Yes, quite often
   - Not very often
   - No, not at all
9. I have been so unhappy that I have been crying*.
   - Yes, most of the time
   - Yes, quite often
   - Only occasionally
   - No, never
10. The thought of harming myself has occurred to me*.
    - Yes, quite often
    - Sometimes
    - Hardly ever
    - Never

Scoring: Response categories are scored 0, 1, 2, and 3 according to increased severity of the symptoms. Items marked with an asterisk – questions 3, 5, 6, 7, 8, 9, and 10 – are reverse scored (i.e. 3, 2, 1, and 0). The total score is calculated by adding together the scores for each of the 10 items.

A score of ≥12 indicates the likelihood of depression, but not its severity.

🚹 The scale indicates how the mother has felt during the previous week and in doubtful cases it may be usefully repeated after 2wk. The scale will not detect mothers with anxiety neuroses, phobias or personality disorder.

Reproduced with permission. © 1987 The Royal College of Psychiatrists. Cox J.L., Holden, J.M., and Sagovsky R. (1987). Detection of postnatal depression. Development of the 10-item Edinburgh Postnatal Depression Scale. *British Journal of Psychiatry*, **150**:782–6.

GMS Contract

Maternity services, including postnatal care, from hospital discharge until 14d. after delivery, but excluding the neonatal check, are provided as an additional service and payment is included in the global sum. 'Opting out' → a 2.1% ↓ in global sum.

Further information

NICE 🖥 www.nice.org.uk
- Antenatal and postnatal mental health: Clinical management and service guidance (2007)
- Postnatal care – due for publication in 2007

Clinical evidence Howard L. Postnatal depression (2006)
🖥 www.clinicalevidence.com

DTB The management of postnatal depression (May 2000) 38 33–6

Cochrane Lawrie TA *et al.* Oestrogens and progestogens for preventing and treating postnatal depression (2000) Accessed via 🖥 www.library.nhs.uk

Lancet Gregoire AJP *et al.* Transdermal oestrogen for treatment of severe postnatal depression (1996) 347 930–3

The neonatal check

A full neonatal check must be carried out <48h. after delivery. Most are carried out by paediatricians in maternity units before discharge but this does not happen if the baby is delivered at home or discharged <24h. after delivery home or to a peripheral unit.

Parental concerns
- Discuss any worries the parent(s) might have about the child.
- Review FH, pregnancy and birth.
- Arrange hepatitis B vaccination if mother is hepatitis B +ve and/or BCG vaccination if mother is sputum smear +ve, the baby is born in an area with high prevalence (>40 cases/100,000 population/y.), or ≥1 parent/grandparent originates from a country of high prevalence.

History: Check the baby has passed urine and meconium.
- *Has the baby passed urine?* If no urine in the 1st 24h., check if there is a palpable bladder. If palpable bladder, may be due to posterior urethral valves. Otherwise suspect either that the baby has passed urine and it has been missed or that there is a renal abnormality. Check for low-set ears, beaked nose and possible limb abnormalities of Potter's syndrome and admit for further investigation. Pink urine/red staining of the nappy due to urinary urates is common and self-limiting.
- *Has the baby passed meconium?* If no meconium in the 1st 24h., suspect meconium ileus (CF), Hirschprung's or anorectal abnormality and admit for further investigation.

Examination: With mother present, lay the baby on a flat surface and check systematically – Table 5.12. Ensure length, weight and head circumference are recorded.

Moro reflex: Support baby's head and shoulders ~15cm from the examination couch. Suddenly allow the baby's head to drop back slightly. The response – extension of the arms followed by adduction towards the chest should be brisk and symmetrical. This reflex disappears by 6mo.

Neonatal bloodspot screening: Discuss – 📖 p.288.

Check vitamin K has been given: Discuss parental concerns.
- Deficiency of vitamin K can → *haemorrhagic disease of the newborn* with potentially serious effects including intracranial bleed and death.
- Vitamin K policies vary widely in the UK. Be aware of local policy.
- Babies at high-risk of bleeding (premature, low birth weight, unwell babies and those who have undergone instrumental deliveries) – routine IM administration of vitamin K is the norm.
- Babies given oral vitamin K at birth – 1 dose doesn't confer full protection. Formula feeds contain vitamin K supplements but breast-fed babies require further doses – ensure they get them.

Health education: Discuss:
- Feeding and nutrition
- Sleeping position – 📖 p.287
- Baby care
- Smoking
- Sibling management
- Crying and sleep problems
- Transport in a car

Table 5.12 Check-list for the neonatal examination

General appearance

Weight – small or large for gestation? Pallor, jaundice or cyanosis (🌑 Slight peripheral cyanosis is normal)	Syndrome? – clusters of features, e.g. features of Downs or Turner's syndrome (📖 p.286)	Oedema Skin – birth marks; meconium staining; purpura; lanugo or evidence of postmaturity

Head and facial features: 🌑 To get babies to open their eyes, try feeding the baby or moving from supine to upright.

Head circumference Caput succedaneum or cephalhaematoma Fontanelles – number (if 3rd ? Down's), size and tension Accessory auricles	Ptosis Conjunctivitis (? Chlamydia/ gonococcus) Subconjunctival haem-orrhage (usually disap-pear in <2–3wk.) Fixation ± following	Cataract/red reflex? Cleft lip/palate; tongue tie Sternomastoid swelling Potter's facies Pierre-Robin jaw (receding jaw with cleft palate) – nurse prone if severe

Mouth: Cleft palate? Profuse saliva – associated with oesophageal atresia. Epstein's pearls (small white spots usually on hard palate – disappear by 2–3wk.)

Arms and hands

Proportion of arms/fingers Number/webbing of fingers	Palmar creases (if single crease look for other abnormalities)	Erb's palsy (waiter's tip) Klumpke's palsy (clawing of hand)

Chest

Breast enlargement ± lactation (witch's milk) – may last several weeks	Shape of chest – dis-tortion, asymmetry Respiratory rate (<60 breaths/min. is normal)	Recession Air entry Added breath sounds

Cardiovascular examination

Pulses (femoral & brachial)	Heart sounds	Murmurs – 📖 p.284

Abdomen

Umbilical infection/ discharge Umbilical hernia – usually resolves by school age	Masses – liver and lower poles of kidneys are palpable; spleen and bladder are never palpable	Anus – patency/position

Genitalia

♂: penis – size and shape; position of urethral orifice; testes (normal, undescended or maldescended), hernia or hydrocoele (small hydrocoeles are common and usually resolve spontaneously)

♀: clitoromegaly; vaginal bleeding (common and self-limiting); posterior vaginal skin tag (common)

Legs and feet: Hips (📖 p.284); proportion; number of digits; club foot

Back: Sacral pit; spina bifida; scoliosis

CNS: Is the baby alert and behaving normally? Is cry normal? Is tone/floppiness normal? Are all 4 limbs moving equally and is the Moro reflex symmetrical?

Murmurs in neonates: Only 44% of cardiac malformations are detected in the first year of life. ~½ the murmurs heard at the neonatal check reflect underlying cardiac malformation. Significant murmurs may not present immediately as pulmonary pressures take several days to ↓.

Common malformations and murmurs heard
● Atrial or ventricular septal defect: pansystolic murmur – persists >7d.
● Patent ductus arteriosus: loud, continuous, 'machinery' murmur in a well baby. Murmur usually disappears in <7d. when the ductus closes.
● Aortic or pulmonary stenosis: ejection systolic murmur – persists >7d.
● Coarctation of the aorta: ejection systolic murmur also heard at the back + absent/delayed femoral pulses.

Management: If there is associated heart failure (poor feeding, tachypnoea or large liver) and/or cyanosis, refer immediately as an emergency if necessary. If a murmur is heard and the baby is otherwise well, review in 1wk. to check the murmur again. If still present refer to paediatrics/paediatric cardiology.

Neonatal screening for deafness: In the UK all newborn babies are now offered a routine hearing screen.
● *Oto-acoustic emission (OAE) screen:* A small, soft-tipped earpiece is placed in the outer part of the baby's ear and quiet clicking sounds played. In a hearing ear, the cochlea produces sounds in response to the clicks which can be recorded and analysed.
● *Automated auditory brainstem response (AABR) screen:* Involves placing small sensors on the baby's head and neck and then presenting quiet clicking sounds through tiny soft headphones (muffs). A computer analyses responses to sounds at and around the brain stem.

Screening a child <3mo. for congenital hip problems: Congenital dislocation of the hip (CDH)/developmental dysplasia of the hip (DDH) affects 3:2000 live births (♂:♀≈6:1) – though 10x that number have unstable hips and even more have 'clicks' detected on routine neonatal screening. Screening tests should be performed in a warm room with the baby undressed and lying on a firm surface. Test each hip separately and only test once as repeated testing can damage the hips.

For both tests: Flex hips and knees to 90° using one hand for each leg with thumbs on the inner side of the baby's knee and ring and little fingers behind the greater trochanters (Figure 5.15).

Ortolani manoeuvre: Gently abduct each hip whilst lifting the greater trochanter forward. As a dislocated hip is abducted a clunk or jumping sensation is felt. It is difficult to tell the difference between a click of a normal hip and a clunk of an abnormal one, so refer any clicky or clunky hips for further investigation (usually USS or orthopaedic review).

Barlow manoeuvre: Holding the legs as described above, gently apply pressure along the line of the femur, pushing it backwards out of the acetabulum. The judder of the femoral head slipping in and out of the acetabulum can be felt if the hip is dislocatable.

🛈 Refer all babies with FH of CDH or after breech presentation for further investigation.

Figure 5.15 Screening for congenital dislocation of the hip (Ortolani test)

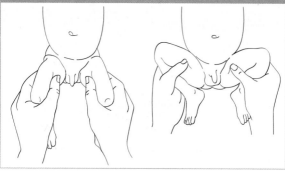

GP Notes: Which babies with jaundice need referral? Refer to paediatrics if:

Jaundice <24h. after birth: Any jaundice in the first 24h. is assumed to be pathological and needs immediate referral back to hospital to determine cause (usually haemolysis or infection) and for treatment with phototherapy or, in rare, severe cases, exchange transfusion.

Significant jaundice within 1wk. of birth: This may be difficult to assess, particularly in a dark-skinned baby. The opinion of midwives who are dealing with neonates daily can be very valuable. If necessary, arrange bilirubin estimation either by asking the community midwife to take a heel-prick sample or by contacting the neonatal SHO. High levels require further investigation and phototherapy. The level at which phototherapy is necessary varies with maturity, age and may differ slightly between paediatric units. Discuss ↑ levels with the neonatal registrar if worried.

Jaundice persisting >10d.: Although physiological jaundice may persist for some time – particularly in breast-fed babies – it is important to rule out pathological causes:

- hypothyroidism
- mild haemolysis
- infection
- liver disease – results in high levels of conjugated bilirubin
- galactosaemia.

Early diagnosis is particularly important in congenital biliary atresia so that surgery can be carried out before the liver is irreversibly damaged.

285

Table 5.13 Structural chromosome problems seen in general practice

Genetic problem	Features
Down's syndrome Trisomy 21 (92%) Translocation (6%) Mosaicism (2%) *Affects 1:600 births*	*Facial abnormalities:* flat occiput; oval face (mongoloid facies); low-set eyes with prominent epicanthic folds *Other abnormalities:* single palmar crease; hypotonia; congenital heart disease Developmental delay Life expectancy is ↓ but ~ ½ live to 60y
Edward's syndrome Trisomy 18 *Affects 1:6000 births* ♀:♂≈2:1	*Facial abnormalities:* low-set malformed ears; receding chin; protruding eyes; cleft lip or palate *Other abnormalities:* short sternum makes the nipples appear too widely separated; fingers cannot be extended and the index finger overlaps the 3rd digit; umbilical/inguinal hernias; rocker-bottom feet; rigid baby with flexion of limbs Developmental delay Life expectancy is ~10mo
Patau's syndrome Trisomy 13 *Affects 1:7500 births*	*Facial abnormalities:* small head and eyes; cleft lip and palate *Other abnormalities:* skeletal abnormalities, e.g. flexion contractures of hands ± polydactyly with narrow fingernails; brain malformation; heart malformation; polycystic kidneys 50% die in <1mo. Usually fatal in the first year
Cri-du-chat syndrome Deletion of short arm of chromosome 5 *Affects 1:50,000 births*	*Facial abnormalities:* microcephaly; marked epicanthic folds; moon-shaped face; alert expression *Other abnormalities:* abnormal cry (cat-like) Developmental delay Usually fatal in the first year
Turner's syndrome XO – deletion of 1 X chromosome. Mosaicism may occur (XO, XX) *Affects 1:2500 births*	Female appearance *Facial abnormalities:* ptosis; nystagmus; webbed neck *Other abnormalities:* short stature (<130cm); hyperconvex nails; wide carrying angle (cubitus valgus); inverted nipples; broad chest; coarctation of the aorta; left heart defects; lymphoedema of the legs; ovaries rudimentary or absent Lifespan is normal
Klinefelter's syndrome XXY or XXYY polysomy *Affects 1:1000 births*	Male appearance Often undetected until presentation with infertility in adult life *Clinical features:* may present in adolescence with psychopathy; ↓ libido, sparse facial hair, gynaecomastia, small firm testes *Associations:* hypothyroidism, DM, asthma *Specialist management:* androgens and plastic surgery may be useful for gynaecomastia.

Child health surveillance 1	Child development checks are offered at intervals consistent with national guide-lines and policy	6 points

GMS practices are expected to perform child health surveillance (excluding neonatal checks) for all children <5y. of age registered with the practice as an additional service. Opting out → a 0.7% ↓ in the global sum payment.

Neonatal checks can be provided by GMS GPs as a national enhanced service (📖 p.6) or by PMS GPs as part of their negotiated services.

Advice for patients: Information for new parents

Reducing the risk of cot death

- Cut smoking in pregnancy and don't let anyone smoke in the same room as your baby.
- Place your baby on his back to sleep.
- Don't let your baby get too hot.
- Keep your baby's head uncovered – place your baby with his feet to the foot of the cot to prevent wriggling down under the covers.
- It's safest to sleep your baby in a cot in your bedroom for the first 6 months. It's dangerous to share a bed with your baby if either parent:
  - is a smoker – no matter where or when he/she smokes
  - has been drinking alcohol
  - feels or has taken any drug which could make him/her drowsy.
- It's very dangerous to sleep together with your baby on a sofa, armchair or settee.
- If your baby is unwell, seek medical advice promptly.

Protecting your baby from accidents and infections

- Keep small objects out of your baby's reach.
- Stay with your baby when he is eating or drinking.
- Make sure your baby's cot and mattress are in good condition and that the mattress fits the cot properly.
- Install at least one smoke alarm and plan a way to escape a fire.
- Never leave your baby alone in a bath or near water.
- Make sure your baby can't reach hot drinks or the kettle or iron flex.
- Immunize your baby.
- Only use toys suitable for your baby's age.
- Never shake your baby – ask for help if crying gets too much.
- Use a properly fitted baby car seat that is the right size for your baby.
- Don't use a baby walker.
- Wash your hands before feeding your baby and make sure your baby's bottle and teats are properly sterilized.

Neonatal bloodspot screening

Neonatal bloodspot screening involves taking a blood sample obtained by pricking a baby's heel. The blood is placed on special filter paper (formerly called the Guthrie card) and sent for analysis. The test is usually carried out by the midwife when the baby is 5–8d. old and the result is available by 6wk.

Aim of bloodspot screening: To identify babies at high-risk of having conditions for which early diagnosis and treatment improves outcome. Screening is not diagnostic and further tests are necessary to confirm diagnosis. When screening tests are positive it is essential that babies are referred quickly for further diagnostic tests/treatment.

Informed consent: As bloodspot screening is performed so soon after birth, it is important that parents have a chance to think about whether they wish their child to be screened for all or any of the conditions covered by the bloodspot screening programme, before the child is born. Where possible, ensure parents are given the national pre-screening leaflet during pregnancy at ~28wk. gestation.

Parents who decline screening: Parents are entitled to decline screening for all or any one of the conditions being screened for. Whilst screening is strongly recommended, parents' decisions must be respected. Discussions with parents and their consent (or decline) to screening should be recorded in the mother's health record. If a parent declines screening, explore the reasons why consent has not been given.

> ⚠ If screening is declined, it is important to flag in the child's notes that the child has not been screened in case the child becomes ill later on.

What conditions does bloodspot testing detect?

- Throughout the UK, babies are screened for phenylketonuria (PKU) and congenital hypothyroidism (CHT).
- Throughout England, babies are screened for sickle cell disease.
- Cystic fibrosis (CF) screening is currently offered in Scotland, Northern Ireland, and some areas of England and will be available throughout the UK by April 2007.
- A pilot study of screening boys for Duchenne muscular dystrophy is underway in Wales and another pilot study of screening for medium-chain Acyl CoA dehydrogenase deficiency (MCADD) is underway in certain areas of England.

Phenylketonuria (PKU): In the UK 1:10,000 babies has PKU (autosomal recessive trait – higher incidence in Ireland). Children are unable to break down phenylalanine, an amino acid present in many foods. The baby appears normal at birth but develops severe developmental delay, learning difficulty and seizures in infancy. Prenatal diagnosis is possible if there is a FH and the bloodspot test is used to detect high levels of blood phenylalanine for all newborns in the UK. Treatment is with lifelong dietary restriction of phenylalanine. With treatment, growth and development are normal.

Advice for patients:

Frequently asked questions about bloodspot screening

What are babies screened for? Bloodspot screening identifies babies who may have rare but serious conditions. Please ask your midwife which conditions are screened for in your area.

Why should I have my baby screened? Most babies screened will not have any of the conditions, but for the few who do, benefits of screening are enormous. Early treatment can improve health and prevent disability or even death.

What does screening involve? When your baby is 5–8 days old, you will be offered a screening test for your baby. The midwife will prick your baby's heel using a special device and collect drops of blood onto a card. The test may be uncomfortable and your baby may cry.

Occasionally the midwife or health visitor will contact you to take another blood sample. This may be because there was not enough blood collected the first time or because the result was unclear. Usually repeat results are normal.

When will I get the result of the screening test? Most babies will have normal results and you should know the result by the time your baby is 6–8 weeks old.

Will screening for these conditions show up anything else? Screening for cystic fibrosis may identify some babies who are likely to be genetic carriers for cystic fibrosis. These babies may need further testing to find out if they are healthy carriers or have cystic fibrosis.

Screening for sickle cell disorders may also identify healthy genetic carriers of sickle cell or other unusual red blood cell disorders. Rarely, other red blood cell disorders are also detected. These disorders may not need treatment or may benefit from early treatment too.

What if my baby has one of these conditions? You will be told any abnormal results by the time your baby is 6 weeks old. Your baby will then be referred to a specialist for further tests to make sure the diagnosis is correct. If the diagnosis is confirmed, the specialist will start treatment and provide you with information and support.

How accurate is screening? Screening is not 100% accurate. Some babies will have a positive result and be referred for further testing and found not to have anything wrong. A few babies will not be detected by screening and their illness will be detected later when they get symptoms which need treatment.

Further information for parents

UK Newborn Screening Programme Centre Leaflets screening for parents ⌨ www.newbornscreening-bloodspot.org.uk
National Society for Phenylketonuria (NSPKU) ☎ 020 8364 3010
⌨ www.nspku.org

289

Congenital hypothyroidism

- In the UK, 1:4000 babies is born with congenital hypothyroidism (5>4).
- Untreated, children with abnormally low levels of thyroid hormone fail to grow properly and have mild–severe mental disability.
- The bloodspot is used to detect low levels of blood thyroxine.
- Treatment with thyroxine replacement results in normal growth and development. Usually thyroxine replacement is needed lifelong.

Cystic fibrosis (CF)

- In the UK, 1:2500 babies is born with CF.
- Early treatment of cystic fibrosis improves outcome and prolongs both quality and quantity of life.
- Screening detects immunoreactive trypsin (IRT) which is ↑ in children with CF. If IRT is ↑, the blood is then DNA tested for the most common gene alterations (Figure 5.16).
- If a child tests positive, it is important that parents and siblings receive genetic counselling and are offered genetic testing for the condition. If both parents are carriers of a CF gene, there is a 1:4 chance of any subsequent children they have together being affected.
- Screening will also detect healthy carriers. This has implications not only for the child but also parents and other siblings. Ensure parents have a full explanation of results and understand their meaning.

❶ As there are many more mutations described than tested for, not all gene mutations will be detected and some affected babies will be missed by newborn screening. Continue to watch for later presentations.

Sickle cell disease

- In the UK, 1:2400 babies is born with a sickle cell disorder (most common in people of Afro-Caribbean or sub-Saharan origin).
- Infants with sickle cell disease are at risk of presenting for the first time with severe overwhelming infections and splenic sequestration crises. Early diagnosis allows prophylaxis with penicillin and vaccines, and parent training to identify children with complications and to present early for treatment. This ↓ complications and deaths in young infants.
- Abnormal haemoglobin is screened for using either high-performance liquid chromatography (HPLC) or iso-electric focusing (IEF). If detected, a confirmatory test is performed on the original spot using a different technique from the initial screening test.
- If a child tests positive, it is important that parents and siblings receive genetic counselling and are offered genetic testing for the condition.
- This test will detect babies with sickle cell trait or other heterozygous states as well as babies with sickle cell disease. It is important that parents understand the meaning and significance of results both for the child and other family members.
- The screening tests will also detect other haemoglobin abnormalities such as haemoglobin E and the thalassaemias. Even if these have no clinical consequences for the child, the current policy is to inform parents of the results. It is essential that parents receive accurate information about what these results mean and the likely implications for the child and other family members.

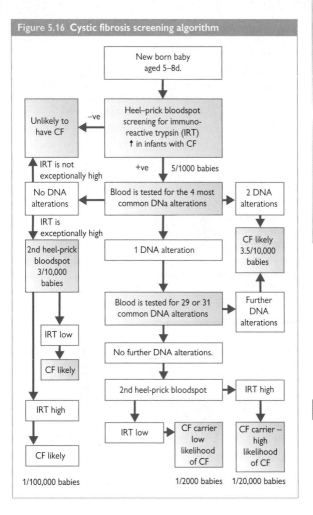

Figure 5.16 Cystic fibrosis screening algorithm

Further information
UK Newborn Screening Programme Centre
💻 www.newbornscreening-bloodspot.org.uk

Feeding babies

Breast feeding: Breast feeding is the preferred way to feed infants from birth until fully weaned or longer. However, ~1:3 mothers who start breast feeding have stopped by 6wk. Most wish to continue, but problems with painful breasts/nipples, concern regarding amount of milk the baby is getting and lack of support are common reasons for stopping.

Breast feeding is something some find natural and others find difficult. Teaching a woman and baby to breast feed takes time and patience. Be supportive and ask a midwife, health visitor or the local breast-feeding advisor to help if needed.

Advantages of breast feeding
- Encourages a strong bond between mother and baby
- More convenient than bottle feeding – the milk is ready warmed and there is no need for sterilized bottles
- Cheaper than bottle feeding
- Protects the baby from infection
- ↓ childhood obesity
- ↓ childhood atopy
- Possible ↓ risk of DM for the baby
- ↓ post-partum bleeding
- Helps the mother ↓ weight after pregnancy
- Protects the mother against breast and ovarian cancer.

Common problems with breast feeding: Table 5.14

Bottle feeding

Cow's milk formula feeds: Prepared from cow's milk altered to simulate the composition of human milk, with added iron and vitamins. Advise parents to choose a formula suitable for their baby and make up the formula exactly as the manufacturer suggests. Feeding bottles and teats should be well washed and, until >6mo. of age, sterilized. Using a cup rather than bottle is advisable from about 6mo. Families on low incomes may be entitled to claim free formula milk for their babies.

Follow-on formula: Not essential unless a child is not taking solids and is >6mo. old. Baby milks suitable from birth can be used until a switch is made to normal cow's milk.

Soya protein-based formula: Available for children with cow's milk allergy – though this group are frequently also intolerant of soya milk. Soya formula is useful for babies who have transient intolerance after gastroenteritis, but be careful – it contains large amounts of glucose syrup and can damage the teeth of babies fed on it long term, and it contains plyto-oestrogens that may be harmful – particularly to male infants. Soya formula is available on NHS prescription.

Special artificial formula: Available for children intolerant to soya and cow's milk formulae – prescribe only on consultant recommendation.

Unmodified cow's milk: Not recommended until the baby is >1y. (semi-skimmed >2y.; skimmed >5y.) old as unmodified cow's milk is less digestible, and contains little iron.

Table 5.14 Common problems with breast feeding

Problem	Possible solutions
Painful breasts and/or nipples	Ensure correct positioning. Treat mastitis or thrush if present – 📖 p.276.
It is difficult to know how much milk the baby is taking at each feed	Encourage demand feeding and tell mothers to exhaust milk supply in one breast before starting the other. Plot weight. If there are concerns about weight gain, consider other causes of failure to thrive.
Breast milk does not contain all the nutrients the baby needs	Breast milk has low levels of vitamin K, D and iron. Ensure babies who have had oral vitamin K at birth receive additional vitamin K supplements. Encourage weaning at 6mo. Lactating mothers and babies from 6mo. can be given vitamin D supplements if needed. Iron drops can be given to babies with low iron reserves (e.g. low birth weight, maternal anaemia).
Only the mother can feed the baby	Mothers who anticipate they will be absent from the baby for a period of time can express milk for someone else to feed to the baby in a bottle whilst they are gone. Advise mothers not to attempt this before breast feeding is well established as the baby might find the 2 techniques confusing. 2 methods are commonly used: • using a commercially available breast pump *or* • by hand into a sterile bowl. Breast milk can be frozen (special bags are available) and defrosted when required. Bottles should be sterilized and the milk warmed in the same way as for bottle feeding.
Disease can be transferred in breast milk	In general, breast milk protects the baby from disease. Some diseases can be transferred in breast milk, e.g. hepatitis B or HIV. Bottle feeding is recommended where uncontaminated water is available.
Drugs taken by the mother may have adverse effects on the baby	Mothers should take medical advice before taking any drugs (including herbal remedies). For most conditions drugs safe for use whilst breast feeding are available. Rarely, breast feeding is contraindicated, e.g. for women taking lithium or on chemotherapy.

293

Advice for patients: Sources of support for breast-feeding mothers

National Childbirth Trust ☎ 0870 444 8708
🖳 www.nctpregnancyandbabycare.com
La Leche League ☎ 0845 120 2918 🖳 www.laleche.org.uk
Baby Café 🖳 www.thebabycafe.co.uk
Association of Breast feeding Mothers ☎ 0870 401771
🖳 www.abm.me.uk
Breast feeding Network ☎ 0870 9000 8787
🖳 www.breast feedingnetwork.org.uk

The 6-week checks

Mother's 6wk. postnatal check
- Discuss any problems in pregnancy or delivery and note for future reference.
- Discuss any current problems the mother has and specifically enquire about persistent vaginal loss, bladder/bowel control and any sex-related problems.
- Discuss any problems with the baby – including worries about hearing/vision.
- Discuss feeding and contraception.

Examination
- BP
- Weight – if overweight discuss weight control – 📖 p.26
- Abdominal examination – uterus should not be palpable per abdomen
- Vaginal examination – only if any problems with tears/episiotomy, persistent vaginal bleeding, pain or overdue cervical smear
- Use NICE screening questions for depression – 📖 p.277.

Investigations
- Cervical smear if required.
- Check Hb if anaemic postnatally.
- Check rubella immunization has been given if not immune antenatally – if not, arrange for vaccination. Check immunity 3mo. after vaccination.

Baby's 6wk. check: Sometimes done at the same visit.

Physical examination
- Weight and head circumference
- Dysmorphic features
- Murmurs
- Red reflexes
- Check for CDH – 📖 p.284
- Testicular descent.

Health education
- Discuss immunizations; feeding; dangers of falls, scalds, and smoking around a baby
- Prevention of cot death – 📖 p.287
- Recognition of illness and advice about what to do.

Developmental screening
Gross motor development
- *Head control (0–3mo.):* Pull the baby gently from a supine position to a sitting position by the hands/wrists. The baby should hold his head upright and steady without wobbling by 6wk.
- *Moro reflex (0–6mo.):* 📖 p.282
- *Ventral suspension (0–10mo.):* Suspend the baby horizontally, face down. The head should be in line with or slightly higher than the body and the hips semi-extended.
- *Prone position (from birth):* Place the baby face down on a flat surface. He should be able to lift his head momentarily from the surface.

Fine motor development and vision

- *Stares (from birth):* Look at the baby's face – he will usually stare back. If not, ask the mother if the baby looks at her while feeding.
- *Follows horizontally to 90°:* Put the child on his back with head turned to 1 side. Move a bright-coloured object 25cm from the child's face from 1 side to the other – the child should follow the object with his eyes ± head across the midline and through ≥90°. If the child's gaze wanders from one side to the other when happy, awake and >6wk. old, suspect a visual problem.

Social behaviour

- Smiles (0–10wk. – mean 5wk.)
- Turns to look at observer's face (from birth).

⚠ **Warning signs**
- Absence of red reflex
- No visual fixation or following
- Failure to respond to sound
- Asymmetrical neonatal reflexes
- Excessive head lag
- Failure to smile.

Figure 5.17 Loss of red reflex in a child with retinoblastoma

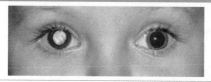

GMS contract

295

Child health surveillance, including the 6wk. check, is provided as an additional service and payment is included in the global sum. 'Opting out' → a 0.7% ↓ in global sum.

Figure 5.17 is reproduced with permission from Childhood Eye Cancer Trust (CHECT), 🖳 www.chect.org.uk

Stillbirth and neonatal death

Those babies born dead after 24wk. gestation. Death may occur *in utero* or during labour. Usually present with a lack of fetal movements and on examination no fetal heart can be detected. If suspected, refer as an emergency to the nearest obstetric unit for confirmation of intrauterine death by USS.

Management: In hospital, mothers of babies who have died *in utero* are usually induced. Samples are routinely taken from mother and baby to try to determine cause of death.

Common causes: Pre-eclampsia; IUGR renal disease; DM; infection; malformation; postmaturity; abruption; knots in the cord. No cause is found for 1:5 stillbirths.

After discharge: Make contact with the parents as soon as possible.

Lactation suppression: Offer carbegoline 1mg as a single dose.

Registration of stillbirth: A certificate of stillbirth is issued by the obstetrician which must be taken to the Registrar of Deaths within 42d. of the stillbirth. Parents are issued with a certificate of burial or cremation and a certificate of registration to keep. The child's name may be entered on the certificate of registration.

Funeral: Parents have the option of a free hospital funeral. Burial is usually in an unmarked multiple occupancy grave. Parents may pay for a single occupancy grave or cremation. Alternatively parents may pay for a private funeral.

Benefits: In the UK all maternity benefits are still payable after stillbirth – 📖 p.203.

Follow-up: Is routinely arranged by the specialist obstetrician to discuss reasons for the stillbirth and implications for future pregnancies. Primary care follow-up is essential. Stillbirth is a huge burden to come to terms with. Parents do not have the regular contact with medical staff a baby brings. Ensure regular follow-up by a member of the primary care team. Broach the issues brought up by the baby's death directly. Offer an open door. Give information about support organizations, e.g. SANDS. Advise waiting 6mo.–1y. before embarking on another pregnancy.

Neonatal death: Death of an infant <28d. old. Rare in the community. If expected, the GP can issue a special death certificate. If unexpected, refer to the police/coroner. Offer lactation suppression and follow up as for stillbirth.

Patient support and information
Stillbirth and Neonatal Death Society (SANDS) ☎ 020 7436 5881
🖥 www.uk-sands.org

Chapter 6

Mental health

Chronic stress *298*
Depression *300*
Suicide and deliberate self-harm (DSH) *308*
Anxiety disorders *312*
Obsessive–compulsive disorder (OCD) *322*
Eating disorders *324*

Chronic stress

The word stress derives from the Latin 'stringere', meaning to 'draw tight', and was first used during the 17th century to describe hardships or affliction. We all suffer from stress and, most of the time, the pressures of everyday life are a motivating force. A problem only arises when those pressures exceed the individual's ability to cope with them.

Causes of stress: Virtually anything we do can cause stress. The most common causes of stress-related morbidity in the UK are:

- Work problems
- Family problems
- Financial problems
- Legal problems
- Exam stress.

The stress epidemic: 105 million working days are lost each year in the UK due to stress (11% of all sickness absence). The Health and Safety Executive estimates that ~½ million people in the UK are experiencing work-related stress at a level they believe is making them ill; up to 5 million people feel 'very' or 'extremely' stressed by their work; and work-related stress costs society >£4 billion every year.

Presentation: Most patients don't consult their GP with stress unless they feel it is affecting their health. Common symptoms include:

- Mood swings
- Anxiety
- Depression
- Low self-esteem
- Poor concentration/memory
- Fatigue and/or lethargy
- Sleep disturbance
- Poor or ↑ appetite
- Other aches and pains for which no cause can be found, e.g. muscular pains, chest pains
- ↑ smoking, alcohol and/or caffeine consumption
- Headaches
- Loss of libido
- Menstrual abnormalities
- Dry mouth
- Worsening of pre-existing conditions, e.g. irritable bowel syndrome, eczema, asthma, psoriasis, migraine.

Management: The GP's role is to:

- Identify that stress is the cause of the presenting symptoms
- Educate about stress and the link between symptoms and stress
- Try to identify the source of the stress
- Provide the patient with self-management strategies (opposite)
- Support the patient
- Treat any medical problems arising out of the stress, e.g. depression
- Provide certification if the stress is so great that the patient is unable to work. ❶ If the stress is work related, consider putting a statement to that effect on the certificate to allow the employer to take steps to alleviate the stress and facilitate return to work.

Advice for patients:

10 tips for chronic stress relief

- Ensure you get enough sleep and rest – avoid using sleeping tablets to achieve this.
- Look after yourself and your own health, e.g. don't skip meals, sit down to eat, take time out to spend time with family and friends, make time for hobbies and relaxation, do not ignore health worries.
- Avoid using nicotine, alcohol or caffeine as a means of stress relief.
- Work off stress with physical exercise – ↓ levels of adrenaline released and ↑ release of natural endorphins which → a sense of well-being and enhance sleep.
- Try relaxation techniques.
- Avoid interpersonal conflicts – try to agree more and be more tolerant.
- Learn to accept what you can't change.
- Learn to say 'no'.
- Manage your time better – prioritize and delegate (see below); create time buffers to deal with unexpected overruns and emergencies.
- Try to sort out the cause of the stress, e.g. talk to line manager at work, arrange marriage or debt counselling, arrange more child care.

Time management made easy: This technique aims to transform an overwhelming volume of work into a series of manageable tasks.
- Make a list of all the things you need to do.
- List them in order of genuine importance.
- Note whether you really need to do the task, what you need to do personally and what can be delegated to others.
- Note a time-scale in which each task needs to be done, e.g. immediately, within a day, within a week, month, etc.

Advice and support for patients

Stress Management Society ☎ 0870 199 3260 🖳 www.stress.org.uk
International Stress Management Association (UK)
☎ 07000 780 430 🖳 www.isma.org.uk

Further information
Health and Safety Executive (HSE) 🖳 www.hse.gov.uk/stress

Depression

2.3 million people suffer from depression in the UK at any time. 1:5 seeking help in primary care have psychological problems; 1:10 suffer from depression and women are twice as likely to suffer as men.

Recognition: ~30–50% cases are not detected, although most of those missed are mild cases, more likely to resolve spontaneously. Diagnosis of mental illness is stigmatizing. Polls show 60% think people with depression would feel too embarrassed to consult their GP. This can lead to 'collusion' between patient and doctor during consultation to avoid any diagnosis of mental health problems, serving interests of doctor and patient but doing little to tackle the problem.

Causes/co-morbidity: Associated with:
- *Psychiatric disorders:* e.g. anxiety disorders, alcohol abuse, substance abuse, eating disorders
- *Physical disorders:* e.g. Parkinson's disease, multiple sclerosis, dementia, endocrine disease (DM, thyroid disorders, Addison's disease), hypercalcaemia, rheumatoid arthritis, SLE, cancer, AIDS and other chronic infections, cardio- and cerebrovascular disease, learning disability
- *Drugs causing symptoms of depression:* β-blockers, anticonvulsants, Ca^{2+} channel blockers, corticosteroids (though prednisolone sometimes used, especially in terminal care, for the artificial 'high' it can give), oral contraceptives, antipsychotic drugs, drugs used for Parkinson's disease (e.g. levodopa)

Definitions

Major depression: 2 key features: depressed mood and/or ↓ interest or pleasure, which must be disabling to the patient.

Diagnosis: ≥1 key feature and ≥5 symptoms from the following list present most of the time for ≥2wk.:
- Change in appetite or weight
- Insomnia or hypersomnia
- Fatigue or loss of energy
- Poor concentration
- Poor appetite or overeating
- Insomnia or hypersomnia
- Low energy or fatigue
- Low self-esteem
- Psychomotor agitation or retardation
- Sense of worthlessness or guilt
- Recurrent thoughts of death or suicide
- Feelings of hopelessness
- Poor concentration or difficulty making decisions.

Mild to moderate depression: Some of the above symptoms (but not enough to make diagnosis of major depression) associated with some functional impairment.

Dysthymia: A chronic form of minor depression. Depressed mood for *most* of the day, for more days than not, for ≥2y. *and* the presence of ≥2 of the above symptoms.

GMS contract			
Depression 1	% of patients on the diabetes register and/or the CHD register for whom case finding for depression has been undertaken on one occasion during the previous 15mo. using 2 standard screening questions *	up to 8 points	40–90%
Depression 2	In those patients with a new diagnosis of depression, recorded between the preceeding 1st April to 31st March, the % of patients who have had an assessment of severity at the outset of treatment using an assessment tool validated for use in primary care	up to 25 points	40–90%

* Screening questions
- During the last month, have you often been bothered by feeling down, depressed or hopeless?
- During the last month, have you often been bothered by having little interest or pleasure in doing things?
A +ve reply to either question requires further mood assessment.

Advice for patients:

Patient experiences of recognition of their depression

Patients say it is difficult to describe their feelings – it was 'terrifying ... I couldn't get across to people how I was feeling'. Unlike a broken leg, outsiders can't directly see depression.

Although some say they are desperate for someone else to notice how bad things are, others want to believe they are stressed or 'run down'. To get a diagnosis people usually have to 'make the first move' and visit their doctor.

Physical ailments associated with depression (e.g. gastric upsets, sore backs, extreme tiredness) can make it even harder to diagnose.

When the seriousness of their depression is not recognized, people can suffer in silence. Those people are often angry about remaining unheard. They feel that an earlier diagnosis and/or recognition of the severity of their condition could have made a real difference to their lives.

Resisting the diagnosis of depression is partly about the stigma attached to depression, but also about trying to avoid the implications.

Sometimes only a crisis (e.g. suicide attempt, inability to work) makes sufferers seek help.

Information and support for patients
Depression Alliance ☎ 020 7207 3293 🖥 www.depressionalliance.org
Royal College of Psychiatrists Patient information sheets
🖥 www.rcpsych.ac.uk

History

- Onset including precipitating events
- Nature of symptoms, severity and affect on life
- Past history of similar symptoms/past psychiatric history
- Current life events – stressors at home and at work
- Family history
- Co-existent medical conditions
- Current medication – prescribed and non-prescribed.

⚠ Sleep disturbance and fatigue have high predictive value for depression and should prompt enquiry about other symptoms.

Cultural considerations: Some cultures have no terms for depression and may present with physical symptoms (somatization) or use less familiar 'cultural-specific' terms to describe depressive symptoms, e.g. 'sorrow in my heart'.

Examination

- *General appearance:* self-neglect, smell of alcohol, weight ↓
- *Assessment of mood:* looks depressed and/or tired, speech monotone or monosyllabic, avoids eye contact, tearful, anxious or jumpy/fidgety, feeling of distance, poor concentration, etc.
- *Psychotic symptoms:* hallucinations, delusions, etc.

Assesing severity of depression: Rapid, self-complete pencil and questionnaires can help determine severity. Significant depression which is likely to need drug or psychological threapy is suggested by:

- A diagnosis of Major Depressive Disorder, with a total score of ≥10 on the Patient Health Questionnaire PHQ-9 (📖 p.306)
- A depression score of ≥11 on the Hospital Anxiety and Depression Scale (HADS) (available from NFER Nelson 🖥 www.nfer-nelson.co.uk) *or*
- A score of ≥14 or more on the Beck Depression Inventory (BDI) (available from Harcourt Assessment 🖥 www.harcourt-uk.com).

⚠ A fee is payable for the use of the HADS or BDI, but not for the PHQ.

Assessment of suicide risk: Ask about suicidal ideas and plans in a sensitive but probing way. It is a common misconception that asking about suicide can plant the idea into a patient's head and make it more likely. Evidence is to the contrary.

Risk factors for suicide	
• ♂ > ♀ • Age 40–60y. • Living alone • Divorced > widowed > single > married • Unemployment • Chronic physical illness	• Past psychiatric history • Recent admission to psychiatric hospital • History of suicide attempt/self harm • Alcohol/drug misuse

Management of depression: Table 6.1

Management of threatened suicide: 📖 p.308

Table 6.1 Summary of management of depression

Presentation	Action
Major depression and dysthymia	Antidepressant therapy (📖 p.304) or cognitive behaviour therapy
Acute milder depression	Education about depression, e.g. information leaflets
	Support, self-help groups and guided self-help
	Simple problem-solving strategies (📖 p.305) or counselling
	Monitor regularly for development of major depression
Persistent milder depression	Trial of antidepressants (📖 p.304)
Milder depression with history of major depression	Consider antidepressants (📖 p.304)
	Monitor closely

Advice for patients: Patient experiences of having depression

Depression is different from just 'not being happy' – there is no joy, life is black, and you can't see a future or remember being happy. Depression is like 'a black pit' or 'trying to run through treacle'.

People feel cut off from their feelings and from other people – like being 'locked in' and isolated behind Perspex or inside a thick balloon. Adding to the isolation, many avoid friends and family in case they are a 'burden'.

Many become tearful and some cry uncontrollably.

Many describe becoming very sensitive to noise, music, and reacting badly to the 'slightest' remark – just wanting to 'sit in a dark cupboard'.

Many also find it becomes very difficult to concentrate and remember things – 'I really couldn't string two sentences together'.

Eating and basic self-care routines such as dressing and applying make-up can seem insurmountable tasks – little details of life (e.g. choosing clothes) can become 'enormous problems you are incapable of dealing with'.

Negative thinking is described as 'things going around in your head, so you don't sleep anymore' and you leap to wrong conclusions, even to the point of paranoia.

People have trouble knowing anything solid about themselves during depression – 'your whole self gets put into the mixer and could come out in any old form'.

Many people talk about feeling 'bad' and guilty as if they have done something terrible.

Many people have trouble sleeping, and variously wake up early, can't get out of bed, and feel like a 'zombie' and/or 'shattered' during the day.

303

Drug treatment: BNF 4.3. Major groups are:

- *Selective serotonin re-uptake inhibitors (SSRIs)*, e.g. fluoxetine 20mg od – usually 1st choice as less likely to be discontinued due to side-effects. Warn of possible anxiety and agitation and advise patients to stop if significant. GI side-effects including dyspepsia are common.
- *Serotonin and noradrenaline re-uptake inhibitors (SNRIs)*, e.g.duloxetine 60mg od, venlafaxine 37.5mg bd. Venlafaxine should not be used in patients with heart disease, electrolyte imbalance or hypertension – monitor BP through use.
- *Tricyclic antidepressants (TCAs)*, e.g. lofepramine 70mg od/bd/tds – titrate dose up from low dose until patient feels it is helping, or until side-effects intrude. Common side-effects include drowsiness, dry mouth, blurred vision, constipation, urinary retention and sweating.
- *Monoamine oxidase inhibitors (MAOIs)*, e.g. phenelzine 15mg tds. MAOIs should not be started until at least 1–2wk. after a tricyclic has been stopped (3wk. in the case of clomipramine or imipramine). Other antidepressants should not be started for 2wk. after treatment with MAOIs has been stopped (3 wk. if starting clomipramine or imipramine).

Specific psychological therapies: e.g. CBT (📖 p.307), behaviour therapy, interpersonal psychotherapy, problem-solving therapy. Possible 1st line therapies in mild/moderate depression though excessive waiting lists are a limiting factor. Simple problem-solving strategies can be tried in the surgery – see Figure 6.1.

Counselling: 📖 p.307

Exercise: Beneficial in mild/moderate depression.

St John's wort: May be effective in mild depression[S] but formulations vary widely in potency. Side-effects include dry mouth, gastrointestinal symptoms, fatigue, dizziness, skin rashes and ↑ sensitivity to sunlight. Interacts with many drugs including antidepressants (especially SSRIs – sweating, shivering, muscle contractions), anticonvulsants (↓ effects), warfarin, oral contraceptives, ciclosporin, digoxin and theophylline.

⚠ Don't use concurrently with prescription antidepressants; discontinue 2wk. prior to surgery due to theoretical risk of interaction with anaesthetic agents.

Referral to psychiatry: U = Urgent; S = Soon; R = Routine
- High suicide risk – U
- Psychotic major depression – U
- History of bipolar disorder – R/S
- Failure or partial response following ≥2 attempts to treat – R

Postnatal depression: 📖 p.277

Essential reading:
NICE Management of depression in primary and secondary care (2004) 🖥 www.nice.org.uk
DTB Mild depression in general practice (2003) 4(8) 60–4

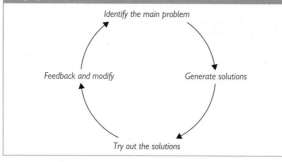

Figure 6.1 Simple problem-solving strategy to use in the surgery

Identify the main problem

Feedback and modify

Generate solutions

Try out the solutions

GP Notes: Frequently asked questions about antidepressants

When should antidepressants be started? Don't prescribe at the first visit as symptoms of depression may improve significantly during 1–3 wks. – 'watchful waiting' (*'Don't just do something, sit there!'*).

What should I tell the patient? Giving patients information ↑ compliance. When starting antidepressant drugs explain reasons for prescribing; time-scale of action – unlikely to have any effect for 2wk., effects build up to max. effect at 4–6wk.; and likely side-effects.

How often should I follow up? Review the patient every 1–2wk. until stable assessing response, compliance, side-effects and suicidal risk.

How long should antidepressants be continued for? Continue treatment for at least 4mo after recovery, and at least 6mo in total. Patients with ≥2 past episodes of major depression should be advised to continue for 2y.[N]

What are discontinuation reactions? These occur once a drug has been used ≥8wk. ↓ risk by tapering dose over ≥4wk. Warn patients about possible discontinuation reactions.

Which discontinuation reactions occur with which drugs?

- *Withdrawal of SSRIs* – headache, nausea, paraesthesia, dizziness and anxiety.
- *Withdrawal of other antidepressants (especially MAOIs)* – nausea, vomiting, anorexia, headache, 'chills', insomnia, anxiety/panic and restlessness

Table 6.2 Patient Health Questionnaire (PHQ-9)

Name		Date				
Over the last 2 weeks, how often have you been bothered by any of the following problems? (use '✓' to indicate your answer)		Not at all	Several days	More than half the days	Nearly every day	
1.	Little interest or pleasure in doing things	0	1	2	3	
2.	Feeling down, depressed, or hopeless	0	1	2	3	
3.	Trouble falling or staying asleep, or sleeping too much	0	1	2	3	
4.	Feeling tired or having little energy	0	1	2	3	
5.	Poor appetite or overeating	0	1	2	3	
6.	Feeling bad about yourself, or that you are a failure or have let yourself or your family down	0	1	2	3	
7.	Trouble concentrating on things, such as reading the newspaper or watching television	0	1	2	3	
8.	Moving or speaking so slowly that other people could have noticed. Or the opposite – being so fidgety or restless that you have been moving around a lot more than usual	0	1	2	3	
9.	Thoughts that you would be better off dead, or of hurting yourself in some way	0	1	2	3	
	Add columns:					
	Total:					
10.	If you ticked off *any* problems, how *difficult* have these problems made it for you to do your work, take care of things at home, or get along with other people?	Not difficult at all				
		Somewhat difficult				
		Very difficult				
		Extremely difficult				

GP Notes: Frequently asked questions about non-drug treatments

What is counselling? There are no universally agreed definitions of the term 'counselling' or 'counsellor' and the distinction between counselling and psychotherapy is often unclear. Usually the key element in counselling is reflective listening to encourage patients to think about and try to resolve their own difficulties. It does not involve giving advice. Most counsellors use brief (time-limited) therapy offering patients a mean of 7 sessions each, usually lasting ~50min.

Who is a counsellor? There is no formal registration requirement in the UK for counsellors or psychotherapists. The GMC advises that GPs should only refer to practitioners who are members of a recognized disciplinary body and thus subject to ethical and disciplinary codes.

Does counselling work? Many patients regard antidepressants as harmful or addictive and are increasingly reluctant to take them. They see counselling as an attractive alternative – a view supported by most GPs. Evidence shows counselling subjectively improves the condition the patient has been referred for, and non-directive counselling is more effective than GP care in reducing anxiety and depression in the short term but not the long term. However, counselling doesn't ↓ drug costs and practices with counsellors make more referrals to 2° care psychiatric services[5]. More research is needed into cost-effectiveness.

Who should be referred? Counsellors see a wide range of patients. ~²/₃ patients referred for counselling have significant levels of anxiety or depression.

What is cognitive behaviour therapy (CBT) used for? CBT is of proven effectiveness in the treatment of mild depression, anxiety disorders, phobias, panic disorder, eating disorders, and for the treatment of delusions and hallucinations in psychotic illness.

How can patients be referred for CBT? CBT is usually provided by highly trained psychotherapists and accessed via psychiatry services. Guided self-help programmes based on CBT are also effective for mild depression and can be delivered:

- using books e.g. Gilbert *Overcoming depression* Constable and Robin (2000) ISBN: 1841191256
- by computer, e.g. *Beating the Blues*© (further information available from ⌨ www.ultrasis.com) *or*
- via the internet, e.g. ⌨ www.psychologyonline.co.uk

Suicide and deliberate self-harm (DSH)

🛈 People who have self-harmed should be treated with the same care, respect and privacy as any other patient.

Deliberate self harm (DSH): Deliberate non-fatal act committed in the knowledge that it was potentially harmful and, in the case of drug overdose, that the amount taken was excessive. 90% DSH is due to self-poisoning and it accounts for 20% of admissions to general medical wards – the most frequent reason for admission for young ♀ patients. Paracetamol and aspirin are the most common drugs used. Self-harm is often aimed at changing a situation (e.g. to get a boyfriend back), a communication of distress ('cry for help'), a sign of emotional distress or may be a failed genuine suicide attempt.

Action: GPs are frequently called to patients who have deliberately self-harmed themselves, are threatening suicide or if relatives are worried about suicide risk.

Algorithm for assessment of patients who have deliberately self-harmed, threatened or attempted suicide – Figure 6.3, 📖 p.310.

Algorithm for management of patients who have deliberately self-harmed, threatened or attempted suicide – Figure 6.4, 📖 p.311.

Suicide prevention: 'Our Healthier Nation' set a target to ↓ death by suicide by 17% by 2010. GPs play a crucial role in achieving this target. The UK suicide rate is 1:6000 and the average GP will have 10–15 patients who commit suicide during a career in general practice. In ♂ <35y. suicide is now the most common cause of death. The National Suicide Prevention Strategy for England sets out 6 goals and objectives:

- To ↓ risk in key high-risk groups
- To promote mental well-being in the wider population
- To ↓ availability and lethality of suicide methods
- To improve reporting of suicidal behaviour in the community
- To promote research on suicide and suicide prevention
- To improve monitoring of progress towards the 'Saving Lives: Our Healthier Nation' target to ↓ suicide.

Support of those bereaved through suicide: Those bereaved through suicide face special problems. Give as much support as possible, try to ↓ stigma, suggest self-help groups and/or counselling.

Further information

NICE Self-harm: the short-term physical and psychological management and secondary prevention of self-harm in primary and secondary care (2004) 🖥 www.nice.org.uk

DoH National Suicide Prevention Strategy for England (2002) 🖥 www.dh.gov.uk

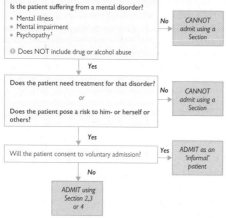

Figure 6.2 Deciding whether a 'section' is needed

Is the patient suffering from a mental disorder?
- Mental illness
- Mental impairment
- Psychopathy[1]

ⓘ Does NOT include drug or alcohol abuse

→ **No** → CANNOT admit using a Section

↓ **Yes**

Does the patient need treatment for that disorder?

or

Does the patient pose a risk to him- or herself or others?

→ **No** → CANNOT admit using a Section

↓ **Yes**

Will the patient consent to voluntary admission? → **Yes** → ADMIT as an 'informal' patient

↓ **No**

ADMIT using Section 2, 3 or 4

1 Personality disorder characterized by inability to make loving relationships, antisocial behaviour and lack of guilt

GP Notes:

What can GPs do to prevent suicide? Early recognition, assessment and treatment of those likely to attempt suicide is the key GP role – many visit their GP just weeks before suicide. Restrict access to lethal agents, e.g. avoid tricyclic antidepressants and monitor repeat prescriptions of antidepressants carefully. Plan follow-up care for those discharged from psychiatric hospital.

What do I do if I need to 'section' someone? In practice, 'sectioning' means calling in the duty social worker and duty psychiatrist. It can be a time-consuming and frustrating business. Always try to obtain voluntary admission – it is better for you and the patient. Keep a supply of forms you might need for sectioning – forms 3, 7 and 10 (GP recommendation for section 2, 4 and 3 respectively) and form 5 (application for section 4 for a 'nearest relative').

ⓘ Deputizing GPs should always try and contact the patient's own GP.

Advice for patients:

Information and support for patients and relatives
Self-injury and Related Issues (SIARI) 🖳 www.siari.co.uk
Samaritans 24h. emotional support via telephone ☎ 08457 909 090
Survivors of Bereavement by Suicide ☎ 0870 241 3337
🖳 www.uk-sobs.org.uk

Figure 6.3 Assessment of patients who have deliberately self-harmed, threatened or attempted suicide

If any self-harm: Assess the situation and admit to A&E as needed

Ask about suicidal ideas and plans: in a sensitive but probing way. It is a common misconception that asking about suicide can plant the idea into a patient's head and make suicide more likely. Evidence is to the contrary.

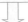

Ask about present circumstances:
- What problems are making the patient feel this way?
- Does she still feel like this?
- Would the act of suicide be aimed to hurt someone in particular?
- What kind of support does the patient have from friends and relatives and formal services (e.g. CPN)?

Assess suicidal risk: Ask patient and any relatives/friends present.
Risk factors:
♂>♀
↑with age
Divorced >widowed>never married >married
Certain professions: vets, pharmacists, farmers, doctors.
Admission or recent discharge from psychiatric hospital.
Social isolation
History of deliberate self-harm (100x ↑risk)
Depression
Alcohol or substance abuse
Personality disorder
Schizophrenia
Serious medical illness (e.g. cancer)

Assess psychiatric state: Features associated with ↑ suicide risk are:
- Presence of suicidal ideation
- Hopelessness -good predictor of subsequent and immediate risk
- Depression
- Agitation
- Early schizophrenia with retained insight – especially young patients who see their ambitions restricted
- Presence of delusions of control, poverty and/or guilt.

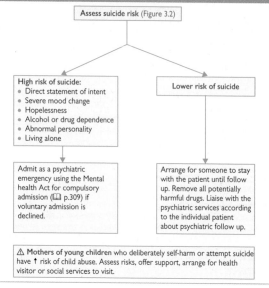

Figure 6.4 Management of patients who have deliberately self-harmed, threatened or at-tempted suicide

Assess suicide risk (Figure 3.2)

High risk of suicide:
- Direct statement of intent
- Severe mood change
- Hopelessness
- Alcohol or drug dependence
- Abnormal personality
- Living alone

Lower risk of suicide

Admit as a psychiatric emergency using the Mental health Act for compulsory admission (📖 p.309) if voluntary admission is declined.

Arrange for someone to stay with the patient until follow up. Remove all potentially harmful drugs. Liaise with the psychiatric services according to the individual patient about psychiatric follow up.

⚠ Mothers of young children who deliberately self-harm or attempt suicide have ↑ risk of child abuse. Assess risks, offer support, arrange for health visitor or social services to visit.

GP Notes: Useful questions for assessing suicidal ideas and plans

- Do you feel you have a future?
- Do you feel that life's not worth living?
- Do you ever feel completely hopeless?
- Do you ever feel you'd be better off dead and away from it all?
- Have you ever made any plans to end your life. (If drug overdose – have you handled the tablets?)
- Have you ever made an attempt to take your own life? – (If so, was there a final act, e.g suicide note?)
- What prevents you doing it?
- Have you made any arrangements for your affairs after your death?

Anxiety disorders

Anxiety is a normal response to an unusual or stressful event; it is the psychological component of the 'flight or fight' response and is only considered abnormal when:
- it occurs in the absence of a stressful event
- it impairs physical, occupational or social functioning
- it is excessively severe or prolonged.

Anxiety disorders are common, particularly amongst women. At any one time, ~5% of adults have an anxiety disorder and ~1:4 will develop an anxiety disorder at some point in their lives.

Diagnosis: Generalized anxiety disorder (GAD) is defined (ICD-10) by symptoms of anxiety present on most days for several consecutive weeks. Two clinical pictures are commonly seen:
- *Acute form:* Sudden onset, usually precipitated by an external event, short course, good prognosis
- *Chronic form:* Fluctuating anxiety over a long period of time.

There is considerable overlap between the anxiety disorders – particularly GAD and agoraphobia, and GAD and panic disorder. Figure 6.5 is a simple algorithm to aid differentiation between generalized anxiety disorder, panic disorder and phobias.

Clinical features of anxiety

Psychological
- Fearful anticipation
- Irritability
- Sensitivity to noise
- Restlessness
- Poor concentration
- Worrying thoughts
- Insomnia
- Nightmares
- Depression
- Obsessions
- Depersonalization

Physical
- Dry mouth
- Difficulty swallowing
- Tremor
- Dizziness
- Headache
- Parasthesiae
- Tinnitus
- Epigastric discomfort
- Excessive wind
- Frequent or loose motions
- Chest discomfort/constriction
- Difficulty breathing/hyperventilation
- Palpitations/awareness of missed beats
- Frequency or urgency of micturition
- Erectile dysfunction
- Menstrual problems.

Associations
- Anxiety often accompanies depression (p.300) and may be a feature of early schizophrenia.
- Other conditions which can cause anxiety and/or mimic symptoms of anxiety include: drug and alcohol withdrawal; caffeine abuse; thyrotoxicosis; hypoglycaemia; temporal lobe epilepsy; phaeochromocytoma.

Figure 6.5 Differentiation of anxiety disorders

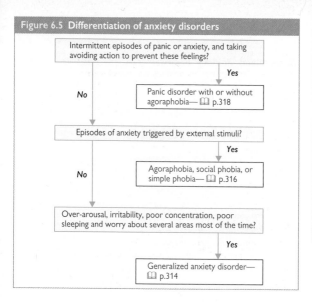

Intermittent episodes of panic or anxiety, and taking avoiding action to prevent these feelings?

→ **Yes** → Panic disorder with or without agoraphobia— ☐ p.318

No ↓

Episodes of anxiety triggered by external stimuli?

→ **Yes** → Agoraphobia, social phobia, or simple phobia— ☐ p.316

No ↓

Over-arousal, irritability, poor concentration, poor sleeping and worry about several areas most of the time?

→ **Yes** → Generalized anxiety disorder— ☐ p.314

GP Notes: Ways of improving outcome

Discuss treatment options: Shared decision making between the individual and health care professionals improves concordance and clinical outcomes.

Provide information: Information in a form suitable to patients and/or carers about the nature, course and treatment of their anxiety disorder – including information on use and likely side-effects of any medication – improves concordance and clinical outcomes.

Advice for patients: Information and support for patients

Anxiety Care Helpline ☎ 020 8478 3400 🖳 www.anxietycare.org.uk
No More Panic 🖳 www.nomorepanic.org.uk
Triumph Over Phobia (TOP) UK Self-help materials and groups
☎ 0845 600 9601 🖳 www.triumphoverphobia.com
Royal College of Psychiatrists Patient information sheets
🖳 www.rcpsych.ac.uk

Generalized anxiety disorder: NICE recommends a stepped approach to management of generalized anxiety disorder (Figure 6.6).

Step 1: Recognition and diagnosis
- Be alert to diagnosis, particularly in patients with unexplained physical symptoms who present frequently to primary care.
- Take a chronological account of symptoms and ask the patient's views and beliefs about nature and cause.
- Ask directly about symptoms of anxiety.
- Consider using an anxiety scale (e.g. Hospital Anxiety and Depression (HAD) Scale) to reinforce diagnosis and give a baseline measure of severity.
- Exclude other potential causes of similar symptoms and associated conditions, e.g. check TFTs to exclude thyrotoxicosis; ask about caffeine ingestion, substance abuse and alcohol consumption; ask about depression.

Step 2: Primary care management
If immediate management of GAD is necessary, consider:
- Support and information
- Problem solving (□ p.305)
- Benzodiazepines, e.g. diazepam 2–5mg tds prn. ⚠ Don't use >2–4wk.

In all cases, discuss and consider longer-term options
- *Psychological therapy* – refer for CBT (□ p.307) – often limited by availability in the community within a reasonable time frame.
- *Drug treatment* – SSRIs, e.g. paroxetine, are drugs of choice (□ p.304). Warn patients that transient ↑ in anxiety on starting treatment and GI side-effects are common, and that they are unlikely to see improvements for 2wk. Minimize initial side-effects by starting at low dose and increasing slowly until there is a satisfactory response. Review <2wk. after starting treatment and at 4, 6 & 12wk. If one SSRI is not suitable, or there is no improvement after 12wk., offer another SSRI (if appropriate) or another form of treatment. If effective, continue treatment for ≥6mo., reviewing every 8–12wk. Minimize discontinuation symptoms by tapering dose over an extended time period.
- *Self -help:* Options are:
  - Bibliotherapy based on CBT principles (□ p.307)
  - Information about support groups
  - Consider large group CBT where available
  - Exercise – may benefit health generally
  - Computerized CBT (□ p.307).

Step 3: Review and offer alternative treatment:
Anxiety scales can be useful in monitoring treatment. If treatment is complete and there has been no improvement, consider trying another type of intervention.

Step 4: Reasons to refer to specialist mental health services:
Significant symptoms despite treatment with 2 different interventions (CBT, medication and/or bibliotherapy).

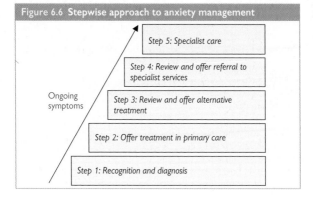

Figure 6.6 Stepwise approach to anxiety management

Step 5: Specialist care

Step 4: Review and offer referral to specialist services

Step 3: Review and offer alternative treatment

Step 2: Offer treatment in primary care

Step 1: Recognition and diagnosis

Ongoing symptoms

Phobias: Patients with phobias have the same symptoms as those with generalized anxiety disorder but symptoms are limited to specific situations. *Features:*
- *Avoidance* of the circumstances that provoke anxiety.
- *Anticipatory anxiety* when there is the prospect of encountering those circumstances.

Simple phobia: Inappropriate anxiety in the presence of ≥1 object/situation, e.g. flying, enclosed spaces, spiders. Common in early life. Most adult phobias are a continuation of childhood phobias. *Lifetime prevalence:* 4% ♂; 13% ♀.

Management: Treatment is only needed if symptoms are frequent, intrusive or prevent necessary activities. Exposure therapy is effective. Obtain directly (via trained psychotherapist), by referral to psychiatry or through the private sector, e.g. British Airways fear of flying course.

Social phobia: Intense and persistent fear of being scrutinized or negatively evaluated by others, causing fear and avoidance of social situations (e.g. meeting people in authority, using a telephone, speaking to a group). Must be significantly disabling, not simple shyness. May be generalized (most social situations) or specific (certain activities only).

Management
- *Drug therapy:* SSRIs – continue ≥12mo. or long term if symptoms remain unresolved, co-morbid condition (depression, generalized anxiety disorder, panic attacks), history of relapse, or early onset.
- *Psychological therapies:* Cognitive behaviour therapy (cognitive restructuring) ± exposure. Obtain directly or via local psychiatric services depending on local arrangements.

Agoraphobia: Onset is usually aged 20–40y. and associated with an initial panic attack. Panic attacks, fear of fainting and/or loss of control are experienced in crowds, away from home or in situations from which escape is difficult. Avoidance → patients remaining within their home where they know symptoms will not occur. Other symptoms include depression, depersonalization and obsessional thoughts.

Management: Difficult to manage in general practice. Diagnosis is often delayed as patients will not come to the surgery and ongoing management is complicated by refusal to be referred to psychiatric services. Prognosis is best when there is good marital/social support. *Options:*
- *Behavioural therapy,* e.g. exposure, training in coping with panic attacks. Available by direct referral or via psychiatric services according to local arrangements. Home visits may be required, but should be resisted as part of therapy.
- *Drug treatment:* SSRIs (citalopram and paroxetine are licensed); MAOIs; TCAs (imipramine and clomipramine are commonly used). Relapse rate is high. Benzodiazepines can be used if frequent panic attacks, particularly if initiating other treatment – but beware of dependence.

Acute panic attacks

Features: Fear, terror and feeling of impending doom accompanied by some or all of the following:

- Palpitations
- Shortness of breath
- Choking sensation
- Dizziness
- Paraesthesiae
- Chest pain/discomfort
- Sweating
- Carpopedal spasm

Differential diagnosis

- Dysrhythmia
- Asthma
- Anaphylaxis
- Thyrotoxicosis
- Temporal lobe epilepsy
- Hypoglycaemia
- Phaeochromocytoma (very rare)

Action

Talking down: Explain the nature of the symptoms to the patient
- Racing of the heart is due to adrenaline produced by the panic.
- Paraesthesiae and feelings of dizziness are due to overbreathing due to panic.
- Count breaths in and out, gently slowing breathing rate.

Rebreathing techniques

- Place a paper bag over the patient's mouth and ask him to breath in and out through the mouth.
- A connected but not switched on O_2 mask or nebulizer mask is an alternative in the surgery.
- This raises the partial pressure of CO_2 in the blood and symptoms due to low CO_2 (e.g. tetany, paraesthesiae, dizziness) resolve. This demonstrates the link between hyperventilation and the symptoms too.

Propranolol: 10–20mg stat may be helpful – DON'T USE for asthmatics or patients with heart failure or on verapamil.

Panic disorder: Panic attacks are very common, but panic disorder is uncommon: lifetime prevalence – 1% ♂; 3% ♀. NICE recommends a stepwise approach to management (Figure 6.6, 📖 p.315).

Step 1: Recognition and diagnosis

Symptoms: Patients experience intense feelings of apprehension or impending disaster. Anxiety builds up quickly and unexpectedly without a recognizable trigger and patients often present with any combination of:

- Shortness of breath and smothering sensations
- Choking
- Palpitations and ↑ heart rate
- Chest discomfort or pain
- Sweating
- Dizziness, unsteady feelings or faintness
- Nausea or abdominal pain
- Depersonalization/derealization
- Numbness or tingling sensations
- Flushes or chills
- Trembling or shaking
- Fear of dying
- Fear of doing something crazy or uncontrolled.

Examination: Obvious distress; sweating; tachycardia; hyperventilation. ↑ BP is common and usually settles when the episode is over. Otherwise examination is normal.

Definitions:
- *Panic attack:* ≥4 symptoms listed above in 1 attack.
- *Panic disorder:* Chronic disorder; initial diagnosis depends on >4 attacks in 4wk. *or* 1 attack and a persistent fear of having more.

Differential diagnosis: Alcohol withdrawal; other psychiatric disorders (e.g. psychosis); hyperthyroidism; temporal lobe epilepsy; cardiac arryhthmia; labyrinthitis; hypoglycaemia; hyperparathyroidism; phaeochromocytoma (very rare).

Associations: Depression (56% patients are depressed); generalized anxiety; agoraphobia; substance abuse; suicide (↑ risk). Panic attacks may predict future panic disorder and depression, especially if the presenting feature is chest pain.

Step 2: Primary care management – consider treatment options

⚠ Don't use benzodiazepines for treatment of patients with panic disorder – they are associated with less good outcome in the long term.

Psychological therapy – refer for CBT (📖 p.307). 🌗 Often limited by availability in the community within a reasonable time frame.

Drug treatment – SSRIs, e.g. escitalopram 5mg od, and TCAs, e.g. clomipramine 10–25mg nocte (unlicensed), are both effective. SSRIs are usually used as first-line treatment.
- Warn patients about possible transient ↑ in anxiety on starting treatment and that they are unlikely to see improvements for 2wk. GI side-effects are common. Minimize initial side-effects by starting at low dose and increasing slowly until there is a satisfactory response.

Advice for patients:

Self-help for panic attacks: One way of tackling panic attacks is to look at the way you talk to yourself, especially during times of stress and pressure. Panic attacks often begin or escalate when you tell yourself scary things, like 'I feel light-headed   I'm about to faint!' or 'I'm trapped in this traffic jam and something terrible is gonna happen!' or 'If I go outside, I'll freak out.' These are called 'negative predictions' and they have a strong influence on the way your body feels. If you're mentally predicting a disaster, your body's alarm response goes off and the 'fight or flight response' kicks in.

To combat this, try to focus on calming, positive thoughts, like 'I'm learning to deal with panicky feelings and I know that people overcome panic all the time' or 'This will pass quickly, and I can help myself by concentrating on my breathing and imagining a relaxing place' or 'These feelings are uncomfortable, but they won't last forever.'

Remind yourself of these FACTS about panic attacks:
• A panic attack cannot cause heart failure or a heart attack.
• A panic attack cannot cause you to stop breathing.
• A panic attack cannot cause you to faint.
• A panic attack cannot cause you to 'go crazy'.
• A panic attack cannot cause you to lose control of yourself.

If it's too hard to think calming thoughts when you're having a panic attack, find ways to distract yourself. Some people do this by talking to other people when they feel the panic coming on. Others prefer to exercise or work on a detailed project or hobby. Changing scenery can sometimes be helpful, too, but it's important not to get into a pattern of avoiding necessary daily tasks. If you notice that you're regularly avoiding things like driving, going shopping, going to work, or taking public transport, it's probably time to get some professional help.

Slow, abdominal breathing (6 breaths per minute) has been shown to stop panic attacks. Learning slow abdominal breathing can be quite difficult and people who have panic attacks are almost always chest breathers. Practise abdominal breathing (moving upper part of tummy to breathe rather than chest wall) when relaxed at home. If you can learn to breathe slowly with your diaphragm, you will not panic!

Cut down on alcohol and caffeine – these can make panic attacks worse. Try relaxation techniques (such as yoga) and exercise regularly – both can help reduce the number of panic attacks people have.

Information and support for patients
Royal College of Psychiatrists Patient information sheets
⊟ www.rcpsych.ac.uk
No More Panic ⊟ www.nomorepanic.org.uk

- Review <2wk. after starting treatment and at 4, 6 & 12wk. If an SSRI is not suitable, or there is no improvement after 12wk., offer imipramine or clomipramine (if appropriate) or another form of treatment.
- If effective, continue treatment for ≥6mo., reviewing every 8–12wk. Minimize discontinuation symptoms by tapering dose over an extended time period.

Self-help: Options are:
- Bibliotherapy based on CBT principles (📖 p.307)
- Information about support groups
- Consider large group CBT where available
- Exercise – may benefit health generally
- Computerized CBT (📖 p.307).

Step 3: Review and offer alternative treatment: If treatment is complete and there has been no improvement, consider trying another type of intervention.

Step 4: Review and offer referral to specialist mental health services: If significant symptoms despite treatment with 2 different interventions (any combination of CBT, medication or bibliotherapy).

Somatization disorder: Chronic condition. History of numerous unsubstantiated physical complaints. Starts at <30y. and often persists many years. ♀:♂≈10:1; lifetime prevalence 0.1–0.2% though mild symptoms are much commoner.

Clinical features
- >2y. history of multiple symptoms with no adequate physical explanation.
- Persistent refusal to be reassured that there is no explanation for the symptoms.
- Impaired social/family functioning due to these symptoms and/or associated behaviour.

Management
- Reattribution – involves acknowledging and taking the symptoms seriously, offering any necessary examination and investigations, enquiring about psychosocial problems, and explaining the link between symptoms and stress.
- Treat co-morbid psychiatric problems (e.g. depression, anxiety, panic). ⚠ Beware of risks of drug interaction – self-medication with multiple OTC (or even prescription) drugs is common.
- Beware of side-effects of medication – patients do not tolerate prescribed drugs well and have a heightened awareness of side-effects.
- Refer to psychiatry if risk of suicide, marked functional impairment, impulsive or antisocial behaviour.

Further reading
NICE Management of anxiety (panic disorder, with or without agoraphobia, and generalized anxiety disorder) in adults in primary, secondary and community care (2004) 🖥 www.nice.org.uk

GP Notes: Heartsink patients

Characterized by:

- Frequent presentation – the top 1% of attenders at GP surgeries generate 6% GP workload.
- Highly complex and often multiple problems – some real, others not.
- Exasperation generated between patient and doctor.

❶ It is a 2-way process. Some GPs report more heartsink patients than others. The problem relates to the GP's perception of patients as well as the patients themselves.

GP risk factors: Perception of high workload; low job satisfaction; lack of training in counselling or communication; lack of postgraduate skills.

Management

- Do a detailed review of notes ± chart of life.
- Agree patient contacts, e.g. limit to one partner, agree frequency of appointments, etc.
- Agree an agenda within consultations, e.g. problem list – only 1 problem/visit
- Employ reattribution techniques (see somatization disorder – on the opposite page).
- Avoid unnecessary investigation and referral.
- Be aware of your own reaction to the patient.
- Acknowledge even heartsink patients can be genuinely ill.
- Consider psychiatric diagnoses – especially chronic anxiety, depression, somatization disorder. Screening questionnaires can be useful.
- Consider referral for cognitive behavioural therapy.

Obsessive–compulsive disorder (OCD)

Common mental illness characterized by recurrent obsessive thoughts and compulsive acts. Lifetime prevalence ~2% though minor obsessional symptoms are much more common. $\male$:$\female$ ≈ 2:3. Onset tends to occur in adolescence (peak 12–14y.) or early adulthood (peak 20–22y.). There is often a family history and identical twin studies show ~90% concordance.

Theoretical basis: Cognitive behavioural theorists suggest obsessive thoughts generate anxiety which is partly relieved by certain actions; anxiety reduction reinforces the actions → development of compulsions.

Presentation: Onset may be acute or insidious and is associated with a precipitating event in 60%. Patients know obsessional thinking comes when what they are thinking or doing is irrational, making them embarrassed to tell anyone. As a result, patients may have had symptoms for years before seeking help. Relatives may highlight the problem rather than the patient. *Features:*

- *Obsessional thinking* – recurrent persistent thoughts ('Have I turned the gas off?'), impulses (e.g. to shout obscenities) and images (often of an obscene/violent nature) causing anxiety or distress.
- *Compulsive behaviour* – repetitive behaviours, rituals (e.g. hand washing, checking doors are locked) or mental acts done to prevent or ↓ anxiety.
- *Other features* – indecisiveness and inability to take action, anxiety, depression and depersonalization.

Diagnosis: For a diagnosis of OCD to be made:

- Obsessive thoughts/compulsive actions must be present on most days for ≥2wk.
- The patient must recognize that the thoughts come from within themselves (i.e. there are no passivity symptoms).
- Obsessive thoughts and compulsive rituals must have been unsuccessfully resisted in the past.
- Thoughts and actions are unpleasant – if only due to repetition.

Differential diagnosis: Obsessive symptoms may occur as a result of a number of psychiatric conditions. It is important to distinguish OCD from such conditions. They are:

- Depression (7–30% of severely depressed patients)
- Schizophrenia – suspect if thoughts or rituals are particularly bizarre
- Tourette's syndrome.

Management: Refer for psychiatric assessment. Treatment involves a combination of patient education, SSRI or clomipramine, and/or CBT.

Prognosis

- Most patients severely affected have a prolonged, steady course with symptoms decreasing slowly with time – 2:3 improve within 1y. of presentation.
- Symptoms worsen with stress.
- 15% have a deteriorating course.
- Bad prognostic indicators also include the presence of an obsessional personality and relative severity of symptoms.

Advice for patients:

Patient experiences of OCD

'I'm afraid of catching something from other people. I fear that the germs that they carry may get on to me and I will become infected. I'm afraid I may also "contaminate" my family by passing these germs on to them. I know it is silly but I feel so tense and anxious if I do touch anyone else or any surfaces – such as door handles that they have touched – that I have to come home and wash my hands many times, then wash my clothes. That makes me feel a lot better until the next contact with others.'

'I fear that I will harm my partner. I know that I don't want to and I love her, but thoughts often come into my head where I can picture myself harming her ... with a knife or by strangling her. I am so upset when I have these thoughts that I have to bring into my mind other "good thoughts" such as "I know I love her very much" and I say these to myself many times to get rid of the bad thoughts. I usually feel a bit better after that, until the next time the awful thoughts come into my head. I have hidden away all sharp objects and knives so that there is no risk of me doing it, and also seeing these objects brings the horrible thoughts to my mind.'

'My whole day is spent checking nothing will go wrong in the house ... I can't get out because I'm never quite sure that I've turned off the gas, electric appliances, water and locked the windows ... I check to see if the gas fire is off. I do this 5 times and then can sometimes go upstairs. At other times it doesn't feel right and I go through the whole "ritual" again. If I don't check I feel so worried I can't bear it ... Its silly, but I keep thinking if something awful did happen, I'd be to blame for being so careless.'

Self-help strategy

- **Carefully recognize** your unwanted thoughts – obsessions – and the actions you take to put them right – compulsions.
- **Gradually** face some of the things you fear. Work out an anxiety ladder to help you do this (i.e. grade a list of unpleasant situations in terms of unpleasantness for you), begin with the easiest step.
- **Do not** carry out any compulsions to reduce or neutralize your anxiety when you are facing the feared situation.
- **Break** the obsession–compulsion cycle.
- **Challenge** gloomy or critical thoughts you may have about yourself.

Information and support for patients

OCD Action ☎ 020 7226 4000 🖳 www.ocdaction.org.uk
Royal College of Psychiatrists Patient information sheets
🖳 www.rcpsych.ac.uk

Further information

NICE Obsessive–Compulsive disorder: core interventions in the treatment of obsessive compulsive disorder and body dysmorphic disorder (2005) 🖳 www.nice.org.uk

Patient experience data and self-help strategy is reproduced with permission from the OCD information sheet available at 🖳 www.gp-training.net

Eating disorders

⚠ Patients who are pregnant or have DM are particularly at risk of complications if they have co-morbid eating disorders. Refer early for specialist support and ensure everyone involved in care is aware of the eating disorder.

Anorexia Nervosa: Prevalence 0.02–0.04%. ♀>>♂. Usually begins in adolescence. Peak prevalence at 16–17y. *Features:*
- Body weight <85% of that expected (BMI <17.5 kg/m^2)
- Intense fear of gaining weight, though underweight
- Disturbed experience of body weight or shape or undue influence of shape on self-image
- Amenorrhoea in women for ≥3mo. and ↓ sexual interest.

Patients tend to have a set daily calorific intake e.g. 600–1000 calories and may employ strategies e.g. bingeing and vomiting, purging or excessive exercise to try to lose weight. Depression and social withdrawal are common as are symptoms 2° to starvation.

Management[N]
- Give ongoing support and information.
- Check electrolytes.
- Refer to a specialist eating disorders clinic (if available) or psychiatry. Treatment involves family therapy for adolescents, psychotherapy, and possible admission for refeeding.

Follow up: Patients with enduring anorexia nervosa not under 2° care follow up should be offered an annual physical and mental health check.

⚠ Many patients with anorexia nervosa have compromised cardiac function. Avoid prescribing drugs which adversely affect cardiac function (e.g. antipsychotics, TCAs, macrolide antibiotics, some antihistamines). If prescribing is essential then follow up with ECG monitoring

Bulimia Nervosa: Prevalence 1–2%. Mainly ♀ aged 16–40y.. *Features:*
- Recurrent episodes of binge eating, far beyond normally accepted amounts of food.
- Inappropriate compensatory behaviour to prevent weight ↑ e.g. vomiting; use of laxatives, diuretics and/or appetite suppressants. Bulimics can be subdivided into those that purge and those that just use fasting and exercise to control their weight.
- Self-image unduly influenced by body shape (see anorexia above).
- Normal menses & normal weight. If low BMI classified as anorexia.

Management
- Give ongoing support and information
- Check electrolytes
- Consider treatment with either and evidence-based self-help programme e.g. Overcoming bulimia - CD-ROM available from Calipso 🖥 www.calipso.co.uk, telephone-based self-help programme run by the Eating Disorders Association - details below; cost ~£200 *and/or* antidepressant medication - fluoxetine 60mg od is the drug of choice
- If unsuccessful, refer to a specialist eating disorders clinic (if available) or psychiatry. CBT may help.

Advice for patients purging

- *Vomiting:* Advise patients to avoid brushing their teeth after vomiting, rinse with a non-acid mouthwash after vomiting, and ↓ acid oral environment (e.g. by limiting acid foods)
- *Laxatives:* Where laxative abuse is present, advise patients to gradually ↓ laxative intake - laxatives do not significantly ↓ calorie absorption.

Binge eating disorder: A pattern of consumption of large amounts of food, even when a patient is not hungry. Common. Usually associated with obsessive feelings about food and body image, feelings of guilt/disgust about the amounts consumed and/or a feeling of lack of control.

Management

- Give ongoing support and information
- Provide an evidence-based self-help programme as a first step and/or antidepressant medication (SSRI is the drug group of choice).
- If unsuccessful refer for specialist help. CBT might be helpful.
- In all cases, provide concurrent advice and support to tackle any co-morbid obesity.

GP Notes: Identification of and screening for eating disorders

Target groups for screening include:

- Young women with low BMI compared with age norms
- Patients consulting with weight concerns who are not overweight
- Women with menstrual disturbances or amenorrhoea
- Patients with GI symptoms
- Patients with symptoms/signs of starvation – sensitivity to cold, delayed gastric emptying, constipation, ↓ BP, bradycardia, hypothermia.
- Patients with physical signs of repeated vomiting – pitted teeth ± dental caries, general weakness, cardiac arrythmias, renal damage, ↑ risk of UTI, epileptic fits, ↓K$^+$
- Children with poor growth
- Young people with type 1 DM and poor treatment adherence

Screen target populations with simple screening questions

- Do you worry excessively about your weight?
- Do you think you have an eating problem?

325

Advice for patients:

Information and support for patient and parents
Eating Disorders Association (EDA) ☎ 0845 634 1414 (Adults)
0845 634 7650 (Youths) 🖳 www.edauk.com

Further information

NICE Core interventions in the treatment and management of anorexia nervosa, bulimia nervosa and related eating disorders (2004)
🖳 www.nice.org

Chapter 7

Miscellaneous topics

Insomnia 328
Tiredness, fatigue and lethargy 330
Fibromyalgia 332
Hirsutism 334
Facial flushing and sweats 336

Insomnia

From the Latin meaning 'no sleep'. Describes a perception of disturbed or inadequate sleep. ~1:4 of the UK population (♀>♂) are thought to suffer in varying degrees. Prevalence ↑ with age, rising to 1:2 amongst the over 65s. It is a serious problem as it can ↓ quality of life; ↓ concentration and memory affecting performance of daytime tasks; cause relationship problems; and ↑ risk of accidents. 10% motor accidents are related to tiredness.

Definition of 'a good night's sleep'
- <30min. to fall asleep
- Maintenance of sleep for 6–8h.
- <3 brief awakenings/night
- Feels well rested and refreshed on awakening.

Causes of insomnia: Numerous – common examples include:
- *Minor, self-limiting:* travel, stress, shift work, small children, arousal
- *Psychological:* ~½ have mental health problems – depression, anxiety, mania, grief, alcoholism
- *Physical:* drugs (e.g. steroids), pain, pruritus, tinnitus, sweats (e.g. menopause), nocturia, asthma, obstructive sleep apnoea.

Management: Evaluate each case carefully. Many don't have a sleep problem themselves but a relative feels there is a problem, e.g. the retired milkman continuing to wake at 4a.m. Others have unrealistic expectations, e.g. they need 12h. sleep/d. Reassurance alone may be all that is required.

For genuine problems
- Eliminate as far as possible any physical problems preventing sleep, e.g. treat asthma or eczema; give long-acting painkillers to last the whole night; consider HRT for sweats; refer if obstructive sleep apnoea is suspected.
- Treat psychiatric problems, e.g. depression, anxiety.
- Sleep hygiene – see opposite.
- Relaxation techniques – audiotapes (borrow from libraries or buy from pharmacies); relaxation classes (often offered by local recreation centres/adult education centres); many physiotherapists can teach relaxation techniques.
- Consider drug treatment – last resort. Benzodiazepines may be prescribed for insomnia 'only when it is severe, disabling, or subjecting the individual to extreme distress'.

Drug treatment: Benzodiazepines (e.g. temazepam), zolpidem, zopiclone and low-dose tricyclic antidepressants (e.g. amitriptyline 25–50mg) are all commonly prescribed to be taken at night for patients with insomnia. Only prescribe a few weeks' supply at a time due to potential for dependence and abuse.

Common side-effects: Amnesia and daytime somnolence. Most hypnotics do affect daytime performance and may cause falls in the elderly. Warn patients about their affect on driving and operating machinery.

GP Notes:

⚠ Beware the temporary resident who has 'forgotten' her night sedation.

Advice for patients: Principles of 'sleep hygiene'

- Don't go to bed until you feel sleepy.
- Don't stay in bed if you're not asleep.
- Avoid daytime naps.
- Establish a regular bedtime routine.
- Reserve a room for sleep only (if possible). Do not eat, read, work or watch TV in it.
- Make sure the bedroom and bed are comfortable, and avoid extremes of noise and temperature.
- Avoid caffeine, alcohol and nicotine.
- Have a warm bath and warm milky drink at bedtime.
- Take regular exercise but avoid late-night hard exercise (sex is OK).
- Monitor your sleep with a sleep diary (record both the times you sleep and its quality).
- Rise at the same time every morning regardless of how long you've slept.

Tiredness, fatigue and lethargy

Almost any disease processes can cause tiredness — whether physical or psychological. Physical causes account for ~9% of cases; 75% have symptoms of emotional distress.

Assessment: Figure 7.1

Common organic causes of fatigue in general practice

- Anaemia
- Infections (EBV, CMV, hepatitis)
- DM
- Hypo – or hyperthyroidism
- Peri-menopausal
- Asthma
- Carcinomatosis
- Sleep apnoea
- Inflammatory conditions, e.g. rheumatoid arthritis.

Management: Treat organic causes. In most, no physical cause is found – reassure. Explaining the relationship of psychological and emotional factors to fatigue can help patients deal with symptoms. If lasts >6–12wk. and symptoms/signs of depression, consider a trial of SSRIs, e.g. sertraline 50mg od. Refer those with chronic or disabling fatigue with no identifiable cause; suspected sleep apnoea; suspected chronic fatigue syndrome; or if referral is requested by the patient.

Chronic fatigue syndrome (CFS, ME): Debilitating and distressing condition affecting up to 1 in 40 of the population. More common in women than men ($\mathcal{Q}:\mathcal{O}^{7} \approx 3:2$). Cause is poorly understood – viral infections ($\approx 10\%$ after EBV), immunization and chemical toxins (e.g. organophosphates, chemotherapy drugs) are all implicated.

Clinical features: Unexplained fatigue of new/definite onset, not resulting from ongoing exertion, nor alleviated by rest, which results in ↓ activity *and* ≥4 of:
- Impaired memory or concentration
- Tender cervical/axillary lymph nodes
- Postexertional malaise lasting >24h.; typically delayed – usually starting 1–2d. after a period of ↑ physical/mental activity and may last weeks
- Headaches of new type, pattern or severity
- Multi-joint pain without swelling
- Sore throat
- Unrefreshing sleep
- Muscle pain.

🚹 Additional symptoms must not have pre-dated fatigue

Other common symptoms/associations
- Postural dizziness
- Vertigo
- Altered temperature sensation
- Paraesthesiae
- Sensitivity to light or sound
- Palpitations
- IBS or food intolerance
- Fibromyalgia
- Feelings of dyspnoea
- Mood swings, panic attacks or depression (60% have no prior psychiatric diagnosis).

Intercurrent infection, immunization, drugs, caffeine, alcohol and stress may → setbacks.

Management: Support and reassurance – explanation, information ± self-help groups. Avoid factors which worsen symptoms, e.g. caffeine, alcohol. Graded exercise is helpful[C]. Treat symptoms, e.g. amitriptyline 10–50mg nocte to help sleep, relieve headache or neuropathic pain; SSRI for depression. Consider referral for specialist care, e.g. CBT (↓ 2° distress and optimizes rehabilitation), specialist CFS clinic.

Prognosis: Variable. Children tend to recover though it may take years. 55% of adults presenting with tiredness have symptoms lasting >6mo. Risk ↑ 3x if there is a history of anxiety or depression. Short duration of fatigue with no anxiety/depression improves prognosis. Only 6% of adults with CFS attending specialist clinics return to pre-morbid functioning.

Figure 7.1 Assessment of patients presenting with fatigue

History:

Onset & duration: short history and abrupt onset suggest post-viral cause or onset of DM, protracted course suggests emotional origin.

Pattern of fatigue: fatigue on exertion which goes away with rest suggests an organic cause whilst fatigue worst in the morning which never goes suggests depression.

Associated symptoms e.g. breathlessness, weight loss or anorexia suggest underlying organic disease. Chronic pain may cause fatigue.

Sleep patterns: early morning wakening and unrefreshing sleep may suggest depression, whilst snoring, pauses of breathing in sleep and sleepiness in the day time suggest sleep apnoea.

Psychiatric history: ask about depression, anxiety, stress; medication. Ask what the patient thinks is wrong and their underlying fears.

⬇

Examination: Full examination unless history suggests cause.
ⓘ Most examinations will be normal.

⬇

Investigations:

Suitable initial investigations are: FBC, ESR, TFTs, blood glucose, U&E, LFTs, Ca^{2+}, monospot test, MSU for M,C&S. ⓘ Viral titres don't help.

Screening questionnaires for depression can be useful.

Further investigations (e.g. autoimmune profile) may be necessary depending on initial test results, clinical findings and course.

⚠ Don't over-investigate: 1:3 patients have ≥ 1 abnormal result in a standard battery of tests—abnormal results are relevant to symptoms in <1:10 of those patients.

Advice for patients: Information and support

ME Association ☎ 0871 222 7824 🖥 www.meassociation.org.uk
Action for ME ☎ 01749 670799 🖥 www.afme.org.uk

Fibromyalgia

Painful, non-articular condition of unknown cause, predominantly involving muscles. Fibromyalgia is common and often results in significant disability and handicap with inability to cope with a job or household activities. Peak age 40–50y. – 90% female.

Clinical picture

- Pain – usually axial and diffuse but may be felt all over.
- Pain is worsened by stress, cold and activity, and associated with generalized morning stiffness.
- Paraesthesiae or dysaesthesiae of hands and feet are common.
- Analgesics, NSAIDs, and local physical treatments are ineffective and may worsen symptoms.
- Sleep patterns are poor – patients tend to wake exhausted and complain of poor concentration.
- Anxiety and depression scores are high.
- Associated symptoms – unexplained headache, urinary frequency and abdominal symptoms – are common.
- Clinical findings are unremarkable.

Investigation: Exclude other causes of pain and fatigue (e.g. hypothyroidism, SLE, Sjögrens, psoriatic arthritis, inflammatory myopathy, hyperparathyroidism, osteomalacia) – check FBC, ESR, TFTs, U&E, Ca^{2+}, CK, PO_4, ANA, Rh.F and immunoglobulins.

Diagnostic criteria

- History of widespread pain (defined as pain on both left and right sides, above and below the waist, together with axial skeletal pain, e.g. neck or back pain), *in combination with*
- Pain in ≥11 of 18 tender points sites (Figure 7.2) on digital palpation

Management: A multidisciplinary approach is helpful – usually accessed through a rheumatology or pain clinic.

- Be supportive – reassurance that there is no serious pathology, explanation and information are vital.
- Low-dose amitriptyline 25–75mg nocte may help with sleep and pain.
- SSRI, e.g. sertraline 25–50mg od, may help anxiety, depression and sleep – stop if no improvement after a month's trial.
- Graded exercise regimes can improve pain, lethargy, mood and general malaise.
- Counselling and learning of coping strategies can be beneficial, as can cognitive behavioural therapy if available locally.
- Some patients benefit from injection of hypalgesic trigger points with steroid or acupuncture to trigger points.

Figure 7.2 Tender points sites for diagnosis of fibromyalgia

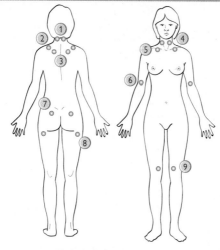

1. Insertion of nuchal muscles into the occiput
2. Upper border of trapezius midportion
3. Muscle attachments to upper medial border of scapula
4. Anterior aspects of the C5, C7 intertransverse spaces
5. 2nd rib space ~3cm lateral to the sternal border
6. Muscle attachments to the lateral epicondyle at the elbow
7. Upper outer quadrant of gluteal muscles
8. Muscle attachments just posterior to the greater trochanter
9. Medial fat pad of the knee just proximal to the joint line

Advice for patients: Information and support

Arthritis Research Campaign (ARC) ☎0870 850 5000
🖳 www.arc.org.uk
Fibromyalgia Association UK ☎ 0870 220 1232
🖳 www.fibromyalgia-associationuk.org

Hirsutism

Excess hair in an androgenic distribution in women – particularly facial hair, hair around the nipples and on the abdomen. Affects 10% women. Psychological impact may be severe even with relatively little excess hair.

Causes
- **Idiopathic** – most cases are idiopathic. There may be a family history. More common in dark-haired individuals and in certain racial groups (e.g. Mediterranean origin). Usually becomes noticeable in teenage years and increases with age.
- **Genetic** – Turner's syndrome
- **Drugs** – phenytoin, corticosteroids, ciclosporin, androgenic oral contraception, anabolic steroids, minoxidil, diazoxide
- **Endocrine**
  - *Adrenal* – congenital adrenal hyperplasia, Cushing's syndrome, virilizing tumours
  - *Pituitary* – acromegaly, hyperprolactinaemia
  - *Ovarian* – polycystic ovarian syndrome (PCOS), virilizing tumours, gonadal dysgenesis.

Assessment
- **History** – long-standing or recent onset, family history, ethnic origin, menstrual history
- **Examination** – distribution of excess hair.

Investigation: Women with long-standing hirsutism (since puberty) and regular periods need no further investigation unless abnormal signs.

Otherwise check
- Serum testosterone – ↑ in PCOS, androgen-secreting tumour, late-onset congenital adrenal hyperplasia
- LH/FSH ratio (>3:1 suggests PCOS)
- Consider pelvic USS if clinical suspicion of PCOS.

Refer to gynaecologist/endocrinologist if
- Recent onset and not a teenager
- Abnormal blood tests
- Virilism
- Galactorrhoea
- Menstrual disturbance
- Infertility and/or
- Pelvic mass.

Management: Treat the underlying cause if possible.
- Cosmetic – bleaching, shaving, plucking, waxing, depilatory creams, electrolysis, ruby laser
- Weight ↓ in obese individuals
- Psychological support
- Drugs – all treatments take ≥6mo. to take effect and none abolish the problem. Relapse follows withdrawal.

Drugs used

- Anti-androgens, e.g. cyproterone acetate – inhibits androgens at peripheral receptors. Often given as a COC pill containing cyproterone (Dianette®) if contraception is required.
- Oestrogen alone or a COC pill without an anti-androgenic progesterone. There is some evidence that COC pills containing desogestrel are most effective.
- Spironolactone – direct anti-androgenic properties.
- Topical 11.5% eflornithine cream – ↓ frequency that physical methods of hair removal are needed. Significantly helps ~1:3 women.
- Flutamide and finasteride are occasionally used under specialist supervision.

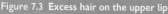
Figure 7.3 Excess hair on the upper lip

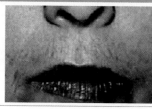

Facial flushing and sweats

Facial flushing and sweating are both common symptoms but can be symptoms of endocrine disease.

Facial flushing: Erythema due to vasodilation. Common and usually benign. Tends to affect face, neck and upper trunk.

Causes
- Physiological: exertion, heat
- Emotion, e.g. anger, anxiety, embarrassment
- Foods, e.g. spices, chillies, alcohol
- Endocrine, e.g. menopause, Cushing's syndrome
- Drugs, e.g. morphine, tamoxifen, danazol, GnRH analogues, clomifene, nitrates, calcium channel blockers
- Dermatological: rosacea (unknown mechanism), contact dermatitis
- Inflammatory: SLE, dermatomyositis
- Infection, e.g. slapped cheek syndrome (5th disease), cellulitis/erysipelas
- Tumour: pancreatic tumours, medullary thyroid cancer, carcinoid, phaeochromocytoma.

Management
- Treat the cause if possible (e.g. avoid alcohol; HRT).
- Embarrassing flushing may be helped with SSRIs (e.g. fluoxetine 20mg od or paroxetine 20/30mg od) or SNRIs (e.g. venlafaxine 75mg od – consultant initiation only). In addition norethisterone 5mg od or megestrol acetate 40mg (vaginal bleeding on withdrawal) may help menopausal flushing.
- If severe and disabling and no response to conservative measures, consider referral for surgery (endoscopic sympathectomy).

Sweating: Sweating, or perspiration, is normal and essential for temperature control. The amount people sweat varies enormously. Usually sweating can be controlled with shop-bought antiperspirants and is only excessive when it cannot be controlled and interferes with the patient's quality of life. Excess sweating is termed *hyperhidrosis* and may be focal or generalized.

Generalized hyperhidrosis: Most likely to occur 2° to other medical conditions. Where possible treat the cause:
- *Physiological* – after and during exercise; hot, humid conditions; emotional response (e.g. anxiety)
- *Menopause*
- *Infection* – can occur with any bacterial or viral infection. Consider malaria if recent history of travel
- *Non-infective* – thyrotoxicosis; phaeochromocytoma; lymphoma; leukaemia.

If no treatable cause can be found, a β-blocker (e.g. propranol 40mg od/bd) or SSRI (e.g. fluoxetine 20mg od) may be effective (both unlicensed uses).

Focal hyperhidrosis: Usually a primary condition though may occur secondary to other medical conditions. Mainly affects the axillae, palms, soles of the feet and/or face. Up to 5% of the population are affected and may run in families. Onset is typically in the teenage years. May be very distressing and socially disabling.

Management

- Give all patients self-help advice (see below).
- Treat topically with 20% aluminium chloride (e.g. Anhydrol Forte®) applied to clean skin every night – wash off the following morning. ↓ frequency of application as symptoms subside.
- Treat local irritation with topical steroid, e.g. hydrocortisone 1%.
- Absorbent dusting powder can be helpful for axillary/plantar sweating.
- Consider a trial of drug therapy, e.g. β- blockers, SSRIs (as above).
- Refer to dermatology or vascular surgery if not responding.

Secondary care treatment options include

- *Iontophoresis* – suitable for isolated palmar or foot hyperhidrosis. A mild electric current is passed through the skin of the hands/feet whilst they are immersed in a warm water bath. Multiple sessions are needed initially (e.g. 6 sessions in the first 3wk.) and then treatments must be repeated every 6wk.–6mo., depending on individual response.
- *Botulinum toxin injections* – suitable for isolated excess sweating of the axillae and/or groins. ↓ sweating but does not stop it completely. Lasts 4–12mo. then repeat injections are needed.
- *Endoscopic transthoracic sympathectomy (ETS)* – 99% effective for relief of palmar hyperhidrosis and, with modification, relieves axillary hyperhidrosis in 80% of people at the same time. A similar procedure can also be used for facial flushing, blushing or sweating – with a success rate of 70% for each side. In all cases patients should expect compensatory hyperhidrosis elsewhere (usually the small of the back).

Advice for patients: Excess sweating

- Avoid clothing and shoes made of lycra, nylon and other man-made fibres.
- Avoid tight clothing.
- Wear colours which don't show the sweat, e.g. white, black.
- Use emollient washes and moisturizers rather than soap.
- Try to identify trigger factors for sweating (e.g. alcohol, crowded rooms) and avoid those situations.
- If sweating comes on in stressful situations, a vicious cycle may start in which you then worry about sweating which in turn increases your level of anxiety and makes you sweat more. Relaxation techniques such as those taught in yoga classes or on relaxation tapes can help.

Chapter 8

Useful information and contacts

Useful information and contacts for GPs *340*
Information and contacts for patients,
   relatives and carers *352*

Useful information and contacts for GPs

General information

DIPEx Patient experience database ▯ www.dipex.org

National Statistics ▯ www.statistics.gov.uk

NICE Referral guidelines for suspected cancer – quick reference guide (2005) ▯ www.nice.org.uk

National Electronic Library for Health ▯ www.library.nhs.uk

Adolescence

BMJ McPherson. Adolescents in primary care (2005) 330 465–7

Alcohol

BMJ Addiction and dependence – II: alcohol (1997) 315 358–60

DTB Managing the heavy drinker in primary care (2000) 38(8) 60–4

SIGN The management of harmful drinking and alcohol dependence in primary care (2003) ▯ www.sign.ac.uk

Antenatal care and antenatal screening

NICE ▯ www.nice.org.uk
- Antenatal and postnatal mental health: Clinical management and service guidance (2007)
- Antenatal care: routine care for the healthy pregnant woman (2003 – due for update in 2007)
- Maternal and fetal nutrition – due for publication in 2007

National Screening Committee Antenatal and newborn screening programme ▯ www.screening.nhs.uk/an

RCOG Amniocentesis and chorionic villus sampling (2005) ▯ www.rcog.org.uk

Anxiety

NICE Management of anxiety (panic disorder, with or without agoraphobia, and generalised anxiety disorder) in adults in primary, secondary and community care (2004) ▯ www.nice.org.uk

Bacterial vaginosis

British Association of Sexual Health and HIV (BASHH) Management of bacterial vaginosis (2001) ▯ www.bashh.org

Breast disease

NICE ▯ www.nice.org.uk
- Referral guidelines for suspected cancer (2005)
- Improving outcomes in breast cancer (2002)
- Classification and care of women at high risk of familial breast cancer in primary, secondary and tertiary care (2004)
- Breast cancer: diagnosis and treatment (due for publication in 2008).

Clinical Evidence ▯ www.clinicalevidence.com
- Stebbing *et al.* Breast cancer (metastatic) (2006)

- Rodger *et al.* Breast cancer (non-metastatic) (2005)
- Bundred N. Breast pain (2005).

Cancer Research UK
- Breast cancer survival statistics
  🖥 http://info.cancerresearchuk.org/cancerstats
- Cancer Research UK Guidelines for referral of patients with breast problems (2003) Available from NHS Response Line ☎ 08701 555 455; e-mail: doh@prolog.uk.com 🖥 www.cancerscreening.nhs.uk
- Breast Screening – UK (2003). Available from
  🖥 http://info.cancerresearchuk.org/cancerstats

NHS Breast Screening 🖥 www.cancerscreening.org.uk

Breech presentation

RCOG The management of breech presentation (2001)
🖥 www.rcog.org.uk

Cochrane Coyle ME *et al.* Cephalic version by moxibustion for breech presentation (2005) Accessed via 🖥 www.library.nhs.uk

Candidiasis – see thrush

Cervical cancer

Cancer Research UK Cervical cancer statistics
🖥 http://info.cancerresearchuk.org/cancerstats

NHS Cervical Screening 🖥 www.cancerscreening.org.uk

NICE Referral guidelines for suspected cancer – quick reference guide (2005) 🖥 www.nice.org.uk

Chlamydia

Department of Health 🖥 www.dh.gov.uk
- National Chlamydia Screening Programme
- National Strategy for Sexual Health and HIV (2001)

British Association of Sexual Health and HIV (BASHH) Management of *Chlamydia trachomatis* genital tract infection (2006)
🖥 www.bashh.org

Combined contraceptive pill
Faculty of Family Planning & Reproductive Health Care (FFPRHC) First prescription of the combined oral contraception (2003)
🖥 www.ffprhc.org.uk

Condoms

FFPRHC male and female condoms (2007) 🖥 www.ffprhc.org.uk

Contraception

Guillebaud J. *Contraception: your questions answered*, 4th edn. Churchill Livingstone (2003) ISBN: 0443073430

Family Planning Association (FPA) ☎ 0845 310 1334
🖥 www.fpa.org.uk

Faculty of Family Planning & Reproductive Health Care (FFPRHC) UK selected practice recommendations for contraceptive use (2002)
🖥 www.ffprhc.org.uk

World Health Organization (WHO) 🖳 www.who.int
- selected practice recommendations for contraceptive use (2004)
- Medical eligibility criteria for contraceptive use (2004).

NICE Long-acting reversible contraception (2005) 🖳 www.nice.org.uk

Coronary prevention

Coronary risk charts Available from 🖳 www.bhsoc.org

DoH National Service Framework: coronary heart disease (2000) 🖳 www.dh.gov.uk

NICE MI: Secondary prevention (2007) 🖳 www.nice.org.uk

JBS2 Joint British Societies' guidelines on prevention of cardiovascular disease in clinical practice (2005) *Heart*, **91** (suppl. 5): vi–52.

Clinical evidence Thorogood *et al.* Cardiovascular disorders: changing behaviour (2003) Accessed via 🖳 www.library.nhs.uk

Depression – see also postnatal depression

NICE Management of depression in primary and secondary care (2004) 🖳 www.nice.org.uk

DTB Mild depression in general practice (2003) 4(8) 60–4

The Patient Health Questionnaire (PHQ-9) 🖳 www.depression-primarycare.org

Diabetes mellitus

NICE Diabetes in pregnancy – due to be published in November 2007 🖳 www.nice.org.uk

Diabetes UK Professional and patient information on the management of pregnant women with gestational diabetes 🖳 www.diabetes.org.uk

Disability and benefits

Citizens' Advice Bureau 🖳 www.adviceguide.org.uk

Department of Work and Pensions (DWP) 🖳 www.dwp.gov.uk

DWP Medical evidence for Statutory Sick Pay, Statutory Maternity Pay and Social Security Incapacity Benefit purposes: a guide for registered Medical Practitioners. IB204. 🖳 www.dwp.gov.uk/medical

Disability Discrimination Act 🖳 www.direct.gov.uk

Jobcentre Plus 🖳 www.jobcentreplus.gov.uk

Domestic violence

DoH Domestic violence: a resource manual for health care professionals. Available from 🖳 www.dh.gov.uk

Home Office 🖳 www.homeoffice.gov.uk/crime-victims/reducing-crime/domestic-violence

RCGP Heath I. Domestic violence 🖳 www.rcgp.org.uk

BMJ Ramsay J et al. Should health professionals screen women for domestic violence? Systematic review (2002) 325 314

Driving
DVLA At-a-glance guide to the current medical standards of fitness to drive for medical practitioners. Available from 🖳 www.dvla.gov.uk

Medical advisors from the DVLA can advise on difficult issues – contact: Drivers Medical Unit, DVLA, Swansea SA99 1TU or ☎ 01792 761119 or e-mail: medadviser@dvla.gsi.gov.uk

Drug abuse
DoH Drug misuse and dependence – guidelines on clinical management (1999) 🖳 www.dh.gov.uk

NICE 🖳 www.nice.org.uk
- Substance misuse interventions (2007)
- Drug misuse: opioid detoxification (2007)
- Drug misuse: psychosocial interventions (2007).

National Treatment Agency for Substance Abuse 🖳 www.nta.nhs.uk

Substance Misuse Management in General Practice (SMMGP) 🖳 www.smmgp.org.uk

RCGP Substance Misuse Unit – provides certificate courses in management of drug abuse 🖳 www.rcgp.org.uk

Drugs and appliances
BNF 🖳 www.bnf.org

Medicines and Healthcare Products Regulatory Agency (MHRA) 🖳 www.mhra.gov.uk

Obtaining steroid cards
- England and Wales: NHS Customer Services ☎ 0161 683 2376/2382
- Scotland: Banner Business Supplies ☎ 01506 448 440

Prescription Pricing Authority Electronic drug tariff 🖳 www.ppa.org.uk

Ectopic pregnancy
RCOG The management of tubal pregnancy (2004) 🖳 www.rcog.org.uk

Emergency contraception
Department of Health CMO Update 35 (2003) 🖳 www.dh.gov.uk

FFPRH Emergency contraception (2006) 🖳 www.ffprhc.org.uk

Endometrial cancer – see uterine cancer

Endometriosis

RCOG The investigation and management of endometriosis (2000)
🖥 www.rcog.org.uk

Epilepsy in pregnancy

NICE The epilepsies: the diagnosis and management of the epilepsies in adults and children in primary and secondary care (2004)
🖥 www.nice.org.uk

SIGN Diagnosis and management of epilepsy in adults (2003)
🖥 www.sign.ac.uk

Exercise

British Journal of Sports Medicine Marshall AL *et al.* Reliability and validity of a brief physical activity assessment for use by family physicians (2005) 39 294–7

NICE Physical activity guidance (2006) 🖥 www.nice.org.uk

DoH The General Practice Physical Activity Questionnaire (2006)
🖥 www.dh.gov.uk

Fibromyalgia

Arthritis Research Campaign (ARC) ☎ 0870 850 5000
🖥 www.arc.org.uk

Fibromyalgia Association UK ☎ 0870 220 1232
🖥 www.fibromyalgia-associationuk.org

Genital herpes

RCOG Management of genital herpes in pregnancy (2002)
🖥 www.rcog.org.uk

British Association for Sexual Health and HIV National guidelines for the management of genital herpes (2001) 🖥 www.bashh.org

Health Protection Agency (HPA) 🖥 www.hpa.org.uk

UK Clinical Virology Network 🖥 www.clinical-virology.org

Genital warts

British Association of Sexual Health and HIV (BASHH) Management of HPV infection (2002) 🖥 www.bashh.org

Gonorrhoea

British Association of Sexual Health and HIV (BASHH) Management of gonorrhoea in adults (2005) 🖥 www.bashh.org

GP contract

NHS Employers Primary care contracting 🖥 www.nhsemployers.org

DoH The GMS contract 🖥 www.dh.gov.uk

BMA The GMS contract, quality and outcomes framework and Read codes 🖳 www.bma.org.uk

Hepatitis

British Association for Sexual Health and HIV National guidelines on the management of viral hepatidides (2005) 🖳 www.bashh.org

Health Protection Agency (HPA) 🖳 www.hpa.org.uk

UK Clinical Virology Network 🖳 www.clinical-virology.org

DoH The Green Book 🖳 www.dh.gov.uk

HIV infection

Medical Foundation for AIDs and Sexual Health HIV in primary care (2004 and revisions 2005) 🖳 www.medfash.org.uk

DoH 🖳 www.dh.gov.uk
- Winning ways: reducing healthcare-associated infection in England (2004)
- National Strategy for Sexual Health and HIV (2001).

British HIV Association 🖳 www.bhiva.org
- HIV Treatment Guidelines (2006)
- Management of HIV infection in pregnant women and the prevention of mother-to-child transmission of HIV (2005).

British Association of Sexual Health and HIV (BASHH)
🖳 www.bashh.org
- National guidelines on HIV testing (2006)
- Guideline for the use of post-exposure prophylaxis for HIV following sexual exposure (2006).

Hormone replacement therapy

Clayton, Monga & Baker. *Gynaecology by ten teachers.* Hodder Arnold (2006) ISBN: 0340816627

RCOG Hormone replacement therapy and venous thromboembolism (2004) 🖳 www.rcog.org.uk

RCP (Edinburgh) Consensus conference on hormone replacement therapy: final consensus statement (October 2003)
🖳 www.rcpe.ac.uk/education/standards/consensus/hrt_03.php

CSM Guidance Further advice on safety of HRT (12/2003)
🖳 www.mca.gov.uk

Million Women Study Collaborators Lancet (2003); 362 419–27

Women's Health Initiative Study 🖳 www.whi.org

Incontinence

Association for Continence Advice Advice for health care professionals
☎ 020 8692 4680 🖳 www.aca.uk.com

Infection in pregnancy

RCOG 🖳 www.rcog.org.uk
- Management of genital herpes in pregnancy (2002)
- Prevention of early-onset neonatal group B Streptococcal disease (2001)
- Chickenpox in pregnancy (2001).

British HIV Association Management of HIV infection in pregnant women and the prevention of mother-to-child transmission of HIV (2005), ⊟ www.bhiva.org

Health Protection Agency (HPA) Guidance on the management of rash illness and exposure to rash illness in pregnancy
⊟ www.hpa.org.uk

DTB Volume 43.
- Chickenpox, pregnancy and the newborn (September 2005)
- Chickenpox, pregnancy and the newborn – a follow-up (December 2005).

Infective endocarditis

British Heart Foundation Factfiles Infective endocarditis (12/2003 &1/2004) ⊟ www.bhf.org.uk

European Heart Journal Horstkotte D. *et al.* Guidelines on prevention, diagnosis and treatment of infective endocarditis (2004) **25**(3) 267–76

Infertility

RCOG Fertility: assessment and treatment of people with fertility problems (2004) ⊟ www.rcog.org.uk

Human Fertilisation and Embryology Authority (HFEA) ☎ 020 7377 5077 ⊟ www.hfea.gov.uk

British Infertility Counselling Association ⊟ www.bica.net

British Fertility Society ⊟ www.britishfertilitysociety.org.uk

Intrauterine devices (including Mirena®)

Letter of competence in intrauterine contraception techniques
☎ 020 7724 5669 ⊟ www.ffprhc.org.uk

FFPRHC The copper intrauterine device as long-term contraception (2004) ⊟ www.ffprhc.org.uk

NICE Long-acting reversible contraception (2005) ⊟ www.nice.org.uk

Labour and intrapartum care

RCOG ⊟ www.rcog.org.uk
- Induction of labour (2001)
- Instrumental vaginal delivery (2000)
- Home birth

NICE ⊟ www.nice.org.uk
- Caesarian section guidelines (2004)
- Intrapatum care – due for publication in 2007.

Lichen sclerosus – see vulval conditions

Lymphoedema

Cochrane Badger *et al.* Physical therapies for reducing and controlling lymphoedema of the limb (2004).

Menopause

Clayton, Monga & Baker. *Gynaecology by ten teachers* Hodder Arnold (2006) ISBN: 0340816627

Menorrhagia

NICE Heavy menstrual bleeding: investigation and treatment (2007)
🖳 www.nice.org.uk

Miscarriage

RCOG 🖳 www.rcog.org.uk
- Management of early pregnancy loss (2000)
- Investigation and treatment of couples with recurrent miscarriage (2003).

Neonatal screening

National Screening Committee Antenatal and newborn screening programme 🖳 www.screening.nhs.uk/an

UK Newborn Screening Programme Centre
🖳 www.newbornscreening-bloodspot.org.uk

Obesity

National Audit Office Tackling obesity in England (2001)
🖳 www.nao.org.uk

NICE 🖳 www.nice.org.uk
- Guidance on the use of sibutramine for the treatment of obesity in adults (2001)
- Orlistat for treatment of obesity in adults (2001)
- Rimonabant for the treatment of overweight and obese patients – in preparation
- Obesity: the prevention, identification, assessment and management of overweight and obesity in adults and children (2006).

National Obesity Forum 🖳 www.nationalobesityforum.org.uk
- Guidelines on the management of adult obesity and overweight in primary care (2002)
- An approach to weight management in children and adolescents (2–18 years) in primary care (2003)

SIGN Management of obesity in children and young people (2003)
🖳 www.sign.ac.uk

Counterweight Project 🖳 www.counterweight.org

Obsessive – compulsive disorder

NICE Obsessive – compulsive disorder: core interventions in the treatment of obsessive – compulsive disorder and body dysmorphic disorder (2005) 🖳 www.nice.org.uk

347

Osteoporosis

NICE 🖳 www.nice.org.uk
- Osteoporosis – secondary prevention (2005)
- Osteoporosis – assessment of fracture risk and prevention in high-risk individuals – due for publication in 2007.

National Osteoporosis Society Primary care strategy for osteoporosis and falls (2002) ⌨ www.nos.org.uk

Royal College of Physicians Osteoporosis: clinical guidelines for prevention and treatment (2003) ⌨ www.rcplondon.ac.uk

Ovarian cancer

Cancer Research UK Ovarian cancer statistics
⌨ http//info.cancerresearchuk.org/cancerstats

Clayton, Monga & Baker. *Gynaecology by ten teachers* Hodder Arnold (2006) ISBN: 0340816627

NICE Referral guidelines for suspected cancer – quick reference guide (2005) ⌨ www.nice.org.uk

Panic disorder – see anxiety

Pelvic inflammatory disease

RCOG Management of acute pelvic inflammatory disease (2003)
⌨ www.rcog.org.uk

British Association for Sexual Health and HIV (BASHH) Management of PID (2005) ⌨ www.bashh.org

Phobia – see anxiety

Pituitary disease

Pituitary Foundation ☎ 0845 450 0375 ⌨ www.pituitary.org.uk

Placenta previa

RCOG Placenta praevia and placenta praevia accreta: diagnosis and management (2005) ⌨ www.rcog.org.uk

Polycystic ovary syndrome

RCOG Long-term consequences of polycystic ovary syndrome (2003)
⌨ www.rcog.org.uk

Postnatal care

NICE ⌨ www.nice.org.uk
- Antenatal and postnatal mental health: clinical management and service guidance (2007)
- Postnatal care – due for publication in 2007.

Postnatal depression

NICE Antenatal and postnatal mental health: clinical management and service guidance (2007) ⌨ www.nice.org.uk

Clinical evidence Howard L. *Postnatal depression* (2006)
⌨ www.clinicalevidence.com

DTB The management of postnatal depression (May 2000) **38** p.33–6

Cochrane Lawrie TA *et al.* Oestrogens and progestogens for preventing and treating postnatal depression (2000) Accessed via 🖳 www.library.nhs.uk

Lancet Gregoire AJP *et al.* Transdermal oestrogen for treatment of severe postnatal depression (1996) 347 930–3

Post-partum haemorrhage

RCOG Management of post-partum haemorrhage (1997 and update 2002) 🖳 www.rcog.org.uk

Pre-eclampsia

APEC Pre-eclampsia community guideline (2004) 🖳 www.apec.org.uk

RCOG Pre-eclampsia – study group recommendations (2003) 🖳 www.rcog.org.uk

Premenstrual syndrome

RCOG PMS guideline currently being updated – will be available on 🖳 www.rcog.org.uk

MeReC bulletin 13(3) Tackling premenstrual syndrome (2003) Accessed via 🖳 www.npc.co.uk/merec_bulletins.htm

Clayton, Monga & Baker. *Gynaecology by ten teachers* Hodder Arnold (2006) ISBN: 0340816627

Puberty – see adolescence

Pubic lice

British Association of Sexual Health and HIV (BASHH) National guideline on the management of *Phthirus pubis* infestation (2001) 🖳 www.bashh.org

Rhesus prophylaxis

RCOG/NICE Use of anti-D immunoglobulin for rhesus prophylaxis (2002) 🖳 www.rcog.org.uk

Scabies

British Association of Sexual Health and HIV (BASHH) National guideline on the management of scabies (2001) 🖳 www.bashh.org

Self-harm and suicide

NICE Self-harm: the short-term physical and psychological management and secondary prevention of self-harm in primary and secondary care (2004) 🖳 www.nice.org.uk

DoH National Suicide Prevention Strategy for England (2002) 🖳 www.dh.gov.uk

Sexual health

British Association of Sexual Health and HIV (BASHH) 🖳 www.bashh.org

DoH 🖳 www.dh.gov.uk
- Winning ways: reducing healthcare-associated infection in England (2004)
- National Strategy for Sexual Health and HIV (2001).

NICE Preventing sexually transmitted infections and reducing under 18 conceptions (2007) 🖳 www.nice.org.uk

Sexual problems
British Association for Sexual and Relationship Therapy
☎ 020 8543 2707 🖳 www.basrt.org.uk

Institute of Psychosexual Medicine 🖳 www.ipm.org.uk

Smoking
Clinical evidence Thorogood et al. Cardiovascular disorders: changing behaviour (2003) Accessed via 🖳 www.library.nhs.uk

NICE 🖳 www.nice.org.uk
- Smoking cessation: brief interventions and referral for smoking cessation in primary care and other settings (2006)
- Nicotine replacement and bupropion for smoking cessation (2002)

Cochrane Accessed via 🖳 www.library.nhs.uk
- Abbot et al. Hypnotherapy for smoking cessation (1998)
- Hughes et al. Antidepressants for smoking cessation (2004)
- Silagy et al. Nicotine replacement for smoking cessation (2004)
- Stead & Lancaster. Group behaviour therapy programmes for smoking cessation (2005).

Thorax Smoking cessation guidelines for health professionals: an update (2000) 55 987–90 🖳 http://thorax.bmjjournals.com

BMJ Russell MAH. Effect of GPs' advice against smoking (1979) 2 231–5

Sterilization
RCOG Male and female sterilization (2004) 🖳 www.rcog.org.uk.

Stress
Health and Safety Executive (HSE) 🖳 www.hse.gov.uk/stress

Syphilis
British Association of Sexual Health and HIV (BASHH)
🖳 www.bashh.org
- Management of early syphilis (2002)
- Management of late syphilis (2002).

Termination of pregnancy
RCOG The care of women requesting induced abortion (2001)
🖳 www. rcog.org.uk

Thromboembolic disease
RCOG 🖳 www.rcog.org.uk
- Thromboprophylaxis during pregnancy, labour and after vaginal delivery (2004)
- Thromboembolic disease in pregnancy and the puerperium (2001).

Thrush
British Association of Sexual Health and HIV (BASHH) Management of vulvovaginal candidiasis (2001) 🖳 www.bashh.org

Trichomonas vaginalis infection
British Association of Sexual Health and HIV (BASHH) Management of *Trichomonas vaginalis* infection (2001) 🖳 www.bashh.org

Trophoblastic disease
RCOG Management of gestational trophoblastic neoplasia (2004) 🖳 www.rcog.org.uk

Uterine cancer
Cancer Research UK Uterine (womb) cancer statistics 🖳 http://info.cancerresearchuk.org/cancerstats

NICE Referral guidelines for suspected cancer – quick reference guide (2005) 🖳 www.nice.org.uk

Vulval conditions
British Association for Sexual Health and HIV (BASHH) National guidelines on the management of vulval conditions (2002) 🖳 www.bashh.org

British Association of Dermatologists Guidelines for the management of lichen sclerosus (2002) 🖳 www.bad.org.uk

RCOG Management of vulval cancer (2006) 🖳 www.rcog.org.uk

NICE Referral guidelines for suspected cancer – quick reference guide (2005) 🖳 www.nice.org.uk

Information and contacts for patients, relatives and carers

General information

DIPEx Patient experience database ⌨ www.dipex.org

Expert Patient Scheme ⌨ www.expertpatients.co.uk

Patient UK Patient information on a range of topics
⌨ www.patient.co.uk

National Electronic Library for Health ⌨ www.library.nhs.uk

NHS Direct ⌨ www.nhsdirect.nhs.uk

Women's Health ☎ 0845 125 5254 ⌨ www.womens-health.co.uk

Alcohol

Drinkline (government-sponsored helpline) ☎ 0800 917 8282

Alcohol Concern ⌨ www.alcoholconcern.org.uk

Alcoholics Anonymous ☎ 0845 7697555 ⌨ www.alcoholics-anonymous.org.uk

Androgen insensitivity syndrome (AIS)

AIS Support Group (UK) ⌨ www.aissg.org/www/ais

Anxiety

Anxiety Care Helpline ☎ 020 8478 3400 ⌨ www.anxietycare.org.uk

No More Panic ⌨ www.nomorepanic.org.uk

Triumph Over Phobia (TOP) UK Self-help materials and groups
☎ 0845 600 9601 ⌨ www.triumphoverphobia.com

Royal College of Psychiatrists Patient information sheets
⌨ www.rcpsych.ac.uk

Benefits

Benefit fraud line ☎ 0800 85 44 40

Citizens' Advice Bureau ⌨ www.adviceguide.org.uk

Department of Work and Pensions ⌨ www.dwp.gov.uk
☎ *Benefits Enquiry Line* – 0800 882200; 0800 243355 (minicom facility);
0800 441144 (for help with form completion).

Government information and services ⌨ www.direct.gov.uk

HM Customs and Revenue ⌨ www.hmcr.gov.uk Tax credit enquiry
line ☎ 0845 300 3900

Jobcentre Plus ⌨ www.jobcentreplus.gov.uk

Pension Service ⌨ www.thepensionservice.gov.uk

Breast cancer

Screening

NHS Cancer Screening 'Be breast aware' leaflet and other information
🖥 www.cancerscreening.org.uk/breastscreen/breastawareness.html

Breast screening – the facts. Available from
🖥 www.cancerscreening.org.uk

Over 70? You are still entitled to breast screening. Available from
🖥 www.cancerscreening.org.uk

Support

Breakthrough Breast Cancer ☎ 08080 100 200
🖥 www.breakthrough.org.uk

Breast Cancer Care ☎ 0808 800 6000
🖥 www.breastcancercare.org.uk

Breast Cancer Campaign 🖥 www.bcc-uk.org

Against Breast Cancer 🖥 www.aabc.org.uk

Cancer Research UK ☎ 0800 226 237 🖥 www.cancerhelp.org.uk

Cancer Backup ☎ 0808 800 1234 (helpline) 🖥 www.cancerbackup.org.uk

Breast feeding

National Childbirth Trust ☎ 0870 444 8708
🖥 www.nctpregnancyandbabycare.com

La Leche League ☎ 0845 120 2918 🖥 www.laleche.org.uk

Baby Café 🖥 www.thebabycafe.co.uk

Association of Breastfeeding Mothers ☎ 0870 401771
🖥 www.abm.me.uk

Breastfeeding Network ☎ 0870 9000 8787
🖥 www.breastfeedingnetwork.org.uk

Cancer

Cancerbackup ☎ 0808 800 1234 🖥 www.cancerbackup.org.uk

Macmillan Cancer Relief ☎ 0808 808 2020 🖥 www.macmillan.org.uk

CancerHelp UK 🖥 www.cancerhelp.org.uk

Choriocarcinoma – see hydatidiform mole

Chronic fatigue/ME

ME Association ☎ 0871 222 7824 🖥 www.meassociation.org.uk

Action for ME ☎ 01749 670799 🖥 www.afme.org.uk.

Cognitive behaviour therapy

Gilbert. *Overcoming depression*. Constable and Robin (2000)
ISBN: 1841191256

Beating the blues© 🖥 www.ultrasis.com
🖥 www.psychologyonline.co.uk

Congenital adrenal hyperplasia
Climb Congenital Adrenal Hyperplasia UK Support Group
☐ www.cah.org.uk

Contraception
Family Planning Association (FPA) ☎ 0845 310 1334
☐ www.fpa.org.uk

Fertility UK ☐ www.fertilityuk.org

Coronary prevention
British Heart Foundation ☎ 0845 708 070 ☐ www.bhf.org.uk

Depression
Depression Alliance ☎ 020 7207 3293 ☐ www.depressionalliance.org

Royal College of Psychiatrists Patient information sheets
☐ www.rcpsych.ac.uk

Diabetes mellitus
Diabetes UK ☎ 0845 120 2960 ☐ www.diabetes.org.uk

British Heart Foundation ☎ 0845 708 070 ☐ www.bhf.org.uk

Domestic violence
Women's Aid ☎ 0808 2000 247 ☐ www.womensaid.org.uk

Action on Elder Abuse ☎ 0808 808 8141 ☐ www.elderabuse.org.uk

Police domestic violence units ☎ 0845 045 45 45

Drug abuse
'Talk to FRANK' (England and Wales) Government-run information, advice and referral service ☎ (24h.) 0800 77 66 00
☐ www.talktofrank.com

Drugscope Information about drug abuse and how to get treatment
☐ www.drugscope.org.uk

Drugs-info Information about substance abuse for families of addicts
☐ www.drugs-info.co.uk

ADFAM Support for families of addicts ☎ 020 7928 8898
☐ www.adfam.org.uk

Ecstasy ☐ www.ecstasy.org

Benzodiazepines ☐ www.benzo.org.uk

Solvent abuse ☎ 0808 800 2345 ☐ www.re-solv.org

Ectopic pregnancy
Ectopic Pregnancy Trust ☎ 01895 238025 ☐ www.ectopic.org

Elder abuse – see domestic violence

Endometriosis
National Endometriosis Society ☎ 020 7222 2781
🖥 www.endo.org.uk

Epilepsy
Epilepsy Action ☎ 0808 800 5050. 🖥 www.epilepsy.org.uk

Epilepsy Scotland ☎ 0808 800 2200 🖥 www.epilepsyscotland.org.uk

Joint Epilepsy Council of the UK and Ireland
🖥 www.jointepilepsycouncil.org.uk

Fibromyalgia
Arthritis Research Campaign (ARC) ☎ 0870 850 5000
🖥 www.arc.org.uk.

Fibromyalgia Association UK ☎ 0870 220 1232 🖥 www.fibromyalgia-associationuk.org

Genetic syndromes
The Genetics Interests Group ☎ 020 7704 3141 🖥 www.gig.org.uk

Down's Syndrome Association ☎ 0845 230 0372 🖥 www.downs-syndrome.org.uk

Sickle Cell Society ☎ 0800 001 5660 🖥 www.sicklecellsociety.org

UK Thalassaemia Society 🖥 www.ukts.org

Tay-Sachs and Allied Disease Association ☎ 01473 404 156

National Society for Phenylketonuria (NSPKU) ☎ 020 8364 3010
🖥 www.nspku.org

Cystic Fibrosis Trust ☎ 0845 859 1000 🖥 www.cftrust.org.uk

Growth disorders
Height Matters 🖥 www.heightmatters.org.uk

Hepatitis
British Liver Trust ☎ 01425 463080 🖥 www.britishlivertrust.org.uk

Department of Health Hepatitis B: how to protect your baby
🖥 www.dh.gov.uk

Herpes
Herpes Association ☎ 0845 123 2305 🖥 www.herpes.org.uk

HIV
NAM Aidsmap ☎ 0207 840 0050 🖥 www.aidsmap.com

National AIDS Helpline ☎ 0800 567 123 (24h. helpline)

Terence Higgins Trust ☎ 0845 1221 200 🖥 www.tht.org.uk

Hydatidiform mole
Hydatidiform Mole and Choriocarcinoma Support Service
🖳 www.hmole-chorio.org.uk

Hysterectomy
Hysterectomy Association 🖳 www.hysterectomy-association.org.uk

Immunization
Immunization NHS website for patients 🖳 www.immunisation.org.uk

Incontinence
Continence Foundation ☎ 0845 345 0165
🖳 www.continence-foundation.org.uk

Infertility
National Fertility Association (ISSUE) ☎ 09050 280 300
🖳 www.issue.co.uk

National Infertility Support Network (CHILD) ☎ 01424 732361
🖳 www.child.org.uk

Human Fertilisation and Embryology Authority (HFEA) ☎ 020 7377
5077 🖳 www.hfea.gov.uk

Lymphoedema
Lymphoedema Support Network ☎ 020 7351 4480
🖳 www.lymphoedema.org/lsn

UKLymph.com Online support network 🖳 www.uklymph.com

Skin Care Campaign 🖳 www.skincarecampaign.org

CancerHelp UK ☎ 0800 226 237 🖳 www.cancerhelp.org.uk

Royal Marsden Hospital 🖳 www.royalmarsden.org.uk

Vascular Society 🖳 www.vascularsociety.org.uk/patient/topics

ME – see chronic fatigue

Menopause
British Menopause Society 🖳 www.the-bms.org

Menopause Amarant Trust ☎ 01293 413000
🖳 www.amarantmenopausetrust.org.uk

Daisy Network For women with premature menopause
🖳 www.daisynetwork.org.uk

Miscarriage
Miscarriage Association ☎ 01924 200799
🖳 www.miscarriageassociation.org.uk

Newborn screening
UK Newborn Screening Programme Centre Leaflets on screening for parents ⌨ www.newbornscreening-bloodspot.org.uk

Obsessive – compulsive disorder
OCD Action ☎ 020 7226 4000 ⌨ www.ocdaction.org.uk

Royal College of Psychiatrists Patient information sheets
⌨ www.rcpsych.ac.uk

Osteoporosis
Arthritis Research Campaign ☎ 0870 850 5000 ⌨ www.arc.org.uk

National Osteoporosis Society ☎ 0845 450 0230 ⌨ www.nos.org.uk

Ovarian cancer
Ovacome ☎ 020 7380 9589 ⌨ www.ovacome.org.uk

Cancerbackup ☎ 0808 800 1234 ⌨ www.cancerbackup.org.uk

CancerHelp UK ⌨ www.cancerhelp.org.uk

Panic disorder and phobias
Anxiety Care Helpline ☎ 020 8478 3400 ⌨ www.anxietycare.org.uk

No More Panic ⌨ www.nomorepanic.org.uk

Triumph Over Phobia (TOP) UK Self-help materials and groups
☎ 0845 600 9601 ⌨ www.triumphoverphobia.com

Royal College of Psychiatrists Patient information sheets
⌨ www.rcpsych.ac.uk

Pelvic pain
Royal College of Obstetricians and Gynaecologists Factsheet
⌨ www.rcog.org.uk

Pituitary disease
Pituitary Foundation ☎ 0845 450 0375 ⌨ www.pituitary.org.uk

Polycystic ovaries
Verity ⌨ www.verity-pcos.org.uk

Well-being of women Leaflet on PCOS ⌨ www.wellbeing.org.uk

Postnatal depression
Royal College of Psychiatrists Information sheet on postnatal depression ⌨ www.rcpsych.ac.uk

Association for Postnatal Illness Support and befriending by women who have suffered postnatal depression/puerperal psychosis
☎ 020 7386 0868 ⌨ www.apni.org

Meet-a-Mum Association Support and information for women with postnatal depression ☎ 0845 120 6162 ⌨ www.mama.co.uk

Pre-eclampsia
Action on Pre-EClampsia (APEC) ☎ 020 8863 3271 🖥 www.apec.org.uk

Pregnancy
National Childbirth Trust (NCT) ☎ 0870 770 3236. Info line 0870 444 8707 🖥 www.nctpregnancyandbabycare.com

Birth Choice UK 🖥 www.birthchoiceuk.com

Mothers 35 Plus 🖥 www.mothers35plus.co.uk

Emma's Diary 🖥 www.emmasdiary.co.uk

NHS Scotland 🖥 www.hebs.nhs.scot.uk/readysteadybaby

Baby World 🖥 www.babyworld.co.uk

Antenatal Results and Choices (ARC) ☎ 0207 631 0285 🖥 www.arc-uk.org

Perinatal Institute 🖥 www.preg.info

Department of Health Testing for down's syndrome in pregnancy booklet. Available from 🖥 www.dh.gov.uk

Group B streptococcus Support 🖥 www.gbss.org.uk

Twins and Multiple Births Association (TAMBA) ☎ 0870 770 3305 🖥 www.tamba.org.uk

RCOG About induction of labour – information for pregnant women, their partners and their families (2001) 🖥 www.rcog.org.uk

Premenstrual syndrome
National Association for Premenstrual Syndrome ☎ 0870 777 2177 🖥 www.pms.org.uk

Puberty
Childline 24h. confidential counselling ☎ 0800 1111 🖥 www.childline.org

Brook Advisory Service Contraceptive advice and counselling for teenagers ☎ 0800 0185 023 🖥 www.brook.org.uk

Sexwise For under 19s ☎ 0800 28 29

Teenage Health Freak 🖥 www.teenagehealthfreak.org

Self-harm and suicide
Self-injury and Related Issues (SIARI) 🖥 www.siari.co.uk

Samaritans 24h. emotional support via telephone ☎ 08457 909 090

Survivors of bereavement by suicide ☎ 0870 241 3337 🖥 www.uk-sobs.org.uk

Sexual health, sexual problems and sexually transmitted diseases
Family Planning Association (FPA) ☎ 0845 310 1334 🖥 www.fpa.org.uk

Society of Sexual Health Advisers ⌨ www.ssha.info

Department of Health Sexual health line ☎ 0800 567 123 (24h.);
Sexwise (for under 19s) ☎ 0800 28 29 30

Brown P, Faulder C. *Treat yourself to sex.* Penguin (1989) ISBN:
0140110186

Smoking
Action on Smoking and Health (ASH) ☎ 020 7739 5902.
⌨ www.ash.org.uk

NHS Smoking helpline ☎ 0800 169 0 169; pregnancy smoking helpline:
☎ 0800 169 9 169 ⌨ www.givingupsmoking.co.uk

Quit Helpline ☎ 0800 00 22 00 ⌨ www.quit.org.uk

Spina bifida
Association for Spina Bifida and Hydrocephalus (ASBAH) ☎ 01733
555988 ⌨ www.asbah.org

Stillbirth and neonatal death
Stillbirth and Neonatal Death Society (SANDS) ☎ 020 7436 5881
⌨ www.uk-sands.org

Stress
Stress Management Society ☎ 0870 199 3260 ⌨ www.stress.org.uk

International Stress Management Association (UK) ☎ 07000 780 430
⌨ www.isma.org.uk

Teenagers
Childline 24h. confidential counselling ☎ 0800 1111 ⌨ www.childline.org

Brook Advisory Service Contraceptive advice and counselling for
teenagers ☎ 0800 0185 023 ⌨ www.brook.org.uk

Marie Stopes International ☎ 0845 300 8090
⌨ www.mariestopes.org.uk

Sexwise For under 19s ☎ 0800 28 29 30 ⌨ ruthinking.co.uk

Teenage Health Freak ⌨ www.teenagehealthfreak.org

Termination of pregnancy
Marie Stopes International ☎ 0845 300 8090
⌨ www.mariestopes.org.uk

British Pregnancy Advisory Service (BPAS) ☎ 0845 730 40 30
⌨ www.bpas.org

Brook Advisory Centres Patients <25y. only ☎ 0800 0185 023
⌨ www.brook.org.uk

Antenatal Results and Choices (ARC) Supports parents faced with
termination for fetal abnormality ☎ 0207 631 0285 ⌨ www.arc-uk.org

Index

A

abdominal mass 93, 99
abdominal pain
  postnatal 276
  in pregnancy 220, 221,
    270–1
abdominal striae 225
abdominal tone, poor
  postnatal 277
abortion see termination
  of pregnancy
abruptio placentae 271
acamprosate 12
accidents, protecting
  babies from 287
achievement payments,
  GMS contract 7
aciclovir 126, 127, 228,
  230
actinomyces-like organisms
  (ALOs) 190
acupressure 210, 222
acupuncture 210
additional services, GMS
  contract 6
adenomyosis 91
adjuvant endocrine therapy
  58
adolescence 342
  see also puberty;
    teenagers
adrenaline 269, 315
adrenal virilism 68, 69
adrenogenital syndrome
  68, 69
advanced HIV 128
agnus castus 75, 77
agoraphobia 314, 317
alcohol
  beneficial effects 10
  cot death 287
  information and contacts
    342, 354
  management strategies
    12, 13
  misuse 10–13
  pre-conception and early
    pregnancy counselling
    200, 201
  pregnancy 210
alcohol-dependent drinkers
  12, 13
alendronate 158, 159
allopurinol 134
α-fetoprotein (AFP) testing
  214, 215, 216
aluminium chloride 339

amenorrhoea 70, 78–9
  COC pill 173
amitriptyline 140, 244, 328,
  332, 334
amniocentesis 216
amniotic fluid embolism
  272
amoxicillin 122, 178, 179,
  239, 278
amphetamines, withdrawal
  effects 21
anaemia in pregnancy 242
anastrozole 58
androgen insensitivity
  syndrome (AIS) 68–9,
  354
Anhydrol Forte® 339
anomalies of normal
  development and
  involution (ANDI) 48
antenatal care 202, 204–11
  domestic violence 39
  information and contacts
    342
antenatal screening 202,
  214–19, 342
antepartum haemorrhage
  (APH) 238
antidepressants 304, 305
antiphospholipid syndrome
  242
anxiety disorders 314–23,
  342, 354
  menopause 146
appendicitis in pregnancy
  221, 270
appliances, information and
  contacts 345
Arimidex® 58
aromatherapy 210
arterial disease 169
artificial formula feeds
  292
asoprisnil 92
aspiration payments, GMS
  contract 7
aspirin 37, 234, 242, 243,
  252, 308
assisted delivery 266, 267
asthma in pregnancy 242–3
atrophic vaginitis 114
atropine 190
automated auditory brain-
  stem response (AABR)
  screen, neonates 284
azathioprine 245
azithromycin 94, 122, 140,
  166, 188

B

baby blues 277
backache in pregnancy
  220
bacterial vaginosis (BV)
  118–20, 342
  in pregnancy 256
barbiturates, withdrawal
  effects 21
barrier contraception 162,
  163, 192
  failure 167
  see also condoms
Bartholin's gland swellings
  116
BCG vaccination, neonates
  282
Beck Depression Inventory
  (BDI) 302
bed covers 143
behavioural therapy
  obesity 30
  phobias 318
  see also cognitive
    behavioural therapy
Behçet's syndrome 116
benefits system
  information and contacts
    344, 354
  pregnancy 202, 203
  stillbirth 296
benign breast disease
  48–51
benign vaginal tumour 114
benzodiazepines,
  withdrawal effects 21
bereavement
  through stillbirth 296
  through suicide 308
Billing's method 192
Binovum® 175
black cohosh 146
bladder training
  programmes 144
bleeding in pregnancy
  232–9
blocked duct 276
bloodspot screening,
  neonates 288–91
body mass index (BMI) 26,
  27
  obesity 26
  ready reckoner 28
bone mineral density
  (BMD) measurement
  154, 155, 156, 159
bottle feeding 292

361

botulinum toxin injections 339
bowel cancer 153
Bowen's disease 117
Braxton-Hicks contractions 264
breakthrough bleeding 176
breast abscess 51
   postnatal 276
breast awareness 42, 43, 52
breast calcifications 47
breast cancer 42, 44, 45, 56–63
   COC pill 169
   HRT 153
   incidence 53
   information and contacts 63, 343, 355
   mortality 53
   prognosis 61
   screening 52–5
   staging 59
breast cross-section 47
breast cyst 50
breast disease
   assessment 42–7
   benign 48–51
   cancer see breast cancer
   information and contacts 342–3
breast feeding 292
   abdominal pain while 276
   COC pill 173
   contraception 275
   diabetes 250
   drugs 244
   epilepsy 248
   hepatitis C 257
   HIV 218, 258
   information and contacts 355
   postnatal depression 277
   problems 276, 293
breast lump 44, 45
breast microcalcifications 47
breast mouse 48
breast pain 44–7
breast problems in breast feeding 293
breast soreness
   postnatal 276
   pregnancy 220
breathing in the newborn 268
breech presentation 262, 343
   congenital dislocation of the hip 284
Brenner tumour 99
Brevinor® 171
Brief Physical Activity Questionnaire 22, 23
broad ligament haematoma 273

bromocriptine 46, 74, 75, 136, 296
bupropion 16, 17

C

Caesarean section (CS) 266, 267
   driving and exercise 274
caffeine 201
CAGE questionnaire 10
calcifications, breast 47
calcitonin 156
calcium, food content 157
calcium supplements 75, 77, 147, 156, 252
cancer
   causes of death 4
   gender differences 5
   information and contacts 355
   see also specific cancers
candidiasis 120–1, 352
   in pregnancy 259
cannabis
   infertility 134
   pre-conception and early pregnancy counselling 200
cap 192
   post-partum 275
carbamazepine 178, 248
carbaryl 128
carbimazole 246
carboprost 239
carcinoma in situ 117
cardiovascular disease (CVD)
   in pregnancy 202, 244
   prevention 32–7
   risk charts 33
carpal tunnel syndrome in pregnancy 220
Carr–Hill allocation formula, GMS contract 7
catheters
   urinary incontinence 143
   urinary tract infection 138
cat litter, and pregnancy 201, 210
cefalexin 259
cefixime 122
Cerazette® 149, 167, 180, 182, 184
cervical cancer 106–8, 109
   COC pill 169
   information and contacts 343
   screening 110–13
cervical caps 192
cervical conditions 106–13

cervical erosion/ectropion 108
cervical incompetence 108
cervical intraepithelial neoplasia (CIN) 106
   screening 110, 112
cervical polyps 108
cervical shock, IUD insertion 190
cervicitis 108
chasteberry 75, 77
chest compressions of the newborn 268
chickenpox 226, 228–30, 231
childbirth see labour; obstetrics
children
   domestic violence 38
   impact on women's employment 2, 3
Child Tax Credit 203
chlamydia 122, 123, 343
   in pregnancy 256
   screening 256
chloasma 225
chlordiazepoxide 12
chloroquine 211
chlorphenamine 243, 315
chocolate cysts 90
cholecystitis in pregnancy 221, 270
choriocarcinoma 102, 236, 358
chorionic villus sampling (CVS) 216
chromosomal problems 286
chronic fatigue syndrome (CFS) 330–2, 355
chronic hypertension in pregnancy 252
ciclosporin 304, 336
Cilest® 171, 172
cimetidine 134
ciprofloxacin 122, 140
circumcision 69
citalopram 318
clap see gonorrhoea
clear cell tumour 99
climacteric 146
clindamycin 120, 130, 256
clomifene 104, 136, 338
clomipramine 304, 318, 320, 322, 324
clonidine 147
clopidogrel 37
clotrimazole 60, 120
co-amoxiclav 122
cocaine
   infertility 134
   withdrawal effects 21
codeine 245
cognitive behavioural therapy (CBT)
   depression 307

fibromyalgia 334
information and contacts
355
OCD 324
panic disorder 320
phobias 317
PMS 75
coitus interruptus 192
colchicines 134
colds in pregnancy 256
combined oral contracep-
tive (COC) patch 168,
172, 174
drug interactions 178, 79
follow-up 178
missed 176
post-partum 275
postponing menstruation
73
after termination of
pregnancy or
miscarriage 196
combined oral contracep-
tive (COC) pill 163,
168–79
adolescents 195
amenorrhoea 79
breast cancer 56
drug interactions 178–9
dysmenorrhoea 84
emergency contraception
167
endometriosis 91
fibroids 92
follow-up 178
hirsutism 337
HRT 151
information and contacts
343
menopause 148, 149
migraine 170
missed 177
ovarian cancer 100
PMS 75
polycystic ovarian
syndrome 104
post-partum 275
postponing menstruation
73
risks and benefits 168,
169
side-effects 174–6
starting routines 172, 173
after termination of
pregnancy or
miscarriage 196
types 171, 172, 175
urethral syndrome 140
Commission for Health-
care Audit and Inspect
8
condoms 163, 192
adolescents 195
post-partum 275
confidentiality for
teenagers 194

congenital adrenal
hyperplasia (CAH) 68,
69, 356
congenital dislocation of
the hip (CDH), neona-
tal screening 284–5
congenital gynaecological
abnormalities 68–9
congenital hypothyroidism
(CHT) 288, 290
consanguineous couples,
pre-pregnancy genetic
screening for 215
consent
neonatal bloodspot
screening 288
teenagers 194
contact tracing 119
contraception 162–5
emergency 166–7, 182,
345
HRT 151
information and contacts
343–4, 356
post-partum 275
pre-conception
counselling 202
after termination of
pregnancy or
miscarriage 196
for women >35y. 149
see also specific types of
contraception
Conveen continence
guard® 142
cord prolapse 272
coronary heart disease
(CHD)
COC pill 169
indicators 36–7
obesity 27
prevention 32, 344, 356
cot death, reducing the risk
of 287
cotrimoxazole 178
coughs in pregnancy 256
counselling
depression 307
pre-conception see
pre-conception
counselling
cow's milk formula feeds
292
Coxsackievirus A, B 230
crab lice 128
cracked nipples, postnatal
276
cramp in pregnancy 220
cranberry juice 140
cri-du-chat syndrome 286
Crinone® 75
cyclical breast pain 44–6
cyclizine 222, 243
cyclophosphamide 245

cyproterone acetate 172,
337
cystic fibrosis (CF) 288,
289, 290, 291
cystitis 138, 139–40
cystocoele prolapse 96
cytomegalovirus (CMV)
230

D

danazol 46, 74, 75, 91, 338
deafness, neonatal
screening for 284
death, causes of 4
deep dyspareunia 86
deep vein thrombosis
(DVT)
COC pill 175
HRT 153
postnatal 278
in pregnancy 247
delayed miscarriage 234
delayed puberty 70
deliberate self-harm (DSH)
308, 310–11
information and contacts
351, 360
delirium tremens (DTs) 13
delivery location choices
212–13
dentistry, free 203
Depo-Provera® 163, 182,
183, 184, 185
adolescents 195
depression 300–7
cardiovascular disease 37
indicators 37
information and contacts
344, 356
menopause 146
postnatal 277–8, 279–81,
350–1, 359
in pregnancy 244
desogestrel 149, 169, 171,
172, 180
developmental dysplasia of
the hip (DDH) 284–5
developmental screening,
babies 294
DEXA scan 154, 155, 156,
159
dextrose 269
diabetes mellitus
cardiovascular disease 35
indicators 35
information and contacts
344, 356
obesity 27
in pregnancy 202, 250–1
dialysis, and pregnancy 245
Dianette® 172, 337
diaphragms, vaginal 163,
192, 193
diazepam 271, 316

diazoxide 336
diet 26
  menopause 146, 147
  obesity 30
  osteoporosis 156, 157
  plate model 29
  PMS 77
  pre-conception and early
    pregnancy counselling
    201
  pregnancy 210
digoxin 304
dipyridamole 37
directed enhanced services,
  GMS contract 6
disability, information and
  contacts 344
disulfiram 12
domestic violence 38–9,
  344–5, 356
domperidone 166, 243
dong quai 146
Down's syndrome 286
  antenatal screening 216,
    217
  risk in relation to age
    of pregnant woman
    217
doxazosin 243, 253
doxycycline
  chlamydia 122
  endometritis 94
  miscarriage 234
  in pregnancy 211, 243
  urethral syndrome 140
driving
  alcohol misuse 13
  drug misuse 19
  information and contacts
    345
  postnatal period 274
drospirenone 171, 172
drug misuse 18–21, 345,
  356
  pre-conception and early
    pregnancy counselling
    200
  in pregnancy 210
drugs 345
  in pregnancy 202, 210,
    243
dual energy X-ray absorp-
  tiometry (DEXA) scan
  154, 155, 156, 159
Duchenne muscular
  dystrophy 288
duct ectasia 51
duplication, gynaecological
  68
dydrogesterone 152
dysfunctional uterine
  bleeding 80
dysgerminoma 102
dysmenorrhoea 84–5
  IUCDs 188

dyspareunia 86–7
  postnatal 276
dysthymia 300, 303
dystocia 265–6, 272–3

E

early HIV 126
early loss of pregnancy
  233
  see also miscarriage
early pregnancy counselling
  200–3
eating healthily see diet
echovirus 230
eclampsia 255, 271
ecstasy, withdrawal effects
  21
ectopic pregnancy 180,
  232, 236, 237
  information and contacts
    345, 356
  IUDs 188, 189
Edinburgh Postnatal
  Depression Scale
  (EPDS) 277, 280–1
education 2
  antenatal care 206
Edward's syndrome 286
eflornithine cream 337
Eisenmenger's syndrome
  244
elder abuse 39
embryonal carcinoma 102
emergency contraception
  166–7, 182, 345
employment 2–3
  and pregnancy 202, 203,
    210
endodermal sinus tumour
  102
endometrial cancer 94–5,
  169, 353
endometrial proliferation
  94
endometrioid tumour 99
endometriomas 90
endometriosis 90–1, 137
  information and contacts
    346, 357
endometritis 94
  postnatal 278
endoscopic transthoracid
  sympathectomy (ETS)
  339
enhanced services, GMS
  contract 6
enterocoele prolapse 96
enteroviruses 230
entonox in labour 265
epidural 265
epilepsy
  IUD insertion 190
  in pregnancy 202, 248–9,
    346, 357

epithelial ovarian cancer
  (EOC) 99–100
Epstein-Barr virus (EBV)
  230
ergometrine 239, 243
erythromycin 122, 178
escitalopram 320
essential hypertension in
  pregnancy 252
essential services, GMS
  contract 6
ethinylestradiol 167, 171,
  172, 175, 177
  drug interactions 179
ethnicity, and
  pre-pregnancy genetic
  screening 215
etidronate 159
etonogestrel 184
etynodiol 180
evacuation of retained
  products of conception
  (ERPC) 234
evening primrose oil
  breast pain 46
  menopause 146
  PMS 75, 77
  pregnancy 210
Evra® 168, 171, 172
exercise 22–5
  amenorrhoea 79
  depression 304
  information and contacts
    346
  obese patients 30
  PMS 75
  postnatal period 274
  pregnancy 210
exercise prescription
  schemes 24
expected date of delivery
  (EDD) calculator 209
extra service payments,
  GMS contract 7

F

facial flushing 338
falls, reducing risk of and
  damage from 157,
  159
fat necrosis 50
fatigue 330–2
  postnatal 278
  in pregnancy 220
feeding babies 292–3
  see also breast feeding
female genital mutilation
  69
female sheath 163
Femodene® 171, 172
Femodene ED® 171
Femodette® 171
Femulen® 180
ferrous sulphate 242

fetal alcohol syndrome
200, 210
fetal distress 272
fetoscopy 216
fibroadenomas 48
fibroids 92–3
in pregnancy 221, 270
fibroma 102
fibromyalgia 334–5, 346,
357
finasteride 337
fine motor development,
babies 295
Flexi-T 300® 187
flu 256
flucloxacillin 51, 276, 278
fluconazole 120, 276
fluid retention in pregnancy
224
fluoxetine 146, 277, 304,
338
flushing
facial 338
menopause 146, 147, 153
flutamide 337
focal hyperhidrosis 339
folate supplementation
infertility 136
pregnancy 211
anaemia 242
diabetes 250
epilepsy 248
pre-conception and
early pregnancy
counselling 200, 201
follicle stimulating
hormone (FSH) 72, 73
follicular cyst 98
follicular phase, menstrual
cycle 72
follow-on formula 292
forceps, assisted delivery
266, 267
formula feeds 292
functional incontinence
144
furosemide 62

G

galactocoele 50
gamolenic acid 46
gardening, and pregnancy
201, 210
gastroplasty 30
generalized anxiety
disorder (GAD) 314,
315, 316–17
generalized hyperhidrosis
338
General Medical Services
(GMS) contract 6–9
alcohol misuse 11
cancer 62, 95, 101, 109,
117

cardiovascular disease
34, 35–7
cervical screening 111
child health surveillance
287, 295
contraception 164, 167
coronary heart disease
indicators 36
depression 37, 301
drug misuse 19
hepatitis B vaccination
125
information and contacts
346–7
intrapartum care 267
IUDs 191
maternity services 207,
281
obesity 29
palliative care 62, 101
postnatal care 275
pre-conception
counselling 203
sexual health services
131
smoking 15, 36
stroke and transient
ischaemic attack
indicators 37
general practitioner
consultations 4
General Practitioner
Physical Activity Ques-
tionnaire (GPPAQ) 22
genetic screening
breast cancer 52, 56, 57
pre-pregnancy 214, 215
genetic syndromes,
information and
contacts 357
genital herpes 126, 127
information and contacts
346, 357
in pregnancy 256
genital mutilation 69
genital ulcers 116
genital warts 130, 131, 346
genito-urinary disease, in
pregnancy 202
genito-urinary medicine
(GUM) clinics 119
germ-cell tumour 102
gestational diabetes 250,
251
gestodene 149, 169, 171,
172, 175
gestrinone 91
ginger 210, 222
ginseng 146
global sum, GMS contract
7
global sum allocation
(GSA), GMS contract 7
global sum equivalent
(GSE), GMS contract 7
glucocorticoids 156

glycosuria in pregnancy
251
gonadal stromal tumour
102
gonadoblastoma 102
gonorrhoea 122, 123, 346
in pregnancy 256
goserelin 46, 88, 91
granulosa cell tumour 102
Graves disease in
pregnancy 246
griseofulvin 178
group B streptococcus
(GBS) 256–7
group therapy 30
growth disorders 357
intrauterine 260–1
Guthrie card 288
gynaecological assessment
66–7
GyneFix® 187
Gyne-T 380® 187

H

Haemabate® 239
haematoma of rectus
abdominis 221, 271
haematuria 139
haemoglobinopathies 218,
219
haemolytic disease 240–1
haemorrhagic disease of
the newborn 282
haemorrhoids
postnatal 276
pregnancy 220
hair loss 276
hallucinogenic drugs,
withdrawal effects 21
headache in pregnancy 220
head control, babies 294
health 4
health promotion for
pregnant women
210–11
healthy eating see diet
hearing checks, babies 295
heartburn in pregnancy
222
heart disease see
cardiovascular disease
heart rate of the newborn
268
heartsink patients 323
HELLP syndrome 253
heparin 234, 242, 243,
246
hepatitis, information and
contacts 347, 358
hepatitis B (HBV) 124
breast feeding 293
immunization 125
drug misuse 20
neonates 257, 282

in pregnancy 257
serology 125
hepatitis C (HCV) 124
in pregnancy 257
Herceptin® 58
herpes simplex virus (HSV)
126, 127
information and contacts
346, 357
in pregnancy 256
hip, congenital dislocation
of the (CDH) 284–5
hirsutism 336–7
HIV see human immuno-
deficiency virus
home births 213
hormone replacement
therapy (HRT) 150–3
amenorrhoea 79
atrophic vaginitis 114
breast cancer 56, 58
cystitis 140
information and contacts
347
menopause 146, 148
osteoporosis 148, 158
post-menopausal
bleeding 93
urinary incontinence 142
Hospital Anxiety and
Depression Scale
(HADS) 302
hospital births 212, 213
hot flushes 146, 147, 153
human immunodeficiency
virus (HIV) 126, 128,
129
antenatal testing 218
breast feeding 293
information and contacts
347, 357
in pregnancy 258
human papilloma virus
(HPV)
testing 110
vaccination 131
hydatidiform mole 236,
358
hydrocortisone 315, 339
hydroxychloroquine 245
hyperemesis gravidarum
222, 244
hyperhidrosis 338–9
hyperplastic vulval
dystrophy 116
hypertension
cardiovascular disease
35
indicators 35
pregnancy 252–5
hyperthyroidism
postnatal 278
pregnancy 246
hypnosis 210
hypoplastic vulval
dystrophy 116

hypotension in pregnancy
222
hypothyroidism
congenital 288, 290
postnatal 278
pregnancy 246
hysterectomy 113, 358

I

ibandronic acid 158
ibuprofen
breast pain 46
cystitis 141
dysmenorrhoea 84, 85
endometriosis 91
genital herpes 127
IUD insertion 190
ovarian hyperstimulation
98
perineal bruising 276
postnatal breast soreness
276
superficial thrombo-
phlebitis 278
illicit drugs see drug
misuse
imidazole 259
imipramine 144, 304, 318,
322
immature teratoma 102
immunization and
vaccination
hepatitis B see hepatitis B,
immunization
human papilloma virus
131
information and contacts
358
neonatal check 282
in pregnancy 211
tetanus 311
imperforate hymen 68
Implanon® 163, 184
Incapacity Benefit 203
income 2
Income Support 203
incomplete miscarriage
234
incontinence 142–5
aids and appliances 142,
143
information and contacts
347, 358
menopause 148
incontinence pads 143
induction of labour 266
indwelling catheters 143
infections
in pregnancy 256–9,
347–8
protecting babies from
287
infective endocarditis 348
infertility 134–7, 348, 358

informed consent
neonatal bloodspot
screening 288
teenagers 194
injectable progestogen
163, 182–4, 185
adolescents 195
emergency contraception
167
menopause 149
post-partum 275
switching to COC pill
173, 174
after termination of
pregnancy or
miscarriage 196
insomnia 328–9
in pregnancy 222
insulin 243, 250
interferon 124, 257
intermittent self-
catheterization 143
interstitial cystitis 140
intraductal papilloma 51
intrapartum care see
labour
intrauterine contraceptive
devices (IUCDs) 163,
186, 187, 188–90
adolescents 195
menopause 149
post-partum 275
switching to COC pill
173
after termination of
pregnancy or
miscarriage 196
intrauterine devices (IUDs)
180, 186–91
emergency contraception
166, 167
GMS contract 164
information and contacts
348
see also intrauterine
contraceptive devices;
intrauterine system
intrauterine growth 260–1
retardation (IUGR) 260
intrauterine pregnancy
190
intrauterine system (IUS)
186, 187, 188–90
emergency contraception
167
post-partum 275
switching to COC pill
173
after termination of
pregnancy or miscar-
riage 196
iontophoresis 339
ipratropium 243
iron, pre-conception
and early pregnancy
counselling 200, 201

iron supplements
anaemia 242
breast feeding 293
postnatal care 274
ischaemic heart disease 148
isotretinoin 243
ispaghula husk 220
itching in pregnancy 222, 223

J

jaundice
neonatal 285
in pregnancy 244
Job-Seekers Allowance 203

K

Kamillosan® 276
kava 146
Keilland's forceps 267
ketoconazole 134
Klinefelter's syndrome 286
K-Y jelly® 192

L

labetalol 243, 253
labour 264–7
delivery location choices 212–13
epilepsy 248
information and contacts 348
see also obstetrics
lactation suppression 296
lamivudine 124
lamotrigine 178
large for dates 260
late menstruation 146
leg cramp in pregnancy 220
leisure 4
lethargy 330–2
levodopa 300
Levonelle® 195
levonorgestrel
COC pill 169, 171, 172, 175
emergency contraception 166
IUDs 186, 187
progestogen-only pill 180
levothyroxine 151
Leydig cell tumour 102
lichen sclerosus 116
lidocaine 86
life expectancy 4, 5
linea nigra 225

lipid cell tumour 102
liquid-based cytology 110, 112
listeriosis 258, 259
lithium 293
Livial® 150
living arrangements 2
Load 375: 187
local enhanced services, GMS contract 6
lochia, persistent 276–7
Loestrin® 171
lofepramine 304
Logynon® 175
Logynon ED® 175
lone parents 2
low calorie diets 30
LSD, withdrawal effects 21
lung cancer 15
luteal cyst 98
luteal phase, menstrual cycle 72
luteinizing hormone 73
lymphoedema 60–2, 63, 348, 358

M

magnesium supplements 75, 77
magnesium trisilicate 222
major placenta praevia 238
malaria 211, 258
Malarone® 211
malathion 128
mammary duct fistula 51
mammography 50, 52–5
Marvelon® 171, 172, 184
mastalgia 44–7
mastitis
periductal 51
plasma cell 51
postnatal 276
maternal postnatal care 274–5
Maternity Allowance (MA) 203
mature teratoma 102
measles 230
meconium-stained liquor 265
medication see drugs
medroxyprogesterone 88, 152
medroxyprogesterone acetate 149, 167, 184, 195
mefenamic acid 82, 84
mefloquine 211
megestrol acetate 146, 338
Meig's syndrome 102
men
breast cancer 56
chlamydia 122, 123
genital warts 130

gonorrhoea 122, 123
infertility 134, 135, 136
osteoporosis 154
sterilization 193
trichomonas vaginalis 130
menopause 146–9, 349, 358
IUDs 190
menorrhagia 80–3, 349
IUDs 188
menstrual cycle 72–3
cervical screening 110, 113
fertility 135, 137
menstrual diary 76, 77, 83, 135
menstruation 72–3
dysmenorrhoea 72, 84–5
IUDs 189
menopause 146
menorrhagia 80–3
merasma 225
Mercilon® 171
mesonephroid tumour 99
metformin 104, 136
methadone 21
methotrexate 236, 245
methyldopa 243, 253
metoclopramide 243
metronidazole
bacterial vaginosis 120, 256
endometritis 94, 278
pelvic inflammatory disease 88
post-partum haemorrhage 239
trichomonas vaginalis 130
vaginal discharge 118
miconazole 276
microcalcifications, breast 47
Microgynon® 171
Micronor® 180
mifepristone 196
migraine
COC pill 170
in pregnancy 220
milk, free 203
minimum practice income guarantee (MPIG), GMS contract 7
mini-pill see progestogen-only pill
minor placenta praevia 238
minoxidil 336
Minulet® 171
Mirena® 163, 166, 180, 186, 187, 189
GMS contract 164, 191
information and contacts 348
menopause 149
post-partum 275

miscarriage 233–5
  COC pill 173, 174
  contraception after 196
  diabetes 251
  information and contacts 349, 358
  missed 234
  threatened 232
missed miscarriage 234
Mittelschermz 72, 86
modafinil 178
'morning after pill' 195
morning sickness 222
  diabetes 251
Moro reflex 282
morphine 338
moxibustion 210, 262
mucinous cystadeno-carcinoma 99
mucinous cystadenoma 99
Multiload Cu250® 187
Multiload Cu250 Short® 187
Multiload Cu375® 187
multiple pregnancy 262–3
murmurs
  in neonates 284
  in pregnancy 244
muscular dystrophy 288
myalgic encephalitis (ME) 330–2, 355

N

nabothian cysts 108
naproxen 84
national enhanced services, GMS contract 6
nausea in pregnancy 222
  diabetes 251
nelfinavir 178
neonatal bloodspot screen-ing 288–91, 349, 359
neonates
  checks 282–7, 294–5
  chlamydia 122
  death 296, 361
  genital herpes 126
  gonorrhoea 122
  life support 268–9
  six-week check 294–5
Neville-Barnes forceps 267
nevirapine 178
nicotine replacement therapy (NRT) 16, 17
nifedipine 243, 253
night sweats 146, 147, 153
nipple discharge 44, 45
nipple problems, breast feeding 276, 293
nitrofurantoin 134, 140
nodular breasts 48
non-cyclical breast pain 46
non-dependent drinkers 12, 13

norelgestromin 171, 172
norethisterone
  COC pill 169, 171, 172, 175
  endometriosis 91
  facial flushing 338
  menopause 146
  menorrhagia 80
  postponing menstruation 73
  progestogen-only pill 180
norethisterone enantate 167, 184
norgestimate 171, 172
Norgeston® 180
Noriday® 180
Norimin® 171
Noristerat® 184, 185
Nova-T 380® 187
nuchal translucency (NT) test 216, 217

O

obesity 26–31, 349
obsessive–compulsive disorder (OCD) 324–5, 349, 359
obstetrics
  antenatal care 204–11
  COC pill after childbirth 173, 174
  emergencies 268–73
  see also labour; pregnancy
obstetric shock 270
oestrogen
  atrophic vaginitis 114
  breast cancer 58
  COC pill 172
  hirsutism 337
  HRT 153
  menopause 148
  menstrual cycle 72, 73
  PMS 74, 75
  postnatal depression 278
  and progestogen implant 184
  urethral syndrome 140
ofloxacin 88, 122
oil of evening primrose see evening primrose oil
older women
  contraception for 149
  pre-pregnancy genetic screening for 215
oligohydramnios 260
oligomenorrhoea 78
opiates, withdrawal effects 21
orgasmic problems 132
orlistat 30, 31
Ortho-Creme 192
Orthoforms 192

Ortolani manoeuvre 284, 285
osteopoenia 154
osteoporosis 147, 148, 153, 154–9
  information and contacts 349–50, 359
oto-acoustic emission (OAE) screen, neonates 284
ovarian cancer 98–101, 102
  COC pill 169
  information and contacts 350, 359
ovarian cyst 98
  dermoid 102
ovarian hyperstimulation 98
ovarian tumour 98–103
  in pregnancy 221, 270–1
Ovranette® 171
ovulation 72, 192
Ovysmen® 171
oxcarbazepine 178
oxybutinin 144
oxytocin 266

P

Paget's disease of the breast 58
pain relief for labour 265
palliative care 62, 101
panic attacks 319, 320–1
  phobias 317, 318
panic disorder 314, 315, 320–2, 359
  see also anxiety disorders
Papanicolou smear (Pap smear) 110, 112
papilloma, intraductal 51
paracetamol
  breast pain 46
  coughs, colds and flu in pregnancy 256
  cystitis 141
  deliberate self-harm 308
  dysmenorrhoea 85
  genital herpes 127
  ovarian hyperstimulation 98
  perineal bruising 276
  in pregnancy 243
  rheumatoid arthritis and pregnancy 245
paroxetine 316, 318, 338
parvovirus B19 infection 226, 227–8, 229
passive smoking 14
Patau's syndrome 286
Patient Health Question-naire (PHQ-9) 302, 306
pelvic floor exercises 142, 145
  postnatal 277

pelvic infection 189
pelvic inflammatory disease
   (PID) 88, 89, 350
   IUDs 188
pelvic mass 93, 99
pelvic muscle tone, poor
   postnatal 277
pelvic pain 86–9, 359
pelvic venous congestion
   88
penicillamine 245
penicillin 60, 290
periductal mastitis 51
perineal bruising 276
perineal infection 278
periods see menstruation
peripheral paraesthesia in
   pregnancy 222
permethrin 128, 211
persistent lochia 276–7
Persona® 192
Personal Medical Services
   (PMS) contract 8
perspiration 338–9
pethidine in labour 265
Phalen's test 220
phenelzine 304
phenobarbital 178
phenobarbitone 248
phenothiazines 134
phenothrin 128
phenylketonuria (PKU)
   288
phenytoin 178, 248, 336
phobias 314, 315, 317–18,
   359
phyllodes tumour 50
pituitary disease 350,
   359
placenta, retained 273
placenta praevia 218, 238,
   350
plasma cell mastitis 51
plate model 29
podophyllin 130
polycystic ovarian
   syndrome (PCOS)
   104–5, 350, 359
polyhydramnios 261
population, UK 2, 3
post-maturity 264
post-menopausal bleeding
   (PMB) 93
   cervical cancer 107
   endometrial carcinoma
   94
postnatal care 274–5
   epilepsy 248
   information and contacts
   350
   six-week checks 294–5
postnatal depression
   277–8, 279–81, 350–1,
   359
postnatal problems
   276–81

post-partum contraception
   275
post-partum haemorrhage
   (PPH) 239, 351
potassium citrate 140,
   141
Potter's syndrome 282
precocious puberty 70
pre-conception counselling
   200–3
   diabetes 250, 251
pre-conception genetic
   screening 214, 215
prednisolone 300
pre-eclampsia (pre-
   eclamptic toxaemia)
   221, 222, 252–5
   antenatal screening 218
   information and contacts
   351, 360
   jaundice 244
   symptoms 219
pregnancy
   additional care, women
   who may need 205
   bacterial vaginosis 119,
   120
   candidiasis 120
   cervical screening 113
   cystitis 141
   domestic violence 39
   ectopic see ectopic
   pregnancy
   epilepsy 202, 248–9, 346,
   357
   exclusion before contraception provision
   165
   genital herpes 127
   genital warts 130
   gonorrhoea 122
   infection 256–9, 347–8
   information and contacts
   360
   intrauterine 190
   pelvic inflammatory
   disease 89
   pre-pregnancy and antenatal care 200–19
   problems 240–63
   rates 134
   smoking cessation in 17
   symptoms 220–39
   teenage 194
   termination see termination of pregnancy
   tests 204
   trichomonas vaginalis
   130
   see also labour; obstetrics
pregnancy-induced
   hypertension (PIH) 252
   and proteinuria see
   pre-eclampsia
Premarin® 190
premature labour 264

premature menopause
   148, 149
   HRT 158
premature rupture of
   membranes (PROM)
   264
premenstrual dysphoric
   disorder (PMDD) 74
premenstrual syndrome
   (PMS) 74–7, 351, 360
pre-pregnancy counselling
   see pre-conception
   counselling
pre-pregnancy genetic
   screening 214, 215
prescriptions, free 203
primary amenorrhoea 70,
   78
primary care trusts (PCOs)
   6
primary dysmenorrhoea
   84
primary HIV 126
primidone 178
probenecid 122
prochlorperazine 243
proctosedyl 276
progesterone
   breast cancer 58
   HRT 153
   menopause 146
   menstrual cycle 72, 73
   PMS 75
progestogen, COC pill
   171, 172
progestogen implant 184
   adolescents 195
   emergency contraception
   167
   menopause 149
   post-partum 275
   switching to COC pill
   173, 174
   after termination of
   pregnancy or
   miscarriage 196
progestogen-only
   contraceptives 180–5
progestogen-only pill
   (POP) 163, 180–2
   emergency contraception
   167
   menopause 149
   post-partum 275
   switching to COC pill
   173, 174
   after termination of
   pregnancy or
   miscarriage 196
progestogen-releasing
   intrauterine device 180
proguanil 211
prolapse 96–7
proliferative phase,
   menstrual cycle 72
prolonged pregnancy 264

propranolol 134, 319, 338
propylthiouracil 246
Protelos® 158
pruritic urticarial papules and plaques of pregnancy (PUPPP) 224
pruritus vulvae (vulval itching) 114, 115
pseudomyxoma peritonei 99
psychiatric illness in pregnancy 218
psychotherapy 307
puberty 70–1, 360
  see also adolescence; teenagers
pubic lice 128, 351
puerperal psychosis 278
puerperal pyrexia 278
puerperium 274, 248
pulmonary embolism (PE) 247, 278
pulmonary hypertension 244
pyelonephritis 138, 139
pyometra 94
pyrexia in pregnancy 222
pyridoxine (vitamin B₆) 75, 77

Q

quality and outcomes framework (QOF), GMS contract 8, 9
quinolone 140

R

raloxifene 158
ranitidine 243
rashes in pregnancy 226–31
raspberry leaf tea 210
rebreathing techniques 319
rectocoele prolapse 96
rectus abdominis, haematoma 271
recurrent miscarriage 234
red clover 146
relaxation
  insomnia 328
  PMS 75
renal disease in pregnancy 245
renal transplant 245
reproductive system 71
resuscitation of the newborn 268–9
retained placenta 273
retinoblastoma 295

rhesus negative women 233, 240–1, 351
rheumatoid arthritis and pregnancy 245
rifabutin 178
rifampicin 178
rifamycin 178, 179
ring pessaries 96, 97
risedronate 159
ritonavir 178
rubella
  postnatal care 274
  and pregnancy 202, 214, 226, 227, 229

S

St John's wort
  COCs 178, 179
  depression 304
  emergency contraception 166
  pregnancy 210
salbutamol 243
scabies 128, 351
sclerosing adenosis 50
secondary amenorrhoea 78–9
secondary dysmenorrhoea 84–5
secretory phase, menstrual cycle 72
'sectioning' 309, 310
selenium supplements 136
self-catheterization 143
self-harm, deliberate (DSH) 308, 310–11
  information and contacts 351, 360
semen analysis 136, 137
sentinel lymph biopsy 59
serous cystadenocarcinoma 99
serous cystadenoma 99
Sertoli cell tumour 102
sertraline 277, 330, 334
sexual ambiguity 68–9
sexual dysfunction 148
sexual health, information and contacts 351, 360–1
sexual intercourse during pregnancy 202
sexual interest, lack of 132
sexually transmitted diseases (STDs) 119, 122–31, 360–1
  contraception 162
sexually transmitted infections (STIs) 131
sexual problems 132–3
  information and contacts 352, 360–1
  teenagers 194

shelf pessaries 96
shingles 226
shoulder dystocia 266, 272–3
sibutramine 30, 31
sickle cell disease
  high-risk groups 219
  neonatal bloodspot screening 288, 289, 290
simple phobia 317
single-parent families 2
six-week checks 294–5
skin changes in pregnancy 222, 224–5
skin infection, postnatal 276
sleep hygiene 329
sleep problems 328–9
  in pregnancy 222
smear tests 110–13
smoking 14–17
  breast disease 51
  cardiovascular disease 34, 36
  cot death 287
  information and contacts 352, 361
  menopause 146
  pre-conception and early pregnancy counselling 200
  in pregnancy 210
social behaviour, babies 295
social phobia 317
society, women in 2–5
sodium bicarbonate 269
sodium citrate 141
sodium valproate 178, 248
solvent abuse 20
somatization disorder 302, 322
sore nipples, postnatal 276
soya protein-based formula 292
special artificial formula feeds 292
speech checks, babies 295
sperm analysis 136, 137
spermicides 192, 193
spider naevus 225
spina bifida 216, 361
spironolactone 75, 337
spontaneous abortion see miscarriage
status epilepticus and pregnancy 248
Statutory Maternity Pay (SMP) 203
Stein–Leventhal syndrome (polycystic ovarian syndrome) 104–5, 350, 359

stepfamilies 2
sterile pyuria 139
sterilization 163, 193, 352
   post-partum 275
steroids, and osteoporosis 156
stilboestrol 234
stillbirth 251, 296, 361
stimulants, withdrawal effects 21
stress 298–9, 352, 361
   amenorrhoea 79
stress incontinence 142, 148
stroke 37
   COC pill 169, 170
   HRT 153
strontium ranelate 158
structural chromosome problems 286
subacute bacterial endocarditis (SBE) 187
sudden infant death syndrome, reducing the risk of 287
suicide 308–12, 351, 360
   prevention 308, 310
   risk assessment 302
sulfasalazine 134, 245
sulphonylureas 250
superficial dyspareunia 86, 87
superficial perineal infection 278
superficial thrombo-phlebitis 278
Sure Start Maternity Grant 203
sweats 338–9
   menopause 146, 147, 153
   pregnancy 222
swelling in pregnancy 224
symphysis pubis dysfunction 224
Synphase® 175
Syntometrine® 232, 243, 273
syphilis 128, 352
   in pregnancy 258
systemic lupus erythema-tosus (SLE) in pregnancy 245

T

tamoxifen
   breast cancer 58
   breast pain 46
   cervical cancer 107
   facial flushing 338
   infertility 136
   menorrhagia 81

post-menopausal bleeding 93
Tanner stages of puberty 71
Tay-Sachs disease 218
teenagers
   consultation with 194
   contraception 195
   information and contacts 361
   pregnancy 194
   see also adolescence; puberty
temazepam 328
tension headache in pregnancy 220
teratoma 102
terbutaline 243
teriparatide 158
termination of pregnancy (TOP) 196–7, 352, 361
   COC pill 173, 174
testicular feminization 68–9
tetanus vaccination 311
tetracycline 120, 243
thalassaemia 219
theca cell tumour 102
thecoma 102
theophylline 304
thiamine 12
threatened miscarriage 232
thromboembolism 246, 352
thrombophlebitis
   postnatal 278
   in pregnancy 224
thrush see candidiasis
thyroid disease in pregnancy 246
thyroxine 151, 243, 246, 278, 290
tibolone 150
time management 299
Tinel's test 220
tiredness 330–2
   postnatal 278
tolterodine 144
topiramate 178
torsion in pregnancy 221, 270–1
toxoplasmosis 259
tranexamic acid 82, 188
transient ischaemic attacks (TIAs) 37
   see also stroke
transitional cell tumour 99
trastuzumab 58
travel and pregnancy 211
Triadene® 175
Trichomonas vaginalis (TV) infection 130, 131, 353

trimethoprim 140, 243, 259
Triminulet® 175
Trinordiol® 175
Trinovum® 175
triplets 262–3
trophoblastic disease 236, 353
T-Safe Cu380 A® 187
TT 380 Slimline® 187
Turner's syndrome 286
twins 262–3

U

ultrasound scan (USS) in pregnancy 214
United Kingdom population 2, 3
unmodified cow's milk, and bottle feeding 292
urethral carbuncle 114
urethral syndrome 140
urethrocoele prolapse 96
urge incontinence 144
urinary fistula 144
urinary frequency in pregnancy 224
urinary incontinence see incontinence
urinary problems in menopause 148
urinary tract infection (UTI) 138–41
   menopause 148
   in pregnancy 259
UT 380 Short or Standard® 187
uterine artery embolization 92
uterine (endometrial) cancer 94–5, 169, 353
uterine height by gestational age 261
uterine inversion 273
uterine leiomyoma 92–3
uterine problems 92–5
uterine prolapse 96, 97
uterine retroversion 92
uterine rupture 271

V

vaccination see immuniza-tion and vaccination
vaginal cancer 114
vaginal caps 192
vaginal cyst 114
vaginal diaphragms 192, 193
vaginal discharge 118–21
   in pregnancy 224
vaginal intraepithelial neoplasia (VAIN) 114

vaginal problems 114
vaginal tumour 114
vaginismus 132
valaciclovir 230
varicose veins in pregnancy 224
Vaseline® 192
vault caps 192
vault smear 113
venlafaxine 304, 338
venous thromboembolism 169
ventouse, assisted delivery 266, 267
verapamil 319
very low calorie diets 30
vision checks, babies 295
vitamin A 201
vitamin B supplements 12, 75, 77
vitamin C supplements 136, 252
vitamin D supplements
  breast feeding 293
  infertility 136

menopause 147
osteoporosis 156
pre-conception and early pregnancy counselling 200
pre-eclampsia 252
vitamin E supplements 77, 136, 146
vitamin K, neonatal check 282
vitamin supplements, free 203
vomiting in pregnancy 222, 251
vulva, anatomy 115
vulval carcinoma 117
vulval conditions, information and contacts 353
vulval dystrophy 116
vulval intraepithelial neoplasia (VIN) 117
vulval itching 114, 115
vulval lumps 114
vulval problems 114–17
vulvodynia 116

W

waist circumference 26, 27
warfarin 31, 146, 243, 246, 304
warts, genital 130, 131
Waterfall® 75
women in society 2–5
work 2–3
Wrigleys' forceps 267

Y

Yasmin® 171, 172
yolk sac tumour 102

Z

zidovudine 218, 258
zinc supplements 136
zolpidem 328
zopiclone 328
Zyban® 16